Archives of Family Practice

Volume II
1981

Archives of Family Practice

Selected Papers and Abstracts Representing
Original Work Advancing the Specialty
of Family Practice

Volume II
1981

Edited by

John P. Geyman, M.D.

Professor and Chairman
Department of Family Medicine
School of Medicine
University of Washington
Seattle, Washington

 APPLETON-CENTURY-CROFTS / *New York*

Prentice-Hall International, Inc., London
Prentice-Hall of Australia, Pty. Ltd., Sydney
Prentice-Hall of India Private Limited, New Delhi
Prentice-Hall of Japan, Inc., Tokyo
Prentice-Hall of Southeast Asia (Pte.) Ltd., Singapore
Whitehall Books Ltd., Wellington, New Zealand

PRINTED IN THE UNITED STATES OF AMERICA
ISBN 0-8385-0325-X

This series is dedicated to family physicians around the world and to the continued refinement of their specialized roles in providing continuing personal and comprehensive health care to their patients and families.

Contents

Abstracts

SECTION TWO: GRADUATE EDUCATION IN FAMILY PRACTICE

Abstracts

Preface

Family practice as a specialty has taken root from general practice and is derived from portions of many other specialty disciplines. Consequently, family practice has lacked its own traditions in education, research and literature. Most of the content of books and journals directed to general/family physicians has been written by specialists in other fields in an effort to distill advances in their various disciplines to what they perceive as the needs of the generalist. Until recently, there has been insufficient research activity in family practice settings to reverse this trend by developing new knowledge advancing family medicine in its own right.

The situation is now changing rapidly as family practice matures as a specialty. In the United States, for example, family practice has entered its second decade of development since the American Board of Family Practice was established in 1969. Family practice teaching programs are operational in about 90 percent of the nation's medical schools, and there is increasing research activity in family practice settings.

The process of specialization in family practice is by no means limited to national boundaries. Whether known as *family practice* or *general practice,* the field is actively involved in many countries in the development of educational programs at undergraduate, graduate and postgraduate levels, improvement of clinical standards, and strengthening of the research base in general/family practice. Although the educational and health care systems may vary considerably from one country to another, there is much that can be learned from the experience of other countries concerning the many common interests in this process.

The literature of record representing original work in general/family practice not only involves parallel efforts in different countries, it is also published in a variety of journals and related publications, many of which are not customarily read by family physicians and others involved in the field. The need, therefore, exists to bring together in a collated form the important work advancing the field.

Archives of Family Practice is unique among existing books in the field as the first to focus *exclusively* on the clinical, educational and research developments of the specialty in its own right and in its own settings. This approach was not possible in the past due to the specialty's relative immaturity as a teachable clinical discipline with an active area of research. The overall goal of *Archives of Family Practice* is therefore to reflect the advancing state of the art in the clinical, educational and research elements of this growing specialty.

As a series of annual volumes, *Archives of Family Practice* includes a collection of papers in both full and abstract form in three general content areas related to (1) the specialty and its clinical application; (2) education for family practice; and (3) research in family practice. Each volume presents 12 to 15 papers and 25 to 50 abstracts in each of three sections. These papers are drawn from the literature of record in numerous journals, reports and related documents. Papers are selected which are considered collectively to best reflect the advancing field within each content area. Where appropriate, authors have been asked to add current comments to update their papers to the year of publication.

This volume will focus on three general content areas: (1) *Family Practice in the Community;* (2) *Graduate Education in Family Practice;* and (3) *Concepts and Methods of Family Practice Research.* Future volumes will deal with such subjects as *Approaches to Patient Care and Clinical Decision-Making, Clinical Research in Family Practice,* and other important areas.

This series is directed primarily to medical students, family practice residents, family physicians and educators involved in family practice teaching programs. *Archives of Family Practice* will also be of interest to others in medicine desiring to better appreciate in a single volume the emerging roles of family practice in medical practice and in medical education.

John P. Geyman, M.D.
Seattle, Washington

Acknowledgments

The papers and abstracts appearing in ARCHIVES OF FAMILY PRACTICE 1981 have been selected from the following journals:

American Journal of Public Health
Australian Family Physician
Canadian Family Physician
Journal of American Medical Association
Journal of Community Health
The Journal of Family Practice
Journal of Medical Education
Journal of Royal College of General Practitioners
Medical Care

I am grateful to Rowena de Saram for her help in preparing the abstracts and other materials for this volume. I am further indebted to Richard Lampert and Gordon Powell of Appleton-Century-Crofts for their diligent efforts in publishing this series. Special thanks are extended to David Stires, President of Appleton-Century-Crofts, for his continued encouragement and early recognition of the vital role of the generalist physician in the health care of families.

John P. Geyman, M.D.

SECTION ONE
Family Practice in the Community

COMMENTARY

THE papers and abstracts in this section have been selected for their importance and comparative value in describing patterns of family practice in the community. Particular attention has been directed to comparisons of general/family practice in different regions and countries in an effort to identify both commonalities and differences. For this reason, it is fitting that the opening paper by Mechanic establishes broad and specific comparisons between practice patterns of primary care physicians (general/family practice, internal medicine, pediatrics, and obstetrics-gynecology) in the United States, England, and Wales based on work carried out about 10 years ago. Other papers provide comparative views of general/family practice in various parts of the United States, Canada, England, Australia, and the Netherlands.

Practice patterns in any clinical specialty are clearly quite variable in response to many factors, such as needs of the community; local and regional customs of medical care; availability of physicians in both primary care and consultant fields; access to hospitals and other clinical resources; third party reimbursement policies; training, experience, and interests of the physician; and attitudes and health seeking behavior of the patient. Many papers and abstracts in this section address one or more of these variables and a "common core" of family practice emerges from all of these descriptions which is likely to be found in any community setting.

Practice patterns naturally may change over time as other changes take place within the health care delivery system. The 1972 paper by Fry is especially interesting not only for the various changes which occurred in his general practice in England over 21 years, but also for the extent of detailed information made available for his practice by an ongoing record and data retrieval system.

The practice patterns and roles of family physicians in several countries are further represented by a group of studies of hospital privileges and referral patterns. Finally, two papers begin to examine the similarities and differences in practice patterns of residency-trained family physicians and general/family physicians who entered practice without formal family practice residency training as established in the United States and Canada during the last 10 years.

1

General Medical Practice:*

Some Comparisons between the Work of Primary Care Physicians in the United States and England and Wales

David Mechanic

Data on comparable questions from national surveys of British general practitioners and American G.P.'s, internists, pediatricians, and obstetricians are compared. British G.P.'s see many more patients in their offices and on home visits. American primary care physicians use a wider array of diagnostic procedures, are more closely associated with professional colleagues, and express less frustration and dissatisfaction. Although American primary care physicians perform more complicated and varied tasks than British G.P.'s, such practices, for the most part, tend to be relatively restricted in dealing with many ordinary primary care problems. This trend is particularly clear among office-based specialists in internal medicine and obstetrics, and the use of paraprofessionals is discussed as a way of broadening these practices. Other differences among types of American doctors and between group and nongroup practitioners are also noted, as well as their perspectives on widely discussed innovations in the organization of medical care.

A major factor in the growing ferment concerning medical care has been the increasing inaccessibility of the general physician. It has been well established that in recent decades the proportion of physicians in primary medical care (including general practitioners, internists, and pediatricians) relative to all physicians has been declining,[7] and consumers frequently complain about the difficulty of finding a primary physician, unwillingness of the doctor to make home calls, and impersonality in health care. It is fully apparent that modifications in the delivery of health services must deal with present difficulties if they are to be reasonably responsive to consumer needs and expectations.

In contrast, the National Health Service of England and Wales has made a concerted attempt to maintain the structure of primary care through its system of general practice. Approximately 40 percent of all English doctors are general practitioners and maintain community practices averag-

ing about 2,500 patients. These doctors practice largely outside the hospital, although a significant proportion of them have access to beds for obstetrics.[10] Difficulties in general practice in England have been widely described,[11] but available evidence also suggests considerable satisfaction among British consumers with general practice and good accessibility to care.[4]

In both countries, there is currently considerable agonizing over the responsibilities of the primary care physician and the types of training that best prepare him for the problems encountered in general practice. There are major differences of perspective among commentators, some of whom are concerned with how to bring the scientific expertise and the latest technology of the teaching hospital to bear on the community practice of medicine, others who feel that the models of practice taught are inappropriate to the needs and proper approach of a generalist practicing in the community. Implicit in the attempts to encourage health center practice in Britain and Health Maintenance Organizations in the United States is a desire to deal with a

* Reprinted by permission from *Medical Care,* 10(5):402–420, September–October, 1972.

greater proportion of medical problems within the context of ambulatory care, making appropriate use of existing technical and ancillary resources. But the proper standards for such practice are themselves in flux, and are likely to undergo considerable modification in the coming years.

As the debate over medical care deepens in the United States, it is likely that comparisons will be made increasingly between our forms of care and those in other countries. Such comparisons are frequently hazardous in that developments of health services in each country tend to occur within a particular historical context influenced by the existing economic system, traditional facilities and forms of professional organization, and the social and cultural patterns of the country. Yet such analyses can be informative if carefully formulated for they provide a perspective and contrast against which each system can evaluate its own practices. Such comparisons also direct us to consider what in fact typical practices are within our diverse system of care, since at present there is relatively little available information on the organization of ambulatory care in the United States and typical work patterns of primary care physicians.

Sources of Data

In 1966, a random sample of general practitioners in England and Wales was selected for the investigation by the Ministry of Health, and each doctor received a long questionnaire. After from one to three communications, 60 percent of the doctors (813) had returned completed questionnaires. On the fourth approach, a much shorter questionnaire was sent, and an additional 13 percent responded, yielding a total response rate of 73 percent (995 doctors) for many key items. Basic demographic data about all general practitioners in England and Wales, as well as all of the doctors designated in our sample, were provided by the Ministry of Health. De-

tailed analyses of the characteristics of the sample in comparison to the population, between responders and nonresponders and between early and later responders, are reported elsewhere.[6] Although the sample obtained had some overrepresentation of younger doctors and those in larger groups, for the most part the respondents were very similar in demographic characteristics to all general practitioners in England and Wales.

While the general practitioner is a structured position in the National Health Service, there is no comparable position in the United States. One way of obtaining a comparable group is to define primary care physicians as doctors of first contact, i.e., office-based doctors that are likely to offer general services on a community basis. Ordinarily, this would include general practitioners, internists, and pediatricians. It is arguable as to whether obstetricians should be included in this definition, but since British general practitioners do a considerable amount of obstetrics, it seemed reasonable to include office-based obstetricians in the population. With the assistance of the American Medical Association, a random sample of office-based general practitioners, internists, pediatricians, and obstetricians was selected with different sampling ratios among group and nongroup practitioners classified by their primary activity code. The population from which the sample was drawn included 82,271 nongroup practitioners and 12,772 group practitioners. Among the nongroup population, 56 percent were general practitioners, 21 percent internists, 14 percent pediatricians, and 9 percent obstetricians. Among group practitioners, comparable percentages were 37, 32, 15, and 16, respectively. A questionnaire similar to, but shorter than, the British questionnaire was sent to each member of our sample between the period October 1970 to March 1971. After five approaches, 1,458 physicians (66 percent of our sample) returned completed questionnaires.

The American Medical Association provided a tape containing information on the entire sample from their Physician's Records Information System. In a preliminary analysis, comparing the data describing physicians who responded to our survey with the total sample on such attributes as year of graduation, sex, state within which the doctor practices, birthdate, license year, National Board year, amount of postgraduate education, source of professional income, present employment, government service, specialty boards and memberships in specialty societies, no differences of significance were obtained. In no case did any category vary by more than 2 or 3 percent in comparing those who responded with the entire sample.

A somewhat sharper picture of possible biases emerges in comparing the minority who did not respond to the survey with those who did. Here we find that nonrespondents include a higher proportion of older doctors (23 percent 61 years or older), those who graduated from medical school in 1935 or earlier (20 percent), and those who were licensed to practice in 1940 or before (23 percent). The comparable figures among respondents were 16 percent, 13 percent, and 18 percent. Nonrespondents were more likely to be in individual fee-for-service practice (53 percent) than respondents (44 percent) and also were more likely to be on full-time salaries (4 percent vs. 2 percent). Nonrespondents were also less likely to have their specialty boards (23 percent) than respondents (33 percent) and were less likely to belong to at least one specialty society (49 percent vs. 34 percent). This selective tendency relative to specialty boards and specialty societies is most pronounced among pediatricians. In sum, although the respondents are characteristic of the entire sample, there was some selective response to the survey. It is noteworthy that the character of this selectivity is similar to that obtained in the British sample. Since we have differentially sampled nongroup and group physi-

cians in the United States, data for these categories will be presented separately.

Before presenting our comparative data, some cautions should be noted. Both surveys depend entirely on doctors' reports of various behaviors and activities, and, for the most part, independent data to assess the accuracy of these reports are not available. Moreover, respondents may frequently answer questions in a fashion which presents them in a favorable light, and they may knowingly and unknowingly distort or exaggerate their responses to promote particular positions. The data from British general practitioners were collected in the midst of a remuneration dispute, and the data from American physicians were collected during a time when there had been considerable discussion of the adequacy of medical organization and medical care. Also, there is a differential of more than 4 years between the two surveys. Finally, although both surveys elicited response rates higher than usual in such surveys of physicians, a significant number of doctors in both samples did not return questionnaires. Although we have attempted to ascertain the impact of nonresponse on various kinds of information available on all physicians, it is impossible to make such estimates for many items of importance for which data are unavailable.

Some Comparative Data

Among the British general practitioners we studied, 19 percent were solo practitioners, 52 percent were in two- or three-man partnerships, 16 percent were in four-man partnerships, and 11 percent were in larger groups. Among American primary care physicians in office-based practice, 13 percent were in groups as their primary activity. Of the remaining 87 percent, 51 percent were in solo practice, 36 percent were in partnerships, 11 percent shared facilities with other doctors but maintained independent practices, and 2 percent had other arrangements. In both countries, solo practice and small partnerships constitute clearly the dominant forms of delivering primary medical services.

Since the roles of British G.P.'s and American primary care physicians vary substantially, we shall concentrate on those aspects common to both. American doctors report spending much more time seeing patients in their offices relative to British doctors and much less time visiting patients in their homes. We asked doctors in both samples to report the amount of time they had spent the day prior to completing our questionnaire seeing patients at their office or, if the prior day had been atypical, during the most recent typical day. Only 6 percent of British G.P.'s reported spending 6 or more hours seeing patients at their offices in comparison to 67 percent of nongroup and 70 percent of group physicians in the American sample. In contrast, only 15 percent of British doctors reported spending less than 2 hours on home calls as compared with 92 percent of nongroup and 99 percent of group physicians in the United States. More than half of the British doctors spend from 2 to 4 hours for home calls, and 32 percent spent more than 4 hours on this activity.

As an examination of Table 1 shows, the vast majority of American doctors made no home calls at all, varying from 52 percent of nongroup G.P.'s to 100 percent of group obstetricians. But even among G.P.'s there is little home visiting; only 9 percent of nongroup G.P.'s and 3 percent of group G.P.'s made three or more home calls. In contrast, two fifths of the British G.P.'s reported 15 or more home calls during the previous day, and only 6 percent reported less than five. We asked similar questions about office consultations and home calls in respect to "a typical day" with comparable results. The most extraordinary aspect of these data concerns the very large number of patients that British G.P.'s

manage to see within the limited time they spend in surgery. The implications of this mode of practice are discussed elsewhere.[12,13,15]

American doctors, in contrast to their British counterparts, also have a great deal of contact with patients through hospital rounds and telephone consultations. Among nongroup physicians, two fifths reported visiting less than five hospital patients during the previous day, two fifths reported making between 5 and 10 visits, and one fifth reported 11 or more such visits. The comparable percentages for group practitioners were 36 percent, 41 percent, and 23 percent. Internists saw the most patients on hospital rounds (28 percent of nongroup and 37 percent of group internists saw 11 or more such patients) and pediatricians saw the least (8 percent of nongroup pediatricians and 5 percent of group pediatricians saw 11 or more). One fifth of general practitioners saw a comparable number of patients on hospital rounds. Relevant to telephone conversations with patients, three fifths of the nongroup physicians and one half of the group physicians reported 10 or more such conversations. Pediatricians clearly reported the most such telephone consultations; 84 percent of the nongroup pediatricians and 64 percent of the group pediatricians reported 10 or more such consultations during the previous day. Approximately one third of the doctors reported seeing patients in other contexts, but, for the most part, the number of patients seen was very small.

We asked each of the doctors in our American sample to give us three estimates for the number of hours they work during a typical week. We then accumulated the time reported in each of these three questions to form an estimate of reported typical workweek, and these data are shown in Table 2. The figures reported cannot be taken on face value without independent validation, and these estimates are at best "rough"; nevertheless, they can be indica-

Table 1. *Number of Reported Patient Visits in Office and Home during Previous Day among British General Practitioners and among Varying Types of American Primary Care Physicians*

	British General Practitioners	General Practitioners		Internists		Pediatricians		Obstetricians	
	N = 813* (percent)	Nongroup N = 599* (percent)	Group N = 111*	Nongroup N = 231* (percent)	Group N = 91*	Nongroup N = 136* (percent)	Group N = 43*	Nongroup N = 150* (percent)	Group N = 58* (percent)
Number of patients seen during previous day at office									
0–10	5⎱	6	6	21	16	2	5	8	7
11–19	⎰	10	5	42	49	9	12	15	12
20–29	12	27	32	24	29	30	36	42	39
30–36	21	23	21	9	5	22	21	20	29
37–43	13	14	16	1	1	13	17	10	7
44–50	20	8	10	1⎱	—	13	2	3	3
51–64	17	8	6	⎰	—	5	7	2⎱	2⎱
65 or more	12	4	3		—	6	—	⎰	⎰
Number of home calls during previous day									
None		52	75	70	82	81	95	96	100
1		26	15	18	11	11	3	1	—
2		13	7	8	5	5	3	—	—
3		5	1	3	1	1	—	1	—
4 or more		4	2	1	1	1	—	3	—

* The sample sizes shown here and in subsequent tables, unless otherwise specified, constitute the full sample available in the analysis. Percentages are calculated only for doctors responding to the specific question, and thus sample size may vary slightly from the base and from one question to another. Percentages do not always equal 100 percent due to rounding errors.

Table 2. *Reported Time Expenditures for a "Typical Week" among American Primary Care Physicians*

	General Practitioners		Internists		Pediatricians		Obstetricians	
	Nongroup N = 599 (percent)	Group N = 111 (percent)	Nongroup N = 231 (percent)	Group N = 91 (percent)	Nongroup N = 136 (percent)	Group N = 43 (percent)	Nongroup N = 150 (percent)	Group N = 58 (percent)
Hours spent during a typical week seeing patients								
Less than 40	29	17	17	22	20	24	41	32
40–49	19	33	27	29	27	33	24	32
50–59	24	24	27	33	25	24	15	21
60 or more	29	27	29	16	28	19	20	16
Additional hours during a typical week devoted to practice management (excluding direct patient contact)								
2 or less	29	41	23	46	28	65	35	45
3–5	32	31	35	22	34	21	33	36
6–10	26	21	30	21	28	9	18	14
11 or more	14	6	12	10	9	5	14	5
Additional hours on activities related to practice such as attending meetings, medical reading, etc.								
2 or less	31	35	19	18	19	19	29	28
3–5	35	31	39	31	42	46	37	33
6–10	28	27	28	40	34	28	26	22
11 or more	7	7	13	11	5	7	8	17
Total reported hours spent during a typical week (sum of three above categories)								
Less than 40	10	6	6	9	7	18	25	12
40–49	14	17	11	13	16	14	15	24
50–59	26	28	26	40	27	32	21	29
60–69	22	26	28	20	28	21	14	17
70 or more	28	23	30	18	23	14	26	17

tive of various trends and variations among the specialties and types of practice. Except for the general practitioners, nongroup practitioners tend to report longer work weeks, with nongroup internists most likely to report a work week exceeding 60 hours. This is attributable, in part, to the tendency of internists to report more time on various aspects of continuing education.

Table 3 reports estimates based on time budgets provided for the previous day by British and American doctors. The items used in the two countries vary, but estimates based on five selected items among the American doctors are roughly equivalent to the British reports. This comparison underestimates the time British doctors spend on telephone work which is small relative to the American situation and underestimates the time American physicians spend on surgery and in delivering babies. The data suggest that a somewhat higher proportion of American doctors report working longer hours on the previous day, although the differences are not particularly large. The proportion of doctors that reported working 12 hours or more during the previous day is highest among nongroup practitioners, but there are only small reported differences between American group practitioners and British G.P.'s. These data suggest that American physicians work somewhat longer hours than British G.P.'s, but that both groups report relatively long days. The major differences appear not so much in the length of the workday, as in the character of daily activities.

Practice Orientations among British and American Primary Care Physicians

One way of assessing, indirectly, the character of the doctor's approach to the patient, is to describe his use of diagnostic fa-

Table 3. *Reported Time Budgets for the Previous Working Day among British and American Primary Care Physicians*

	British General Practitioners* (Specified items)† N = 772 (percent)	American Primary Care Physicians			
		Nongroup (first five items)‡ N = 1148 (percent)	Group (first five items)‡ N = 310 (percent)	Nongroup (all items)§ N = 1148 (percent)	Group (all items)§ N = 310 (percent)
Less than 6 hours	4	3	4	2	1
6 hours or more but less than 8 hours	12	10	9	3	3
8 hours or more but less than 10 hours	42	26	33	13	16
10 hours or more but less than 12 hours	29	34	37	33	37
12 hours or more	14	26	18	49	44

* Part of our analysis of British doctors is based on a data tape that excluded 41 doctors because they failed to respond to 10 percent or more of our questions. In remaining cases, where data on a particular question were missing, the respondent was assigned to the mean response of those replying to the question. The demographic profile of this sample was almost identical to the profile of all respondents.
† Items include seeing patients at surgery, domiciliary visits and travel, other work relevant travel, administrative and paper work, and hospital work.
‡ Items include seeing patients at office, talking with patients or other doctors on phone, house calls and related travel, hospital rounds and related travel, and administrative and paper work.
§ Includes five items above, and also doing surgery, delivering babies, continuing education, and other professional duties.

cilities and his social orientation to medical care. We asked American respondents to report whether they had used each of 14 diagnostic procedures in the previous 2 weeks, 13 of which were identical to those we presented to our British sample. As an examination of Table 4 shows, in every case American doctors were more likely to use these procedures than their British counterparts. As might be expected, internists and general practitioners, on the average, were more likely to use these procedures than obstetricians and pediatricians. American doctors in group practice are more likely to use each of these diagnostic procedures regardless of speciality, although this factor only accounts for modest differences. Having 14 procedures and four subgroups of doctors allows 56 comparisons between nongroup and group practitioners. In 48 of these comparisons,

doctors in group practice were more likely to use the given procedure, although the average difference between solo and group practitioners was only 7 percentage points. Significant deviations by specialty included the tendency of obstetricians to be less likely to use full-size chest x-rays, bone or joint x-rays, erythrocyte sedimentation rate, prothrombin activity, serum cholesterol, blood culture, liver function tests, radioactive iodine uptake, and electrocardiogram; the tendency of pediatricians to be less likely to use glucose tolerance, blood sugar, prothrombin activity, serum cholesterol, liver function tests, radioactive iodine uptake, protein-bound iodine, and electrocardiograms; and the tendency for general practitioners to be less likely to use blood cultures.

American doctors are clearly dependent on the clinical laboratory to a point which

Table 4. *Reported Use of Various Diagnostic Procedures among British and American Primary Care Physicians*

	Reported Use in Previous Weeks		
		American Primary Care Physicians	
Procedure	British General Practitioners N = 813 (percent)	Nongroup N = 1148 (percent)	Group N = 310 (percent)
Full-size chest x-rays	67	91	94
Bone and joint x-rays	57	81	79
Bacteriologic examination of urine	57	78	91
Glucose tolerance tests	15	65	68
Erythrocyte sedimentation rate	48	67	74
Blood sugar	21	90	92
Prothrombin activity	20	64	66
Serum cholesterol	15	71	73
Blood culture	4	35	40
Liver function tests	16	67	75
Serum electrolytes	10	71	77
Radioactive iodine uptake	3	29	32
Protein-bound iodine	*	71	75
Electrocardiogram	15	83	84
Hemoglobin	80	*	*
Reb blood cell count	70	*	*
White blood cell count	67	*	*
Routine urinalysis	53	*	*

* Not asked.

Table 5. *Comparisons of Various Aspects of the Work of Primary Care Physicians in Britain and in the United States*

Aspects of Work	British General Practitioners N = 772 (percent)	Kern Data* British GP's in Health Centers N = 95 (percent)	British GP Cartwright Survey, 1963‡ N = 157	British GP Cartwright Survey, 1967§ N = 442	General Practitioners Non-group N = 599 (percent)	General Practitioners Group N = 111 (percent)	Internists Non-group N = 231 (percent)	Internists Group N = 91 (percent)	Pediatricians Non-group N = 136 (percent)	Pediatricians Group N = 43 (percent)	Obstetricians Non-group N = 150 (percent)	Obstetricians Group N = 58 (percent)
Use of diagnostic procedures during previous two weeks†												
5 or less	70	24 }			8	6	3	—	29	32	46	29
6–7	15				9	2	5	—	26	20	21	26
8–9	6	19			20	12	15	7	25	20	17	29
10–12	7	57 }			52	66	56	66	20	22	14	16
13	1				10	14	22	28	1	7	1	—
Reports uses of following procedures on occasion or more frequently‖												
"Tape" (strap)#												
sprains			91	98	86	88	56	42	78	71	16	12
Excise simple cysts			62	62	94	90	20	11	28	19	87	93
Open abscesses			89	94	99	95	56	46	92	73	97	95
Suture lacerations (stitch cuts)			93	94	98	95	37	31	85	80	62	65
Do proctoscopic or sigmoidoscopic							89	91	40	39	43	33

Procedure									
...and interpret your own electrocardiograms (perform electrocardiography)	3	††	69	81	98	97	24	43	76	16
Do vaginal exam with a speculum	††	88	99	98	96	92	30	39	99	100
Use a laryngoscope	††	35	48	62	30	27	58	71	20	26
Do uncomplicated obstetrics	25‡‡	20§§	59	58	—	—	3	—	97	100
Do well-baby care	††	††	91	83	7	1	97	100	14	11
Do simple psychotherapy	22‖	††	96	99	95	93	93	95	88	93
Do pap smears	††	††	98	94	94	92	7	5	99	100
Set simple fractures	††	††	80	77	6	3	50	32	5	2
Do major general surgery	††	††	35	37	1	—	5	—	74	74
Take and interpret selected x-rays in your office	††	††	.57	87	53	73	31	64	17	41

* Kern[9] obtained data from 96 of a sample of 140 general practitioners in 24 health centers in England, Wales, and Scotland. The study was restricted to centers housing at least four general practitioners in communities of 50,000 or less.

† This scale includes only those diagnostic procedures included in the questionnaires in both countries.

‡ A representative two-stage sample of 195 general practitioners of whom 157 responded (Cartwright[3]).

§ Patients interviewed in 12 areas of England and Wales named their doctors, resulting in 552 names. Of those who were sent questionnaires, 442 responded (Cartwright[4]).

‖ The data are reported using identical categories in Mechanic's survey and in Cartwright.[4] In Cartwright,[3] data are reported as the "proportions who said they carry out these procedures."

Wording on some of the items varied. British wording given in parentheses.

** British doctors were only asked about proctoscopic exams.

†† Question not asked.

‡‡ These data come from Mechanic's survey and are in response to the question, "Do you do domiciliary obstetrics?"

§§ This is the estimated proportion of doctors with 50 or more obstetric cases in previous 12 months (Cartwright[4]).

‖‖ These data are from Mechanic's survey and are in response to the question, "Do you do any regular psychotherapy with patients?" This question obviously has different meaning than the one posed to American physicians.

some commentators regard as excessive, while it is generally agreed that the average primary care physician in Britain does not do sufficient laboratory work. Younger British doctors and those in group practice are more likely to use diagnostic aids, and some recent data on doctors practicing in health centers reported by Kern[9] show very strong evidence of increased use. Kern's data include many younger doctors who tend to be more likely to use diagnostic aids, but even this sample has a lower rate of diagnostic use than either American G.P.'s or internists. It should be noted, however, that a good deal of the diagnostic work which characterizes American practice is performed in British hospital outpatient departments, where patients are readily referred by general practitioners.

Table 5 also provides some comparative data on the performance of various tasks. There are only four items in the British and American surveys where the questions were sufficiently similar to argue for comparability (tape sprains, open abscesses, excise simple cysts, and suture lacerations). These are all relatively simple procedures which one might expect a primary care physician to perform. Relevant to three of these procedures, British G.P.'s are comparable to American G.P.'s and pediatricians. There is more variability in reports of excising simple cysts, where both American G.P.'s and obstetricians are relatively likely to perform the procedure, and pediatricians and internists relatively unlikely. British G.P.'s fall between these two groupings. Cartwright[3] has queried British doctors about other procedures, and has found only small proportions performing them: administering intravenous fluids (37 percent), aspirating chest (22 percent), injecting piles (19 percent), cauterizing cervix (17 percent), reducing simple limb fractures (15 percent), lumbar puncture (7 percent), sigmoidoscopy (3 percent), electrocardiography (3 percent), ligating varicose veins (3 percent), estimating hemoglobin with a hemoglobinometer (27 percent), and use of a laryngoscope (35 percent). An exception was doing a vaginal exam with a speculum which was reported by 88 percent of the British G.P.'s. These data support the general impression of observers that British G.P.'s function as generalists but in a relatively restricted manner. In contrast, American general practitioners have a much wider range of practice. The fact that more than a third of American generalists report doing major general surgery suggests that this may have some disadvantages.

The data presented in Tables 4 and 5 show considerable variability in the work of G.P.'s, internists, pediatricians, and obstetricians. To some extent, such differences reflect expected varying case mix, but they also suggest that the tendency to classify all these types as primary care physicians in assessing physician distribution may be somewhat misleading. These types of practitioners are usually categorized together with the implication that they perform as generalists and maintain a very wide scope of practice. But these data suggest that a large proportion of such practices are more restricted than generally believed.

Table 6 provides some fragmentary data on the doctors' social orientations, their satisfaction and degree of frustration. These measures appear to have validity, and they are discussed in greater detail elsewhere.[6,13] Contrary to general belief, these data support the notion that American doctors are more socially oriented to medical care than their British counterparts who are also less satisfied and more frustrated. These data must be viewed with some caution since the social orientation questions all involved items as to whether it is appropriate for persons with varying kinds of problems to seek the assistance of physicians. British doctors tend to have very heavy workloads, and since they are paid on a capitation system they have little incentive to encourage "marginal" consultations. In contrast, in the American case, there is usually an economic incentive for additional patient visits. However, there were only trivial differences between American group and nongroup physicians

Table 6. *Comparison of British and American Primary Care Physicians on Measures of "Social Orientations to Medical Care," "Frustration," and "Satisfaction"*

	British General Practitioners N = 772 (percent)	American Primary Care Physicians			
		General Practitioners		All Nongroup N = 1148 (percent)	All Group N = 310 (percent)
		Nongroup N = 599 (percent)	Group N = 111 (percent)		
Social orientation to medical care*					
High (scores of 1 to 3)	24	43	47	38	40
Medium high (scores 4–5)	39	38	38	38	35
Medium low (scores of 6–7)	27	16	14	19	19
Low (scores of 8 or 9)	10	4	1	6	5
Index of frustration; percent of patient visits estimated as trivial, unnecessary, or inappropriate					
Less than 10 percent	12	33	28	36	36
10 percent or more but less than 25 percent	29	35	36	35	35
25 percent or more but less than 50 percent	35	23	24	22	19
50 percent or more	24	9	13	7	10
Satisfaction†					
Very satisfied	10	53	56	51	52
Fairly satisfied	41	42	41	44	43
Not very satisfied	35	4	3	4	4
Quite dissatisfied	14	—	—	1	—

* The items used are the propriety of consulting the doctor for family financial troubles, disobedience of children, marital difficulties, handling behavior in a relative such as drunkeness, children's poor school performance, birth control advice, problems with drinking too much, general feelings of unhappiness, anxieties about child care, and obesity. Also included was a correlated question: "Some medical commentators have recently argued that there is a growing tendency for people to bring less serious disorders to doctors and more readily seek help for problems in their family lives. In general, do you feel that this is a good or bad trend, given present conditions of medical practice?"

† There was a significant variation in the way the question was worded in the two countries. In the British case, the question asked was "In general, how satisfied are you with general practice?" In the American case, the question referred to "your practice." We gathered considerable data on satisfaction, and we have examined the internal consistency of these data. We feel confident that these two questions are reasonably comparable.

despite the fact that one third to one half of group physicians reported receiving salaries as the major component of their remuneration, while nongroup physicians depended largely on fee for service. This is an important issue, and we shall examine it in detail in a later report.

As an examination of Table 6 also shows, American doctors express less frustration, as reflected in their estimates of trivial and inappropriate consultations, than their British counterparts, and also

report considerably greater satisfaction. The British data reflecting dissatisfaction may be somewhat exaggerated by the political dispute over remuneration and terms of service that were concurrent with the survey, but it is unlikely that these events could account for the magnitude of observed differences. In both countries, doctors were most dissatisfied about time —being able to devote sufficient time to each patient, total amount of time devoted to one's practice, and the limited leisure time available. But unlike British general practitioners, American doctors are far more satisfied with their income, status, incentives, and professional arrangements. Some improvements have been made in remuneration and other conditions of work since the British survey was completed.

One aspect of the British pattern of general practice that has frequently been commented upon is the professional isolation of the general practitioner from his peers. We asked doctors in both countries a very similar question regarding the frequency with which they seek advice from other medical men concerning some aspect of their practice. The question asked of American doctors was somewhat more rigorous in its criterion since it referred to *specifically* contacting other doctors to seek advice in comparison to the British version which asked "How frequently do you seek advice . . . ?" Yet despite this, American doctors report that they much more frequently seek such advice, with 43 percent of the nongroup practitioners and 56 per-

cent of the group practitioners indicating that they seek such advice several times a week, in contrast to only 16 percent of the British doctors.

It is possible that this type of contact might be influenced by friendship patterns and social customs generally rather than the way in which professional practice is structured. We also asked two identical questions of doctors in both countries concerning social contacts and friendships among doctors. In both cases, as Table 7 shows, the distributions were very similar suggesting that the patterns of professional advice seeking probably cannot be attributed to different types of social relationships in the two countries.

Attitudes toward Medical Practice and Government

In both countries, we asked doctors a series of attitudinal questions concerning government involvement in medical affairs, the role of self-sacrifice in being a

Table 7. *Professional and Social Contacts among Primary Care Physicians in Britain and the United States*

	British General	American Primary Care Physicians	
Measures of Contact	Practitioners N = 772 (percent)	Nongroup N = 1148 (percent)	Group N = 310 (percent)
Frequency of seeking advice from other medical men concerning some aspect of practice*			
Several times a week	16	43	56
Every week or so	28	21	19
Couple times a month	17	12	8
A few times a year or less	40	24	17
Frequency of social contact with other physicians in homes			
Every week or so or more	17	10	11
A couple of times a month	19	23	24
A few times a year	43	45	50
Hardly ever	21	22	15
Number of three closest friends who are doctors			
None	24	27	23
One	35	36	37
Two or three	41	37	40

* A slight wording difference is discussed in the text.

doctor, and uncertainty in carrying on a general practice. Table 8 provides data on those items which are to some extent comparable. There was only one item where we asked a clearly comparable question concerning the role of government, and this statement dealt with whether it is proper for government physicians to attempt to evaluate the quality of care in general practice. About three quarters of the British doctors agreed that this was proper, but only 26 percent of American nongroup practitioners, and 35 percent of group practitioners agreed. Although this is only a single item, it does suggest considerably more receptivity to government auditing among British general practitioners than among their American counterparts. As the data in Table 9 relevant to controls show, the vast majority of American doctors approve of peer review of medical work in the hospital, but their enthusiasm is dampened when the review is to be carried out by physicians from outside their own community. These data suggest that American doctors remain quite suspicious of controls by government, or even physician groups outside their immediate community. Pediatricians and internists are least resistant toward outside controls.

In respect to attitudes toward sacrifice, we found no consistent differences between British and American doctors. Among American physicians, doctors in group practice were less likely to endorse sacrificing attitudes, but such differences were relatively modest and have limited practical significance. The third set of items concerned uncertainty about the nature of knowledge underlying decisions that the general practitioner has to make. In my observations of British doctors, I was impressed that such uncertainties were widely prevalent and contributed to the crisis in role definition of the general practitioner.[11] There was only one instance where the identical question was asked in both countries, and this item concerned whether general practice decisions are based upon well-established knowledge. On this item, British general practitioners express much greater uncertainty than American general practitioners, but, in general, American internists and obstetricians respond very much as the British doctors do. The American pediatricians fall between these two extremes. The American general practitioners also express less uncertainty than other American subgroups on a question concerning the doctor's certainty in making many of the assessments for which he is called upon.

In considering these responses, we should note that the questions were addressed to "general practice" and thus general practitioners were probably responding more in terms of their conceptions of their own practices than the other subgroups. American general practitioners seem to have made a better adaptation to feelings of uncertainty than their British counterparts, and this is probably due to the wider scope of their practice, their greater dependence on modern technology and laboratory aids, and their closer tie to hospital work. From the point of view of physicians with more restricted practices, however, general practice appears more vague and ill defined.

Table 9 shows physicians to be relatively evenly divided on many of the major innovations currently under discussion. These attitudinal items are of a very general nature, and a doctor may generally approve of an innovation until it encroaches on his practice or demands that he change his accustomed habits; and, similarly, there are data that indicate that doctors' cooperation with a new program may be relatively independent of their initial attitude toward it.[5] These attitudes, however, suggest trends which are reviewed within the context of other findings in the discussion that follows.

Discussion and Conclusions

The types of data presented in this paper are descriptive rather than evaluative, and implications for public policy do not naturally flow from them. Nor do they pertain

Table 8. *Attitudes of Primary Care Physicians in Britain and the United States toward Various Aspects of Medical Practice*

Percent Agreeing On Various Attitudes	British General Practitioners N = 772 (percent)	American Primary Care Physicians							
		General Practitioners		Internists		Pediatricians		Obstetricians	
		Nongroup N = 599 (percent)	Group N = 111 (percent)	Nongroup N = 231 (percent)	Group N = 91 (percent)	Nongroup N = 136 (percent)	Group N = 43 (percent)	Nongroup N = 150 (percent)	Group N = 58 (percent)
Government auditing									
It is quite proper for government physicians (the N.H.S.)* to attempt to evaluate the quality of care patients receive (provided in general practice)	74	20	30	34	41	38	41	29	29
Sacrificing orientation									
One should not become a doctor unless he is willing to work long and irregular hours	76	88	76	89	78	83	76	89	88
One should not become a doctor unless he is willing to sacrifice his own needs to those of the general welfare	67	56	37	58	42	50	51	51	54
Uncertainty in medical decision-making									
In general practice, one's decisions often are not based on well-established knowledge	58	28	21	45	54	38	38	46	53
Given the conditions of general practice, the doctor is not really in a position to make many of the assessments he is called upon to make	†	19	20	33	40	35	33	38	43
Given the conditions of general practice, the doctor isn't really in a position to make the evaluations necessary for issuing medical certificates	41	†	†	†	†	†	†	†	†

* Differences in wording on the British questions are noted by parentheses.
† Question not asked.

Table 9. *Attitudes of American Primary Care Physicians toward New Features of the Organization of Medical Care*

Proportion Responding that They Strongly Approve or Moderately Approve	General Practitioners		Internists		Pediatricians		Obstetricians	
	Nongroup N = 599 (percent)	Group N = 111 (percent)	Nongroup N = 231 (percent)	Group N = 91 (percent)	Nongroup N = 136 (percent)	Group N = 43 (percent)	Nongroup N = 150 (percent)	Group N = 58 (percent)
Financing								
Concept of government financing of medical care as in the Medicaid Program in your state	38	44	44	57	45	51	39	51
Federal financing of medical care through some system of National Health Insurance	32	44	41	51	43	54	39	41
Practice organization and innovations								
Community health centers such as those established by the Office of Economic Opportunity	52	59	69	78	68	80	60	66
Prepaid group practice such as the Kaiser Permanente Plan or the Health Insurance Plan of New York	40	61	54	65	61	86	45	76
Doctors working on a salaried basis	37	54	50	57	54	68	39	66
Controls over medical work								
Peer review of medical work in the hospital	83	90	88	96	93	100	85	90
Peer review of medical work in the doctor's office	44	57	67	77	69	78	54	64
Review of hospital work by physicians from outside one's community	35	44	54	57	51	60	44	34
New practitioners								
The use of specially trained physician's assistants who work under the doctor's supervision in his practice	78	85	79	87	82	93	74	88
The training of non-M.D. associates who work independently to some extent in underdoctored areas	51	72	62	75	63	68	55	65
Multiphasic health testing								
Multiphasic health screening as part of a doctor's or clinic's practice	75	79	79	82	80	86	73	81
Autonomous programs of multiphasic automated health testing	60	70	57	63	64	69	61	68

directly to the major problems we confront in maintaining primary health care services, in excessive specialization and subspecialization, in the maldistribution of physicians and in maintaining coordinated and comprehensive health care services. Moreover, they speak to doctors' orientations and responses and not to those of their clients, and the interests of these two groups are clearly different. However, when viewed in a larger context, these data provide some appreciation of the advantages and difficulties of primary care practice in the two countries.

Unlike Britain, which directs doctors into general medical practice through organizational means, the American system presently has no mechanism to keep physicians in primary medical care. Our data suggest, however, that it may be incorrect to regard internists and pediatricians as modern replacements of traditional practitioners in that the scope and character of their practice diverges markedly in many respects from the more traditional doctor. Should the trend continue, and we have every reason to believe it will, then the distress of patients concerning the availability of a comprehensive family physician is likely to continue well into the future. Those American doctors who continue to maintain a practice of wide scope appear to function with greater gratification than their British counterparts, who have a much narrower general orientation which seems to exaggerate the disparity between the scientific orientation of medical schools and their own daily practice. They express greater uncertainty about what they are doing, more disillusionment with their role, and they seem more isolated from the mainstream of medicine than is true of their American counterparts.

It appears that the British general practitioner still offers certain advantages that seem to be disappearing in the United States. Within the limits we have described, British G.P.'s take on a wide variety of routine functions which patients expect doctors to perform, and which account for much of the demand on the doctor's time.

Our data indicate that an American patient, with his own internist or pediatrician, has no assurance that such routine functions will be performed by his own doctor if needed. Simple procedures such as suturing lacerations, excising simple cysts, taping strains, etc., may be referred to the local emergency room or some other doctor. Similarly, it seems regrettable that the physician home visit is now defunct in the United States. Certainly given the shortage of physician manpower, the costs of medical care, and the expense of educating new physicians, it would be wasteful to attempt to replicate the high prevalence of home visiting characteristic of the British situation, and even there home visiting is decreasing with time. But it is also difficult to believe that the current situation where home visiting has become a rarity is a particularly desirable pattern. The primary care physician can learn a great deal about a patient and his difficulties by visiting the home from time to time, and the modern form of practice has perhaps gone too far. Yet, it seems unlikely that the current trend can be turned back and, given the pressures on medical care, it seems apparent that alternatives will be necessary.

If, indeed, primary care physicians of the future are to be internists and pediatricians, and perhaps some family doctors as well, then it would be prudent to encourage such physicians to enlarge the scope of their practices so that they can encompass routine problems of care as well as those more complicated. It seems apparent that one way of doing this is to make use of trained assistants and technicians who can expertly carry out certain procedures that the doctor is unwilling to do himself. These procedures would include handling simple trauma, dealing with problems of behavior and child care, simple surgery, health education, etc. It is reasonably clear from our data that physicians support the use of such assistants, but thus far there is no evidence that they are widely or effectively used. Nurse practitioners and others might also be helpful in reviving the institution of home visiting which, if well organized, can contribute to a more comprehensive pattern of primary care than is now evident. Such goals as increasing the scope and comprehensiveness of practice perhaps may best be fulfilled within the context of prepaid group practice, and certainly such practices facilitate the effective use of technology and ancillary workers, but at least one major study has suggested that such practices may be less responsive to the social and psychological aspects of the doctor-patient relationship.[8]

Although we have not examined such issues as the doctor-patient relationship directly, the data we have provide a mixed picture in respect to the issue of the relative merits of group vs. nongroup practice. Nongroup doctors are more likely to make homecalls, however few, but there are no differences between group and nongroup doctors in their orientations to medicine. Doctors in groups appear to do somewhat more diagnostic work, have more professional contact with colleagues, and are generally more receptive to a variety of innovations in practice organization (Table 9). We have no way of assessing to what extent these differences are a product of group practice, or the result of a selection process in which persons with certain characteristics have chosen one or the other type of activity. Although some have suggested that group practice is less satisfying than an independent one, our data suggest that at least those doctors already in group practice are no less satisfied than their counterparts in nongroup practice.

Although our data are rather gross relative to time budgets, they suggest that nongroup practitioners work longer hours than those in groups. Given the extremely long hours worked by physicians, this is a mixed blessing, but these data do support Bailey's concern[1,2] that group practice may lead to a more limited workweek, thus minimizing already scarce physician manhours. Of course, our data do not exclude the possibility that physicians who are somewhat less oriented to long workweeks are presently selected into group practice,

or that incentives can be developed to increase the workweek among group practitioners if this was seen as desirable.

In sum, our data indicate that primary medical practice in the United States and Britain are radically different types of practice,[14] and that within the United States the concept of the primary care physician involves varied orientations and patterns. There is little doubt that an effective system of health care services depends on a viable system of delivering and coordinating primary care, and it is clear that we still have much work to do in developing viable future models of primary health services that make use of modern developments in medical technology and knowledge, but that are also responsive to the needs and human dilemmas of those who seek the care of a physician.

This study was supported, in part, by Grant No. CH 00404, National Center for Health Services Research and Development, Health Services and Mental Health Administration, United States Department of Health, Education, and Welfare.

REFERENCES

1. Bailey R: Economies of scale in medical practice. In Klarman HE (ed.): Empirical Studies in Health Economics. Baltimore, Johns Hopkins Press, 1970, pp 255–277
2. ———: Philosophy, faith, fact and fiction in the production of medical services. Inquiry 7:37, 1970
3. Cartwright A: General practice in 1963: its conditions, contents and satisfactions. Med Care 3:69, 1965
4. ———: Patients and Their Doctors: A Study of General Practice. London, Routledge and Kegan Paul, 1967
5. Colombotos J: Physicians' responses to changes in health care: some projections. Inquiry 8:20, 1971
6. Faich R: Social and Structural Factors Affecting Work Satisfaction. Dissertation in the Dept. of Sociology, University of Wisconsin, 1969
7. Fein R: The Doctor Shortage: An Economic Analysis. Washington, D. C., The Brookings Institution, 1967

8. Freidson E: Patients' Views of Medical Practice. New York, Russell Sage Foundation, 1961

9. Kern D: Survey of communication patterns between general practitioners and consultants: a preliminary report. Unpublished manuscript, Harvard Medical School

10. Mechanic D: General practice in England and Wales: results from a survey of a national sample of general practitioners. Med Care 6:245, 1968

11. ———: General medical practice in England and Wales: its organization and future. N Engl J Med 279:680, 1968

12. ———: Practice orientations among general medical practitioners in England and Wales. Med Care 8:15, 1970

13. ———: Correlates of frustration among British general practitioners. J Health Soc Behav 11;87, 1970

14. ———: The English National Health Service: some comparisons with the United States. J Health Soc Behav 12:18, 1971

15. Mechanic D, Faich R: Doctors in revolt: the crisis in the English National Health Service. Med Care 8:442, 1970

Twenty-One Years of General Practice —Changing Patterns*

John Fry

The form and character of medical care are never static. There must be constant change to adapt to new medical and social situations. Planning for the future should be based on a continuing evaluation of data to ensure the best use of available resources.

General practice, or primary medical care, is an essential part of any system of health care. Its form may be influenced by local and national philosophies but it must be present otherwise the other parts of the health services are unable to function effectively.

Since the introduction of the National Health Service in 1948 there have been some major changes in the organisation of general practice. More changes are projected for the future. If these are to be beneficial to the public and the profession, recent developments in general practice during this period should be taken into account. A review of 21 years work in one general practice is presented to stimulate discussion.

The Practice

The practice is over 50 years old and I began single-handed 25 years ago. It is now a two-man practice supported by a nurse, health visitor, midwife and secretary-receptionists. The area is a middle-class South-east London suburb about ten miles from the centre of the city.

Since 1947 continuous records of work patterns have been kept. The 21-year pe-

* Reprinted by permission from the *Journal of the Royal College of General Practitioners*, 22:521–528, 1972.

riod 1951–1972 has been selected for review and analysis to allow for the introductory period in the early days of the National Health Service.

Standard records are available for the population at risk; the changes in personnel and methods within the practice; the work load; the use of hospital facilities; and the attendance rates for the main clinical groups.

Data for practice population were available for all the patients registered with the practice through the National Health Service. There have been virtually no private patients.

The work carried out by the general practitioners has been recorded by doctor-patient consultations in the consulting room and at home visits.

Records have been kept of all referrals for direct radiological or pathological investigations and also of all those referred to hospital specialists for outpatient consultation or admission.

Details of the clinical diagnosis were made by classifying the general practitioners' work into clinical groups. This was done to help recording. It was not possible to record and analyse all attendances with the *International Classification of Disease*.

Results

Practice Population

The population at risk during the period under review is shown in Table 1. Two general practitioners can care for almost 9,000 people as there is a partnership with two other practitioners with relatively small lists and therefore there is a maxi-

Table 1. *Practice Population 1951–1972*

	1951	1952	1953	1954	1955	1956	1957	1958	1959	1960	
Practice population	4400	4658	5065	5411	5551	5741	5853	6365	6663	6801	
	1961	1962	1963	1964	1965	1966	1967	1968	1969	1970	1971
Practice population	7082	7578	7843	7831	7902	8241	8480	8784	9022	9020	9007

mum allowance of up to 4,500 per doctor. Nevertheless it has been possible for two doctors to provide a good standard of care.

Work Patterns—Consultations and Home Visits

The rates for consultations and home visits are shown in Table 2 measured by the average attendance rates per person per year.

Some trends can be noted. First, there has been an overall reduction of work during the 21 years, particularly with home visits. It has also occurred with consultations.

Secondly, the changes were related closely to external influences. The workload increased when extra doctors were first introduced into the practice in 1955–1959, when the first assistant was em-ployed, and in 1960–1963 when three doctors worked in the practice. The workload began to decrease from 1963 when a full appointment system was introduced, when a health visitor was first attached and when more secretarial-receptionist staff were employed.

Thirdly, since 1964 there have been active and positive efforts to reduce unnecessary work. Patients were encouraged to come to the consulting rooms rather than receive home visits. Revisiting by the doctors was reduced and some delegated to the practice nurse and health visitor. The number of visits they carried out were 500 –600 per year. [0.05 per person].

Better methods of care, for example, better antibiotics for infections, better diuretics for congestive cardiac failure, better drugs for the management of asthma, arthritis, depression, anxiety and skin conditions have all made it possible to

Table 2. *Work Patterns—Consultations and Home Visit Rates Per Person Per Year*

	1951	1952	1953	1954	1955	1956	1957	1958	1959	1960
Consultations	2.7	2.5	2.5	2.4	2.6	2.7	3.1	2.9	2.8	3.0
Home visits	0.6	0.7	0.7	0.7	0.7	0.8	0.8	0.7	0.8	0.7
Total	3.3	3.2	3.2	3.1	3.3	3.5	3.9	3.6	3.6	3.7

NOTE: 1951–5 : one doctor   1955–1961 : two doctors
1960–1972 : two consulting rooms

	1961	1962	1963	1964	1965	1966	1967	1968	1969	1970	1971
Consultations	3.2	3.0	2.7	2.7	2.5	2.6	2.5	2.2	2.2	2.2	2.0
Home visits	0.6	0.6	0.6	0.5	0.3	0.4	0.4	0.2	0.1	0.1	0.1
Total	3.8	3.6	3.3	3.2	2.8	3.0	2.9	2.4	2.3	2.3	2.1

NOTE: 1961–3 : three doctors   1963–1970 : two doctors
1962–1972 : Full appointment system
1962–1972 : Health visitor attached
1968–1972 : Practice nurse

reduce the number of times patients have to be seen.

For many reasons the work-load in the practice has been reduced appreciably during the 21 years. Overall, there has been a 46 percent reduction from the peak to now and an 87 percent reduction in home visits with a 31 percent reduction in surgery consultations.

Work Patterns—per Session, Day, and Week

Alternatively, it is possible to calculate the amount of work as shown by the number of consultations and home visits per doctor during each week, each day, and at each working session (Table 3).

The total work in the practice reached its peak in 1960–63, but has fallen since. Personally, I was busiest in the 1950s and I am now seeing almost 100 fewer patients per week than at my peak in 1954 for almost the same number of people at risk.

The number of consulting sessions per week has risen from ten in 1951 to 25 in 1971. All are now by appointment and five are special clinics including antenatal and child care.

What is not shown in the table and what has made life much easier for me has been the rota system with another group for night and weekend work. With the appointment system, I now finish my practice work by 1800 hours instead of 2000 or 2100 hours, as in the pre-appointment period.

Table 3. *Work Patterns—Consultations and Home Visits per Day, Session, and Week for Each General Practitioner*

	Practice Total per Working Day		Daily Total per General Practitioner			Weekly Total per General Practitioner	
Year	Consulta-tions	Home Visits	Consulta-tions	Home Visits	Per Consulting Session	Total Consultations and Home Visits	Hours per Week in Contact with Patients
1951	40	9	40	9	24	285	39.3
1952	39	10	39	10	23	280	
1953	42	11	42	11	25	305	
1954	44	9	44	9	24	309	43.0
1955	47	9	31	6	24	275	
1956	53	11	35	7	26	275	
1957	60	14	40	9	30	260	
1958	62	13	42	9	25	270	
1959	65	15	44	10	26	275	
1960	69	15	35	8	20	250	
1961	76	14	30	5	21	250	
1962	77	14	30	5	21	245	
1963	71	15	35	8	19	235	
1964	71	11	35	5	19	235	
1965	65	10	33	5	17	235	
1966	72	10	36	5	19	230	
1967	71	11	35	5	17	225	
1968	66	6	33	3	16	225	
1969	67	5	34	2	16	220	
1970	65	4	33	2	16	215	27.1
1971	61	3	30	2	15	210	

Table 4. *Timetable*

Day	Morning		Afternoon		Night
	08:30–11:30	*11:30–13:00*	*14:00–15:00*	*15:30–17:30*	*17:30–07:30 next day*
Monday	Consultations	Home visits	Antenatal clinic	Consultations	FREE
Tuesday	Consultations	Home visits	Child care clinic	Consultations	ON CALL
Wednesday	Consultations	Home visits	Consultations*	Consultations*	FREE
Thursday	FREE DAY				FREE
Friday	Consultations	Home visits	Consultations	Consultations	ON CALL one in four
Saturday	Consultations*	Home visits	ON CALL ONE IN FOUR		
Sunday	ON CALL ONE IN FOUR				

* Some weeks only.
Note: In addition about three to four hours a week are spent on administration including letter writing.

My life in general practice is now very much easier, more planned and controlled, and less stressful than 20 years ago. I believe that I am providing a much better service for my patients.

Other work, outside the practice, was carried out during this period. During 1951–1960 two, weekly sessions, as a hospital clinical assistant, were undertaken and since 1960 at least one day per week has been spent on a variety of extra-practice professional activities (Table 4).

Referrals to Hospital

The referral system to hospital specialists makes the British general practitioner an important influence on the number of people treated in hospital. During 1951–1972 the rates of hospital referrals fell in this practice by one half (Table 5) (Fry, 1971).

Referral for Radiography and Pathology

Full access to direct radiography and pathology have been available at local hospitals. The rates of referral shown in Table 6 show fairly constant levels during the 21 year period.

Clinical Groups

The attendances for various clinical groups and the rates of attendance for 13

Table 5. *Hospital Referrals per 100 Patients 1951–1972*

	1951	1952	1953	1954	1955	1956	1957	1958	1959	1960	
Patients referred to hospital (%)	10.5	10.3	9.0	8.7	8.5	8.3	7.5	6.5	6.5	6.7	
	1961	1962	1963	1964	1965	1966	1967	1968	1969	1970	1971
Patients referred to hospital (%)	7.2	6.6	6.0	5.2	5.0	5.5	5.0	5.0	4.8	5.2	4.0

selected groups of conditions were calculated for each year (Table 7).

There were falls in rheumatic, gastro-intestinal, cardiovascular, central nervous system, respiratory and dermatological groups. There were increased rates of attendance for obstetric, gynecological and immunization groups. No marked changes were noted in upper respiratory infections, psychiatric, ear, nose and throat, and urological conditions. Dramatic psychosocial emergencies have all but disappeared.

It would appear that the main reduction in work has been with the degenerative conditions associated with ageing and that increase in work has occurred with those groups in which positive preventive activities have been a feature. It is of interest that the rates of attendance for psychiatric conditions have remained constant in spite of the advent of the newer psychotropic drugs.

Discussion

It is agreed that general practice or its equivalent is an essential part of our National Health System. It is also accepted that our general practitioners should continue as personal and family doctors acting as generalists. To provide good care on a continuing basis, the general practitioner must have the right tools, including education, premises and staff and access to diagnostic and therapeutic facilities at local hospitals.

General practice is a highly personal field and the individual doctor should be free to plan and organise his work as he feels best for his patients. Nevertheless there are many common features and even a highly personalised review of one practice in one area by one particular, and perhaps peculiar, general practitioner may pose questions for the future.

This review of 21 years in one practice raises some fundamental queries which suggest some long held beliefs should be reviewed.

It is clear that in this particular practice it is possible for two practitioners to cope with twice as many patients as average in ways that, apparently, are satisfactory to both patients and doctors. If this is so in one practice, is it possible in others?

The volume of work in the practice, by several measurements, has fallen considerably during the 20 year period. This has been particularly noteworthy in the home visiting role which has been reduced eightfold.

Among many factors the most important have been the organisation of the work and the attitudes of patients, doctors and staff, who through collaboration and co-operation have made it possible for the same number of doctors to care for more people.

The increased work in the preventive field suggests that the National Health Service is making it possible for general practice to move towards a *health* service rather than a disease service. There were reductions in attendances for the more chronic and degenerative conditions, possibly be-

Table 6. *Radiography and Pathology Referrals per 100 Patients*

	1951	1952	1953	1954	1955	1956	1957	1958	1959	1960	
Radiography	6.9	5.9	5.9	5.5	6.0	7.2	5.2	5.5	6.7	6.2	
Pathology	5.7	5.1	5.4	6.9	8.2	5.8	5.4	4.5	5.9	5.5	
	1961	1962	1963	1964	1965	1966	1967	1968	1969	1970	1971
Radiography	8.3	7.4	7.1	5.3	6.0	6.1	5.3	4.7	6.1	6.0	5.5
Pathology	8.2	6.6	6.4	5.5	5.6	8.8	5.8	6.1	6.4	6.8	6.2

Table 7. *Attendance Rates per 100 Patients by Clinical Groups*

	Rheumatic	Gastro-intestinal	Cardio-vascular	Central Nervous System	Respiratory	Upper Respiratory Infections	Pregnancy	Gynae-cology	Skin	Psychiatric	Immunizations	Ear, Nose, and Throat	Urological
1951	22.7	27.3	12.8	9.0	22.7	36.3	7.7	8.0	26.1	29.5	3.9	14.8	4.8
1952	23.4	36.2	21.3	8.1	30.8	48.5	6.8	6.5	30.7	30.7	4.2	15.9	6.5
1953	21.0	28.0	18.0	12.0	30.0	66.0	7.5	7.0	30.0	30.0	5.0	18.0	5.0
1954	24.1	29.9	18.5	15.5	23.7	41.0	7.5	7.5	31.5	23.5	7.7	16.7	5.6
1955	22.5	30.4	17.9	13.4	25.0	50.0	7.5	7.3	31.2	23.0	9.0	17.9	7.3
1956	27.5	33.3	21.8	13.2	30.0	54.2	10.5	7.0	33.3	27.3	8.7	17.5	7.0
1957	27.1	30.5	23.6	13.6	30.5	71.2	9.3	9.3	33.6	30.5	16.0	16.8	6.8
1958	28.1	28.1	26.5	12.5	26.8	51.5	9.4	7.8	32.8	28.1	32.5	16.2	6.3
1959	26.9	31.4	25.3	11.2	29.9	55.2	11.8	11.0	35.4	23.8	25.2	17.7	6.5
1960	32.3	36.8	26.5	13.3	28.0	45.6	13.3	13.5	33.0	32.3	31.0	22.1	5.8
1961	30.0	35.5	25.5	14.3	22.5	50.0	17.7	13.5	33.0	34.0	31.5	18.5	8.0
1962	27.8	32.8	26.3	11.8	27.5	42.1	17.0	11.8	29.0	30.5	29.0	18.4	8.0
1963	24.3	32.1	21.2	10.3	28.2	47.5	15.4	10.5	27.0	30.8	14.2	19.3	6.5
1964	27.0	29.5	23.0	14.1	23.0	35.8	15.6	12.8	28.3	32.3	11.6	18.0	6.6
1965	22.8	27.8	19.0	10.5	22.8	43.4	15.2	13.3	27.0	25.8	10.5	17.8	6.7
1966	23.2	29.5	18.3	9.7	22.4	41.4	15.0	15.0	24.3	28.0	18.3	18.3	7.5
1967	22.3	23.5	16.5	9.4	20.0	35.3	14.4	13.0	24.8	30.6	9.5	15.3	5.9
1968	20.5	20.6	14.2	8.0	17.3	30.7	10.2	14.0	20.5	28.3	9.7	15.3	5.6
1969	20.0	21.2	11.2	7.2	16.6	33.3	10.5	11.2	22.2	26.7	8.8	15.6	5.6
1970	19.0	19.0	10.0	9.9	15.6	27.8	11.2	11.3	20.0	25.6	11.2	14.5	5.6
1971	18.9	20.5	10.0	7.8	14.5	27.8	10.2	12.2	16.6	26.7	14.0	12.5	6.1

cause of better therapeutic methods or because of changing attitudes of the doctors in seeing these persons less frequently.

There were no great changes in the rates of use of the diagnostic radiological and pathological facilities but there was a remarkable two-fold reduction in the rates of referrals to hospital specialists including domiciliary consultations. Perhaps with more experience, more confidence and better therapeutic resources the general practitioners are better able to cope with the more serious diseases outside hospital?

The major question is how many general practitioners are needed in the future? Have we perhaps a surfeit now? Should we be trying to induce more and more young doctors to enter general practice?

These are important national and public issues that can be answered only by a much larger national analysis and studies of the work patterns of both general practitioners and of hospital specialists as well.

Before this study is dismissed as biased and irrelevant because it is from one single practice, the findings in other practices of work patterns as shown in *The Report from General Practice No.* 13 (1970) should be consulted. Similar trends are shown here. The facts show indisputable changes in this practice; if they can be repeated in others then we may have to revise our manpower policies for the future.

Summary

A review of the patterns of work and care in one general practice in South London over 21 years (1951–1972) raises some fundamental questions on the use of manpower resources in the future.

It has been found possible for two general practitioners to provide sound care for a population of over 9,000—twice the national average.

The volume of work, expressed in annual doctor-patient consulting rates and home visits, has fallen by more than one third during the 20 year period, particularly for home visits. Expressed in another way, the author is now seeing 100 patients fewer and working 16 hours a week less with approximately the same number of patients.

Increases in rates of work are shown for preventive procedures such as immunization, antenatal care, cervical cytology and child welfare, with decreases for degenerative conditions including rheumatic, cardiovascular and central nervous systems and those affecting the skin and the gastrointestinal tract. Referrals to specialists fell by half.

While acknowledging that these findings are those derived from one particular single practice, nevertheless the results merit urgent national studies to test the hypothesis that perhaps there are already enough general practitioners. Similar studies are needed to examine the work-patterns of hospital consultants.

Addendum

The number of patients booked per hour at surgery consultations is as follows:
Normal consultation
     session . . . . 9–10 per hour
Antenatal session . . . . . . 12 per hour
Child care session . . . . . . 12 per hour
    Home visits are done at a rate of 4–5 per hour.

Acknowledgment

Since 1960, Dr John B Dillane has been my partner and colleague and his great help has been gratefully acknowledged.

Author's Update

It is interesting to note how the "changing patterns" have become stabilised and relatively unchanging since 1972.

The volume of work has remained at a constant level for a practice population of the same size, and the referral rates to specialists, and the use of radiological and pathological sciences have remained constant, too.

It is concluded that, unless major external forces alter the practice routine, the work rate will remain constant. If this is so, then it is possible to predict and forecast future needs of resources and manpower in a practice.

REFERENCES

1. Fry J: Lancet 2:148, 1971
2. Report from General Practice No. 13. (1970). Present State and Future Needs. Second edition. London: J R Coll Gen Pract

The Work Content of General Practice*

Based on a Survey of Selected Procedures Performed by Victorian General Practitioners in 1978

Ian L. Rowe, Neil E. Carson

Much has been spoken about the changing nature of general practice, although little documental evidence is available to identify the nature of these changes. Such changes are said to include provision of some diagnostic services, diminishing involvement in surgical and obstetrical procedures, and a lessening of GP involvement in the hospital care of patients.

Information about the range of services provided by the average general practitioner is essential knowledge required by planners of undergraduate, vocational and continuing education programmes. In view of the anticipated rapid increase in general practitioner numbers in the near future, further changes in the nature of the discipline are predicted.

A survey of general practitioners was therefore proposed by four bodies concerned with medical education relevant to general practice, viz.—the Victorian Medical Postgraduate Foundation, the Monash University Department of Social and Preventive Medicine (Section of Community Practice), the Royal Australian College of General Practitioners (Victoria Faculty) and the Victorian Academy for General Practice Limited.

Method

A combined list of general practitioners was constructed from the mailing lists of a commercial firm and *Australian Family Physician*. This list was distributed to all area coordinators of the RACGP Family Medicine Programme, who corrected the list to conform to their local knowledge. The resultant mailing list comprised 2418 doctors. Information from the Medical Board survey was not available because of its confidentiality.

A letter was then mailed to each doctor, together with a questionnaire and reply paid envelope, seeking information on procedures personally performed by the doctor in the previous two years, investigations on site, hospital access in 1977–78, and background data on year of graduation, sex, number of years full time hospital experience and location of practice.

The data were analyzed as a whole and no identification with individual doctors was made.

* Reprinted by permission from *Australian Family Physician*, 9:177–183, March, 1980.

Response

Altogether 1420 completed forms were returned. Despite efforts to eliminate errors, 131 doctors declared themselves ineligible for a variety of reasons, such as specialization or restriction of their practice, and seven were deceased. Deletion of these 138 names reduced the original list to 2280. Such inaccuracies demonstrate the difficulty of maintaining an accurate up-to-date list of GPs. The response of 1420 to 2280 was 62 percent.

Results

Year of Graduation

Graduates in the decade 1951–60 were more numerous than in any other decade (see Figure 1), and accounted for 469 (33 percent) of respondents. The decade 1961–70, however, accounted for 402 (28 percent). This is particularly significant when one notes that graduates of the University of Melbourne numbered 1445 in 1951–60

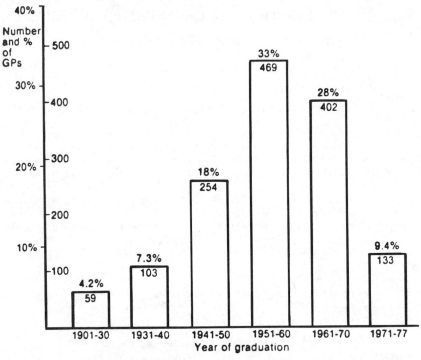

Fig. 1. Percentage of graduation by decade.

and, with the addition of a small number from Monash University, rose to 1929 in 1961–70. These figures are consistent with expressed views that too many graduates in the 1960s sought specialist training and too few sought a career in general practice.

Sex

Male general practitioners comprised 89.5 percent of respondents and female general practitioners 10.5 percent.

Hospital Experience

Following graduation, the average mean number of years of full time hospital experience was three years, and the median was 2.5 years. Table 1 details the length of this experience. Fifty-four respondents (3.9 percent) failed to answer this question, whereas non responses to questions on

year of graduation, sex and local government area were 0, 27 and four respectively.

Location

Melbourne statistical division, which includes Werribee, Melton, Whittlesea, Dandenong and the Mornington Peninsula, ac-

Table 1. *Hospital Experience following Graduation*

Number of Years	Number of Doctors	Percentage of Total
0 years	9	0.6
1 year	259	18.0
2 years	406	29.0
3 years	290	20.0
4 years	153	11.0
5 years and more	249	17.5

counted for 977 (69 percent) and country divisions 443 (31 percent). This distirbution of respondents is slightly different from that found in the Medical Manpower Survey 1977,[1] where country divisions accounted for 26 percent. The response of country GPs was higher in this survey of general practitioners, possibly because of the greater involvement of country GPs, compared with city GPs in the scope of work under investigation (see later).

Details of Work Content

Table 2 summarizes the findings related to GP involvement in a range of minor surgical procedures, and Table 3 lists some 'major' surgical procedures. The percentage of general practitioners now performing major surgery is very small.

Obstetrics is still practised by two thirds of general practitioners, with an additional 14 percent providing antenatal and postnatal care only. Table 4 refers to some obstetric and family planning services performed by GPs.

Approximately half the GPs gave anaesthetics (40 percent) ranging from 12 percent still performing open ether anaesthetics, to halothane (20 percent) and those using relaxants (35 percent).

Table 5 lists the various diagnostic procedures performed by the general practitioners on site. Pathology testing was completely absent in many practices, and only

Table 3. *GP Surgery*

'Major' Surgical Procedures	% of GPs
Appendicectomy	27
Herniorrhaphy	16
Cholecystectomy	7
Hysterectomy	8
Perforated duodenal ulcer	5

55 percent performed on site microurine examinations.

Half the GPs reported that they held hospital appointments of different types—honorary appointments (18 percent); paid sessional (10 percent); part-time salaried (three percent); part-time hospital superintendent (two percent); but the majority being medical staff fee-for-service (32 percent). Nearly all GPs had access to hospital beds for private patients (86 percent) but only half had access to beds for standard ward patients (52 percent)

Work Content and Decade of Graduation

The work content varied with the decade of graduation. Tonsillectomy, D and C, major surgery, fracture manipulation under GA and complicated obstetrics were done by a higher proportion of graduates from 1951–60 than from other decades. On the other hand, the work of graduates of 1971–76 included a higher proportion than other decades, of minor surgery, fractures requiring POP only, ECG and

Table 2. *GP Surgery*

'Minor' Surgical Procedures	% of GPs
Suturing of wounds	95
Removal of sebaceous cysts	88
D and C	54
Tonsillectomy	33
Fracture management (Plaster only)	87
Fracture management (Plus manipulation under general anaesthetic)	46

Table 4. *Obstetrics and Family Planning*

Procedure	% of GPs
Full obstetric care	64
Surgical induction	58
Manual removal of placenta	48
Caesarean section	13
Sexual counselling	83
IUD insertion	64
Vasectomy	24
Tubal ligation	22

Table 5. *On Site Diagnostic Procedures*

Radiology	% of GPs	Pathology Tests	% of GPs	Others	% of GPs
Extremities	49	Pregnancy	78	ECG	61
Chest	16	Microurine	55	Spirometry	31
IVP	4	Haemoglobin	33		
		Biochemical estimations	8		

spirometry, confinements, sex counselling, IUD insertion and anaesthetics.

Hospital appointments were held by a higher proportion of graduates of 1961–70 than from other decades.

Work Content and Sex

The work content varied markedly with sex. Male doctors recorded a higher proportion of every item of work on the questionnaire except for three things—antenatal care only, antenatal and postnatal care but not confinement, and paid sessional hospital appointments.

Work Content and Hospital Experience

The work content also markedly related to the number of years full-time hospital experience. Doctors with three or more years hospital experience recorded a higher percentage of nearly all items on the questionnaire. Only in halothane and relaxant anaesthetics and microurine were the doctors with two years' hospital experience able to surpass those with three or more years of experience.

Melbourne and Country

The work content by country GPs exceeded that of Melbourne GPs in nearly every item. The exceptions were paid sessional or part time salaried hospital appointments, which involved only a small number of practitioners, and radiology and pathology on site, in which there was no significant difference between country and Melbourne.

The difference between country and Melbourne was not related to years of hospital experience, nor to the year of graduation. There was no significant difference in hospital experience and year of graduation between country and Melbourne GPs. The proportion of female doctors was lower among country GPs (eight percent female) than Melbourne GPs (11 percent female), but the difference was not sufficient to account for the increased work content of country GPs.

Some of the more interesting differences are demonstrated in Table 6.

Hospital Experience and Year of Graduation

There was an interesting correlation between hospital experience and year of graduation. Graduates of 1971–77 had a longer average hospital experience than did earlier decades; for example, 47 percent had two years hospital experience and 31 percent had three years hospital experience. The next longest average hospital experience was demonstrated in the 1961–70 graduates, who had 29 percent with two years hospital experience, and 23 percent with three years.

Table 6. *Number and Percentage of GPs Performing Various Services in Melbourne and the Country*

Scope of Work	Melb. GPs		Country GPs		All GPs	
Tonsillectomy	268	27%	205	47%	474	33%
D and C	470	48%	296	67%	768	54%
Appendicectomy	171	18%	211	48%	383	27%
Fracture manip. GA	377	39%	280	64%	659	46%
Blood transfusion	337	34%	307	70%	646	45%
ECG on site	526	54%	339	77%	866	61%
AN confinement and PN	537	55%	370	84%	911	64%
Surg. induction labour	492	50%	332	76%	828	58%
Caesarian section	69	7%	111	25%	182	13%
Ectopic preg. op.	68	7%	94	21%	163	12%
Tubal ligation	154	16%	162	37%	317	22%
Vasectomy	180	18%	156	36%	337	24%
Anaesthesia	365	37%	275	63%	642	45%

Hospital Experience and Sex

Another interesting correlation was between hospital experience and sex. Female GPs had a shorter average hospital experience than did male GPs. One year was the duration of full time hospital experience for 29 percent of female GPs and 17 percent of male GPs, whereas two years was the duration for 26 percent of female GPs and 30 percent of male GPs, and the percentage of males was higher for three or more years of hospital experience.

This could partly account for the more limited work content of female GPs.

Discussion

Previous Studies

The percentage of practices providing pathology and special investigations was consistent with the Australia-wide findings of Carson[2] in 1973. The investigations provided by the highest percentage of practices were pregnancy test, ECG, microurine and haemoglobin, in that order, in both the 1973 and 1978 surveys.

Similarly, the percentage of practices providing on site radiology services was consistent with that found by Farrell[3] in 1976, when approximately half the practices providing x-rays of extremities also took chest x-rays and only a minority took IVP and barium x-rays.

Kelly's[4] survey of 1971 revealed a higher percentage of practices providing surgical, obstetrical, transfusion and anaesthetic procedures (see Table 2), than the present survey. Kelly's published paper revealed Australia-wide data, but the figures quoted in Table 7 are his unpublished data on his sample of 281 Victorian GPs. This confirms the often stated opinion that general practice surgery, obstetrics and anaesthetics have been taken over by specialists.

Provision of radiology on site, on the other hand, was much the same in 1978 and 1971. Comparison of pathology services revealed opposite trends for two important tests—haemoglobin estimation was provided by fewer practices in 1978 (33:68), whereas microurine was provided by more practices in 1978 (55:42). ECG and spirometry were provided by more practices in 1978 (ECG 61:45, spirometry 31:10). The overall percentage of GPs with hospital appointments was much the same.

Kelly's survey also revealed that surgical and obstetric services were provided by a higher percentage of country GPs than capital city GPs in all Australian States.

Similar differences between country and

Table 7. *Percentage of GPs Performing Various Services, 1971 and 1978*

Scope of Work by GPs	% of GPs 1971	% of GPs 1978
Tonsillectomy	56	33
D and C	67	54
Haemorrhoidectomy	43	18
Appendicectomy	38	27
Herniorrhaphy	26	16
Cholecystectomy	10	7
Hysterectomy	9	8
Perforated ulcer	8	5
Normal confinement	81	64
Surgical induction labour	72	58
Caesarian section	15	13
Ectopic pregnancy operation	20	12
Anaesthetics	65	45
Blood transfusion	74	46
X-rays—extremities	45	49
—chest	19	16
Microurine	42	55
Haemoglobin	68	33
Culture and sensitivities	6	8
Biochemical estimations	11	8
ECG (on site)	45	61
Spirometry (on site)	10	31

city were demonstrated in New South Wales by Andersen[5] in 1966 and Chancellor and Andersen[6] in 1974–75.

GP Surgery

The role of GPs in major surgery is obviously diminishing, as specialist surgeons become more numerous, more readily available and no more expensive to the patient than GP surgeons as a result of the differential rebate provisions of the National Health Service. Even for major emergency surgery in the country, improving patient transport will enable a patient to be brought to a major city or provincial hospital or at other times enable a specialist surgeon to travel to a country hospital.

GPs with adequate training and experi-

ence in surgery will probably continue to perform surgical operations for many years, especially in the country, but opportunities for such training and experience have diminished markedly and this partly explains why young graduates are not performing the range of surgical services provided by graduates of the 1950s.

One can predict therefore that the present trend will continue.

GP Obstetrics

The percentage of GPs performing obstetrics is still high; though not as high as several years ago. Here the situation is different from surgery, and this may be due to the provision of training opportunities for GPs in obstetrics. Whereas the Royal Australasian College of Surgeons encourages the transfer of all operative surgery from GPs to surgeons, the Royal College of Obstetricians and Gynaecologists has joined with the Royal Australian College of General Practitioners in acknowledging the important role of GPs in providing obstetrical services, and has cooperated in the provision of training posts for GPs in obstetrics and in the establishment of a Diploma of Obstetrics for GP obstetricians.

The situation is therefore evolving whereby GPs will be able to choose whether or not to add obstetrics to their range of services.

Anaesthetics

As with surgery, the role of the GP is diminishing with regard to the giving of anaesthetics. However, it may surprise many that 45 percent of respondents gave anaesthetics, and most of these used halothane and relaxants.

One can detect a similar trend to that pertaining to GP obstetrics. GPs are making a deliberate choice as to whether to give anaesthetics or not.

The survey revealed that a higher percentage of 1970–76 graduates gave anaesthetics than did older graduates. This suggests that the GP anaesthetist will not be replaced by the specialist anaesthetist, and both will continue to play their part in the provision of anaesthetic services.

Radiology on Site

Nearly half the practices provided x-ray services as in 1971. Obviously, it is convenient for patient and doctor to have these services on site. Since there has been no change since 1971, it would appear likely that many GPs will continue to provide such services for simple x-rays, and that the provision of more complicated x-rays will be provided only by large groups which include a radiologist or employ a radiographer, as was demonstrated by Farrell in 1976.

Pathology on Site

The provision of facilities for microurine by only 55 percent of practices would appear to be a matter for criticism, although it has increased since the previous survey.

The simplicity, low cost and usefulness in patient management of microscopy of urine appears to be poorly understood by many general practitioners. Similarly, the falling number of GPs providing haemoglobin as an on site test to only 33 percent, needs to be examined further.

ECG

It is also surprising that only 61 percent of GPs provided ECG on site, although this has increased considerably in the period between surveys. It is likely that the need to acquire additional skills is a barrier that older GPs are not prepared to overcome. The younger generation of GPs are likely to solve this problem in time.

Family Planning

Sex counselling was provided by 83 percent of GPs, and IUD insertions by 64 percent. Obviously, a great majority of GPs regard family planning as an integral part of general practice.

But the lack of involvement by a significant number of GPs in this area supports the contention that family planning clinics are required to meet a need not fully met by family doctors.

Hospital Appointments and Access

Only 14 percent of GPs do not have access to hospital beds for private and intermediate patients. Fifty-two percent have hospital appointments with access to hospital beds for standard patients. These data are not consistent with complaints by GPs of lack of access to hospitals.

Conclusion

A significant percentage of Victorian GPs perform major surgery, complicated obstetrics, modern anaesthetics and a wide range of investigatory services, especially in the country. However, the percentage of GPs performing major surgery has diminished markedly, especially by more recent graduates, and this trend can be expected to continue.

On the other hand, the percentage of GPs performing obstetrics and anaesthetics, although diminished, is 64 percent and 45 percent respectively and higher among 1970–76 graduates, thus indicating the likelihood of continued involvement of many GPs in obstetrics and anaesthetics.

The percentage of practices providing appropriate on site pathology, ECG and spirometry was low. The attention of medical educators is drawn to these areas.

Future surveys at intervals are recommended to monitor trends, and to guide those persons concerned in the education of general practitioners.

Acknowledgments

We wish to acknowledge with grateful thanks the grant from the Victorian Academy for General Practice Limited, which has enabled this study to be done. We also wish to thank the following for their assistance: the members of the Research Committee, Victoria Faculty, and area coordinators, Family Medicine Programme, Royal Australian College of General Practitioners; Professor LJ Opit and Miss DB Mercer, Department of Social and Preventive Medicine, Monash University; Mr. N. Webster and other staff members of the Hospitals Computer Service; and finally, the general practitioners who returned the completed survey forms.

REFERENCES

1. Rowe IL, Carson NE: Medical manpower in Victoria, 1977. Med J Aust (Specl. Supp.), 1979
2. Carson NE: Survey into on site pathology services in general practice. Aust Fam Physician 3:36, 1974
3. Farrell TWO: Survey into on site radiology services in general practice. Aust Fam Physician 6:1585, 1977
4. Kelly KM: Survey of general practice–1971. Aust Fam Physician 5:1396, 1976
5. Andersen NA: An assessment of the structure of general practice in NSW: Report of a survey. Med J Aust Supp 2:155, 1968
6. Chancellor AH, Andersen NA: General practitioners in three regions of New South Wales—a survey report. RACGP Research Committee NSW Faculty, January, 1977

Differences in Morbidity Patterns among Rural, Urban, and Teaching Family Practices: A One-Year Study of Twelve Colorado Family Practices*

Larry A. Green, Frank M. Reed, Carlos Martini, Perry S. Warren, Roger L. Simmons, and Julie A. Marshall

An analysis of one year's data from family practices in Colorado tested the hypothesis that there are no significant differences in the proportion of patients with problems in each of the 18 major International Classification of Health Problems in Primary Care (ICHPPC) categories among visiting patients in rural, urban, and teaching family practices. Four rural, three urban, and five residency practices participated in the study from January 1, 1978, through December 31, 1978. Transient patients were excluded. There were 25,525 patients included in the study. Each setting was compared with the other two settings in each of the 18 ICHPPC categories. More than half of the comparisons differed at the .001 significance level, and the setting with a significantly greater proportion of visiting patients with diseases in a given category was identified. These differences may have implications for disease surveillance, the planning for delivery of primary health care in different settings, and the preparation of health care providers for practice.

When family physicians discuss practice, they frequently indicate dissimilarities between practicing in rural, urban, and teaching settings. This belief, that there are differences in rural, urban, and teaching family practices, is sufficient to influence health care planning and family medicine education despite uncertainty about the essential meaning of the words urban and rural. Studies describing morbidity patterns for specific diseases in practices in different settings have been reported,[1-3] but studies contrasting morbidity patterns in urban, rural, and teaching family practices are scarce.[4]

This paper reports the results of an analysis of one year's morbidity data collected using the Family Medicine Information System (FMIS)[5] to test the hypothesis that, when adjusted for age and sex, there

is no difference between the proportions of persons with particular types of illnesses visiting rural, urban, and teaching family practices.

Methods

Data Collection

The data reported in this study were collected from January 1, 1978, to December 31, 1978, on encounter forms completed at the time care was received in 12 family practices using the FMIS. These data were coded by physicians or staff and entered into the FMIS by their staff through terminals located at the physicians' offices. Error detection mechanisms in the FMIS check that each patient visit recorded includes at least one problem or diagnosis and that the problem code be contained in the rubrics of the International Classification of

* Reprinted by permission from *The Journal of Family Practice*, 9(6): 1075–1080, 1979.

37

Health Problems in Primary Care (ICHPPC), version I. The data are stored on magnetic discs in a medical record file whose structure is patient and practice oriented. Each patient visit thus results in an entry in the patient's record of the date of visit and the ICHPPC problems for which the patient was seen during that visit.

The computer program, to count patients seen and sort diagnoses and problems into the 18 ICHPPC categories, was checked by two programmers for accuracy. The initial data display totaled the data in two ways so that totals could be verified by inspection. In addition, the accuracy of the computer program was checked by listing for a small portion of the patient population the medical record file and hand calculating the totals and categories to assure that these results matched those produced by the program.

Data Organization

Definitions proposed in a glossary of primary care[6] were used to define the terms urban, rural, and transient patients. Although the three urban and four rural practices are occasionally involved in teaching, for this study only five family medicine center practices associated with family medicine residencies were defined as teaching practices. A visiting patient was defined as a patient who personally received services from one of the study practices during the study period of one year.* Transient patients, as identified by office staff, were excluded. The major ICHPPC categories are those listed by roman numerals in the ICHPPC 1975 edition with the addition of the Supplementary Classification as an 18th category.

The data were organized for three set-

* A Glossary for Primary Care does not define visiting patient for practices registering by family. The definition used for a visiting patient corresponds to the glossary's definition of attending patient proposed for practices registering by patient.

tings: rural, urban, and teaching. The total number of visiting patients was determined for each setting and stratified by sex and 15 age groups (denominator). Then, for each major ICHPPC category the number of patients identified as having had a problem in that category was determined by age and sex groups (numerator). A patient may have had more than one problem and, consequently, may be included in the numerator for more than one ICHPPC category. Ratios were then calculated for each setting by dividing the number of patients of a particular age and sex within an ICHPPC category by the number of visiting patients from the same setting and in the same age and sex group. Thus, the proportion of persons of a particular age and sex (eg, 25–29 year old females) receiving care in a particular setting (eg, urban) having a problem classified into a major ICHPPC category (eg, respiratory) was determined (38.4 percent).

Data Evaluation

Each of the 18 ICHPPC categories was analyzed separately. To reduce the number of calculations, the 15 age groups were reduced to nine groups: <1, 1–4, 5–9, 10–19, 20–29, 30–39, 40–49, 50–59, ≥60. Age-sex adjusted rates for each setting were calculated using the direct method of adjustment with the age-sex distribution of the combined urban, rural, and teaching groups as the standard.

Since patients can be included in more than one of the 18 ICHPPC categories, the disease categories are not mutually exclusive and, thus, were not combined into one multidimensional contingency table. Furthermore, by considering each disease category separately, differences and the direction of differences between settings could be identified. However, by doing three pairwise analyses instead of one overall analysis, the probability of finding a difference that occurred merely by chance was increased. Therefore, a P value of .001 was used rather than .01 or .05.

Statistical analysis was performed using the Mantel-Haenszel technique of multiple 2 × 2 tables, controlling for age and sex, giving an adjusted chi square.[7] The extension of this test described in 1963 requires that the considered variable (in this instance, setting) be orderable. As setting is nominal and not ordinal data, this more recent technique was not used. Another statistical tool, the logistic model, was considered, but rejected because it requires the assumption of linearity in the log scale. Such an assumption seemed premature at this stage of data analysis.

Age and sex were considered important concomitant factors, and adjustments were made for them as indicated. Since the intent of the study was not to describe demographic characteristics of rural, urban, and teaching settings, no further age-sex analysis was done.

Results

After 6,076 transient patients and 479 patients for whom no age was recorded were excluded, 25,525 patients comprised the study group, as shown in Table 1.

Of the 54 possible comparisons of the proportions of patients seen among urban, rural, and teaching settings, 28 were found to be significantly different at the .001 significance level. The only categories for which no significant differences were observed among urban, rural, or teaching family practices were: diseases of the genitourinary system, diseases of the musculoskeletal system, and congenital abnormalities.

The proportion of patients seen in each setting significantly exceeded the other two settings in certain ICHPPC categories:

Teaching Practices

There were four disease categories in which teaching practices exceeded rural practices: mental, circulatory, pregnancy, and the supplementary classification.

There were three disease categories in which teaching practices exceeded urban practices: mental, pregnancy, and the supplementary classification.

Table 1. *Patients Seen from January 1, 1978 through December 31, 1978*

Age (Years)	Rural		Urban		Teaching		Total
	Male	*Female*	*Male*	*Female*	*Male*	*Female*	
<1	104	103	52	51	323	315	948
1–4	316	268	158	136	694	645	2,217
5–9	321	280	164	170	462	430	1,827
10–14	247	260	167	151	398	389	1,612
15–19	251	374	180	231	522	898	2,456
20–24	230	410	263	441	492	1,297	3,133
25–29	225	383	399	704	599	1,050	3,360
30–34	213	312	414	502	406	611	2,458
35–39	149	188	241	255	273	429	1,535
40–44	102	117	111	134	244	315	1,023
45–49	89	114	84	133	202	272	894
50–54	78	127	94	141	215	277	932
55–59	77	115	80	113	169	222	776
60–64	85	116	63	78	164	193	699
≥65	180	267	96	155	397	560	1,655
Subtotal	2,667	3,434	2,566	3,395	5,560	7,903	
Total	6,101		5,961		13,463		25,525

Rural Practices

There was only one category in which rural practices exceeded urban practices: pregnancy.

There were four categories in which rural practices exceeded teaching practices: neoplasms, nervous system, respiratory, and injuries.

Urban Practices

There were seven categories in which urban practices exceeded rural practices: infectious and parasitic, endocrine, blood, circulatory, skin, perinatal, and signs and symptoms. There were nine categories in which urban practices exceeded teaching practices: infectious and parasitic, endocrine, blood, nervous system, circulatory, respiratory, digestive, skin, and signs and symptoms.

The data are summarized in Tables 2 and 3.

Discussion

This study assesses morbidity patterns not by counting problems or encounters but rather by counting *persons* who have certain types of disease and who get at least some of their care from a rural, urban, or teaching family practice. A measure of morbidity is suggested by the proportion of all patients visiting the physician who have certain types of disease rather than problems or illnesses defined by specific ICHPPC rubrics. This study analyzes major disease groupings following the maxim of "looking at the forest before the trees." The temptation to reorganize ICHPPC into more homogenous categories was resisted, in favor of maintaining standardization of data organization and reporting.

Although it is not the purpose of this descriptive study to explain fully the findings, some conjecture as to possible rea-

sons for the apparent differences in morbidity patterns among rural, urban, and teaching family practices is appropriate. There are several reasons why the apparent differences may be *real:*

1. Disease prevalence may differ for the populations studied. For example, blood diseases appeared with greater frequency in urban practices in both sexes and showed a peak prevalence in the very old. The distribution for teaching and rural practices paralleled this morbidity and while not different from each other were significantly different from urban practices. Patients receiving care in urban practices may have blood diseases more often than patients receiving care in teaching and rural practices, but these data do not prove it.
2. Service patterns may differ for the population studied. It may be unlikely that more neoplastic disease occurs in rural areas; however, it may be likely that family physicians care for more of these patients for geographic or economic reasons.
   The lower prevalence of pregnancy in urban practices may be related to the relatively large number of obstetricians in urban areas and resulting referral patterns.
3. Unmeasured characteristics of the patients studied may determine the apparent differences in morbidity. For example, the predominance of pregnancy in the teaching practices could reflect a lower socioeconomic status of patients within these practices producing a patient preference for less expensive care.

There are several reasons why the apparent differences may be *artifact:*

1. There may be increased recording and coding of all diagnoses in some practices not related to increased morbidity. Indeed, the practices in the three settings differed ($P < .0002$—Fisher Exact Probability Test) when compared to

Table 2. *Morbidity Comparisons: Rural, Urban, and Teaching Practices with Age/Sex Adjusted Rates per 1,000 Persons**

Disease Categories	Rural 6,101 Patients Seen		Urban 5,961 Patients Seen		Teaching 13,463 Patients Seen	
	Patients	*Age/Sex Adjusted Rates*	*Patients*	*Age/Sex Adjusted Rates*	*Patients*	*Age/Sex Adjusted Rates*
I. Infective and parasitic diseases	1,035	163	1,323	232	2,223	165
II. Neoplasms	192	32	164	28	309	23
III. Endocrine, nutritional, and metabolic diseases	398	67	645	108	901	67
IV. Diseases of the blood and blood forming organs	78	12	139	28	199	14
V. Mental disorders	327	56	416	63	1,014	78
VI. Diseases of the nervous system and sense organs	1,027	159	877	167	1,500	107
VII. Diseases of the circulatory system	625	100	843	144	1,661	124
VIII. Diseases of the respiratory system	2,279	364	2,061	355	3,719	276
IX. Diseases of the digestive system	399	67	502	83	760	57
X. Diseases of the genitourinary system	769	135	929	147	1,828	136
XI. Pregnancy, childbirth, and the puerperium	127	25	77	13	724	53
XII. Diseases of the skin and subcutaneous tissue	624	101	721	125	1,207	89
XIII. Diseases of the musculoskeletal system and connective tissue	575	96	587	95	1,167	88
XIV. Congenital anomalies	80	13	84	16	144	11
XV. Perinatal morbidity and mortality conditions	12	2	22	7	65	4
XVI. Physical signs, symptoms, and ill-defined conditions	1,134	186	1,562	259	2,309	173
XVII. Accidents, poisonings, and violence	1,185	191	1,135	186	2,255	170
XVIII. Supplementary classification	2,584	434	2,336	425	6,802	496

* Adjusted by direct method using the total group (Rural + Urban + Teaching) as the standard.

each of the other two in terms of the number of problems per encounter. Urban practices coded 1.38 problems per encounter, rural practices coded 1.32 problems per encounter, and teaching practices coded 1.19 problems per encounter.

2. There may be different levels of interest by participating practices in some problems leading to increased or decreased problem recognition. For ex-ample, the high rate of disorders in the supplementary classification in teaching practices may occur because of the current teaching emphasis on identifying and treating these problems.

3. Coding preferences may influence the group into which a problem is classified. For example, a practice participating in a study about patients complaining of tiredness may code "fatigue" in the signs and symptoms category rather

Table 3. *Morbidity Comparisons: Significant Differences (P < .001)* among Rural, Urban, and Teaching Practices*

ICHPPC Category	Rural vs. Urban	Urban vs. Teaching	Teaching vs. Rural
I. Infective and parasitic diseases	U > R	U > T	—
II. Neoplasms	—	—	R > T
III. Endocrine, nutritional, and metabolic diseases	U > R	U > T	—
IV. Diseases of the blood and blood forming organs	U > R	U > T	—
V. Mental disorders	—	T > U	T > R
VI. Diseases of the nervous system and sense organs	—	U > T	R > T
VII. Diseases of the circulatory system	U > R	U > T	T > R
VIII. Diseases of the respiratory system	—	U > T	R > T
IX. Diseases of the digestive system	—	U > T	—
X. Diseases of the genitourinary system	—	—	—
XI. Pregnancy, childbirth, and the puerperium	R > U	T > U	T > R
XII. Diseases of the skin and subcutaneous tissue	U > R	U > T	—
XIII. Diseases of the musculoskeletal system and connective tissue	—	—	—
XIV. Congenital anomalies	—	—	—
XV. Perinatal morbidity and mortality conditions	U > R	—	—
XVI. Physical signs, symptoms, and ill-defined conditions	U > R	U > T	—
XVII. Accidents, poisonings, and violence	—	—	R > T
XVIII. Supplementary classification	—	T > U	T > R

R = Rural; U = Urban; T = Teaching; — "No significant difference."
* Mantel-Haenszel technique of multiple 2 × 2 tables.

than "depression" in the mental disorders category, despite a clinical impression that the patient was depressed.

If the differences reported in this paper are real and not artifact, the distinction between statistically significant and clinically significant must be considered. With large numbers of patients in the study groups, relatively small differences may be statistically significant without appearing clinically significant to the individual practitioner.

If confirmed, results of this study have significant implications for both teaching and researching family medicine. Residents anticipating practice in an urban or rural setting may want to tailor their residency curriculum to accommodate the special needs of an urban or rural practice. Urban and rural family physicians may benefit from specially designed continuing education courses. Studies derived from family medicine residency populations may not be applicable to family practice in the urban or rural setting. Therefore, it becomes important for the practicing physician, teachers of family medicine, epidemiologists, and data analysts to work cooperatively to more fully understand family medicine.

REFERENCES

1. Hart RD: Anaemia and diabetes mellitus in general practice. J R Coll Gen Pract 19:248, 1970
2. Shephard M: The prevalence and distribution of psychiatric illness in general practice. J R Coll Gen Pract 23(2):16, 1973
3. Stewart LC, Gehringer GR, Byars VG Jr, et al: Patient problems in the office practice of six family physicians in Louisiana. J Fam Pract 5:103, 1977
4. Johnson SE, Eaumler WL, Carter RE, et al: The family physician: A comparative study of Minnesota and Wisconsin family physicians practicing in rural and urban communities. Minn Med 56:713, 1973
5. Green LA, Simmons RL, Reed FM, et al: A family medicine information system: The beginning of a network for practicing and resident family physicians. J Fam Pract 7:567, 1978
6. A glossary for primary care. Report of the North American Primary Care Research Group (NAPCRG). J Fam Pract 5:635, 1977
7. Mantel N, Haenszel W: Statistical aspects of the analysis of data from retrospective studies of disease. J Natl Cancer Inst 22:719, 1959

Hospital Privileges for Family Physicians: A Comparative Study between the New England States and the Intermountain States*

David N. Sundwall, David V. Hansen

Coincident with the training of increasing numbers of family physicians over the past decade, there has been concern that these new specialists are being limited in utilizing hospital facilities. In 1976, a survey was conducted of hospital administrators throughout eight Rocky Mountain states, and it was determined there were few restrictions placed on family physicians in this area. To determine if there are regional differences this survey was repeated for 242 hospitals in the New England states.

The results showed 80 percent of urban hospitals would very likely extend staff privileges to family physicians (board certified). Specific data on the likelihood of family physicians utilizing surgical, obstetric, intensive care unit, and coronary care unit facilities indicated significant restrictions as compared with the western states surveyed. This study documents presumed regional differences, and raises questions regarding the role of family physicians in hospitals in some parts of the country.

The specialty of family practice is now a decade old, having become the 20th recognized specialty by the American Board of Medical Specialties in 1969. However, in spite of what appears to be dramatic changes in medical education, the role of the family doctor in the modern hospital seems unsettled and in the state of evolution. This is particularly true in urban areas. In fact, reports from various medical news media have indicated that in certain parts of the United States family physicians have indeed been restricted from utilizing certain hospital facilities.

Those involved in family medicine education, both predoctoral and residency training, have been aware that this is a growing concern which may have a negative influence on career choice of prospective primary care physicians. Many medical students interested in pursuing careers as family physicians, and some family practice residents, have expressed fears that

they may not be able to obtain hospital privileges. In fact, faculty and housestaff in other disciplines seem to advise students accordingly, that they should "at least" become board certified as an internist or pediatrician if they hope to become adequately trained primary care physicians and to be able to utilize hospital facilities. Such concern is not limited only to prospective family physicians, but probably dissuades many students from all primary care specialties. Petersdorf stated in a recent article:

. . . perhaps the most important determinant that motivates young physicians to a sub-specialty, however, is the apprehension that some accrediting body, and probably the government, will limit the practice privileges of the internist who is not certified in a sub-specialty. For example, the fear that only certified cardiologists will be able to work in a coronary care unit or to interpret electrocardiograms or echocardiograms, that only pulmonary specialists will be able to attend to patients in intensive care units, and that only certified gastroenterologists will be permitted to perform liver biopsies.[1]

* Reprinted by permission from *The Journal of Family Practice*, 9(5):885–894, 1979.

Some concern over hospital privileges by the national representatives of the specialty of family practice is evidenced by the American Board of Family Practice (ABFP) assigning a long-range planning committee to study this problem. In March 1976, they took a major stand on hospital privileges by stating,

. . . a diplomat of the ABFP should be accorded the same basic consideration in regard to hospital privileges as given to diplomats of other specialty boards. The diplomat's hospital privileges should be commensurate with training, experience, and demonstrated abilities. Within the hospital staff, the diplomat should be eligible for full privileges in the Department of Family Practice, in conformity with the department's bylaws.[2]

The American Academy of Family Physicians has also firmly stated their position— "the Academy's position in brief opposes any arbitrary qualifications for appointment to hospital staff other than those of demonstrated ability and competence and [supports the position] that the final responsibility should rest with the Chairman of the Department of Family Practice and other specialty departments involved."[3]

In spite of the efforts of the American Academy of Family Physicians and the American Board of Family Practice to ensure that family physicians have privileges based on their abilities, there has been resistance from other national specialty organizations. In fact, the President of the American College of Surgeons in 1977 expressed categorical opposition to the training of family physicians in surgery, and their subsequent utilization of surgical facilities in hospitals. His comments were made public in the December issue of the *American College of Surgeons Bulletin*, which quoted the surgical leader as follows: "It is obvious that there is a coordinated effort by Family Practice for surgical privileges in hospitals, and for surgical knowledge and competency necessary for the generalist." Furthermore, "it is time for us to drop the unwarranted politeness we have accorded a movement dedicated to lowering the quality of surgical care."[4]

It is remarkable how little data are available to support these concerns. A review of the literature in this area is most impressive in the paucity of information. Regional studies have shown that there are apparently few restrictions on family physicians in the state of Washington and the Intermountain West.[5,6] A statewide survey of New Jersey hospitals in 1977 revealed that over 90 percent would commonly grant all family physicians general admitting privileges, but significant limitations were imposed on specific clinical areas (eg, routine obstetrics, coronary care unit, etc).[7]

In an attempt to gain current information regarding the status of family physicians in the hospital setting a survey was conducted in 1976 of hospital administrators (not physicians), throughout the Intermountain West (Census Division Region VIII, Figure 1).[6] The survey included 176 hospitals by mailing a two-page questionnaire to the administrators; 93 percent responded either by mail or by telephone. Hospitals were classified as urban or rural, and information was obtained regarding general staff privileges and specific clinical areas (eg, surgery, obstetrics, intensive care unit, and coronary care unit). All of the urban hospitals were surveyed and a random selection of rural hospitals was included. Criteria for extending staff privileges, consultation requirements, and number of family physicians applying for privileges were also studied. The results showed that 88 percent of urban and 98 percent of rural hospitals stated that it would be very likely that a board certified family physician would obtain full staff privileges. Specific data on the likelihood of a family physician utilizing the ICU, CCU, surgical, and obstetrics departments indicated some restriction in urban areas, although it was not as much as expected. The results were encouraging, and suggested that family physicians in the Intermountain West have access to the majority of hospital facilities, even in urban areas.

Although the initial study provided data which might help dispel fears of students and resident physicians that they would be limited in utilizing hospitals in the Intermountain West in 1976, it is obvious that these data are not reflective of any other part of the country. As indicated above, isolated reports from various parts of the United States have given publicity to the fact that family physicians have been restricted from hospital facilities. One disturbing example is of a young board certified family physician who was trained in a university based residency program in the West, had documented considerable obstetrical training, and yet was refused obstetrical privileges in a Massachusetts hospital.[8]

Recognizing the initial study of Region VIII states had geographic limitations and represented a relatively small number of the nation's family physicians, the current study of New England states was undertaken to gain further data to document the status of family physicians in the hospital setting.

Methods

To obtain current data about hospital privileges in the New England area, a survey of hospital administrators was again conducted. The area included Census Division Region I, the states of Connecticut, Rhode

Island, Massachusetts, Vermont, New Hampshire, and Maine (Figure 1). Hospitals were divided into urban and rural areas, based on their location within or not within a standard metropolitan statistical area (SMSA).*

The hospitals studied were limited to those classified by the American Hospital Association as follows: (1) control: nongovernmental, not for profit; (2) services: general medical or surgical; and (3) stay: short stay, ie, 50 percent of all patients stay less than 30 days.[9] A total of 242 hospitals have been so classified in this area. Of these, 137 (57 percent) were within an SMSA, and classified as urban, and 105 (43 percent) were not within an SMSA and were classified as rural.

In the summer of 1978, a two-page questionnaire was sent to the administrators of each hospital along with a cover letter from the Division of Primary Care and Family Practice at Harvard Medical School, which supported the need for this survey and requested cooperation from the hospitals.† The hospital administrator

---

* An SMSA is defined as county or group of counties containing at least one city with a population of 50,000 or more, plus any adjacent counties which are metropolitan in character and economically and socially integrated within the central county or counties.
† The authors are indebted to Dr. Anthony Bower (Instructor in Preventive Medicine, Harvard Medical School) for his cooperation and efforts to solicit assistance from the hospital administrators of the New England area.

Region VIII-1976
States
1. Arizona
2. Colorado
3. Idaho
4. Montana
5. Nevada
6. New Mexico
7. Utah
8. Wyoming
SMSAs-13

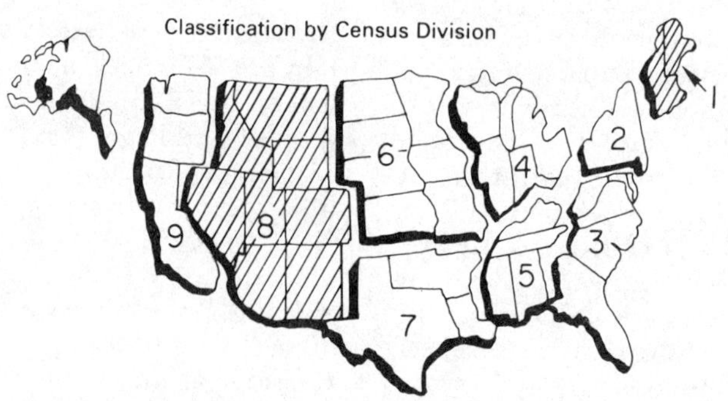

Classification by Census Division

Region I-1978
States
1. Connecticut
2. Maine
3. Massachusetts
4. New Hampshire
5. Rhode Island
6. Vermont

SMSA's-26

Fig. 1. Area used in research.

was then requested either to return the completed questionnaire by mail or to provide the information via a toll-free telephone call. If no response was received within three weeks, the administrator was contacted by telephone. Forty-one percent of those who provided data mailed the questionnaire within the expected time. Six percent telephoned in the data. When the three-week period from the time the questionnaire was mailed had elapsed, the remaining hospitals were contacted directly by telephone. Another 18 percent mailed the questionnaire and 35 percent provided their data over the telephone. Data was obtained from 200 hospitals, representing 83 percent of all those surveyed.

Questions were asked regarding general staff privileges, use of specific departmental or clinical areas, and changes over the past five years in requests for hospital privileges. Other hospital characteristics considered in the analysis were occupancy rate, presence of a clinical department of general or family practice, and the ratio of general practitioners and/or family physicians to the total active staff. The data obtained in Region I are compared to that of Region VIII which were obtained in the initial study in 1976. Differences were compared by chi-square test with a standard significance level set at $P < .05$.

Results

The questionnaires sent to the hospital administrators listed a series of questions designed to assess current and future status of hospital privileges for family physicians. The response rate from the urban and rural hospitals was nearly identical. Of the 137 urban hospitals polled, 112 (82 percent) responded; for the rural hospitals, 88 of the 105 hospitals polled responded (84 percent). Total response rate was therefore 83 percent.

As shown in Table 1, the administrators of urban and rural hospitals in both regions stated that board certified family physicians would generally be able to get hospital privileges. However, it was shown that the non-board certified general practitioner would be less likely to get privileges in Region I than in Region VIII.

When questioned concerning how they based their decisions on granting privileges, administrators of rural hospitals in Region VIII relied more heavily on medical experience than did those of rural hospitals in Region I, suggesting that board certification is less important in the rural West. Administrators of urban hospitals in both Region I and Region VIII, 93 percent and 85 percent respectively, indicated that a combination of documented medical ex-

Table 1. *Likelihood that a Family Physician/General Practitioner Would Be Able To Obtain Hospital Privileges**

	Region	Very Likely	Probable	Possible	Unlikely
Family physician					
Urban	I	80	9	8	3
	VIII	88	8	2	2
Rural	I	94	5	1	—
	VIII	98	2	—	—
General practitioner†					
Urban	I	49	27	17	7
	VIII	76	19	3	2
Rural	I	59	33	7	1
	VIII	90	8	2	—

* All figures in percentages.
† Differences between Region I and VIII hospitals for the general practitioner significant at $P < .005$.

Table 2. *Extent of Privileges Granted to Family Physicians in Specific Clinical Areas**

		Region I			Region VIII			
		Full	*Some*	*None*	*Full*	*Some*	*None*	**P Value†**
General surgery	Urban	—	46	54	7	82	11	<.005‡
	Rural	—	65	35	32	64	4	<.005
Nonsurgical obstetrics	Urban	14	45	41	24	71	5	<.005
	Rural	30	55	15	76	24	—	<.005
Surgical obstetrics	Urban	—	27	73	11	60	29	<.005
	Rural	—	17	83	36	52	12	<.005
Intensive care unit	Urban	19	60	21	30	61	9	NS
	Rural	35	60	5	54	45	1	<.03
Coronary care unit	Urban	18	59	23	27	59	14	NS
	Rural	35	60	5	54	44	2	<.04

* All figures in percentages.
† Difference between Regions I and VIII.
‡ P value <0.05 is statistically significant.
NS = Not significant.

perience and board certification was most important.

When the extent to which privileges would be granted in specific areas was probed, differences between Region I and Region VIII became more apparent. Table 2 summarizes the responses of Region I and Region VIII hospital administrators regarding privileges granted to family physicians in the areas of obstetrics, surgery, and the medical intensive care units. In each case, the Region I hospitals were significantly more limiting in their granting of privileges to family physicians in surgery and obstetrics. However, there was remarkably little difference in restrictions in the use of ICU and CCU facilities in the urban hospitals of each region, both areas indicating limitations. The data also show that the rural ICU and CCU in Region I were not as significantly limited as the areas of surgery and obstetrics, in rural as well as urban areas. However, the family physicians currently may utilize the ICU/CCU with proper supervision or use of consultation.

All of these data are clearly illustrated in Figures 2 and 3, indicating differences in

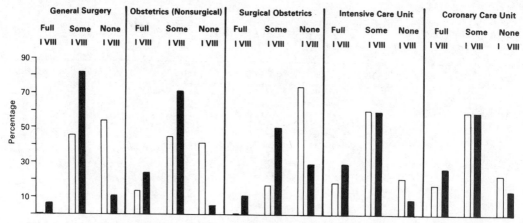

Fig. 2. Privileges granted to family physicians in specific clinical areas of urban hospitals.

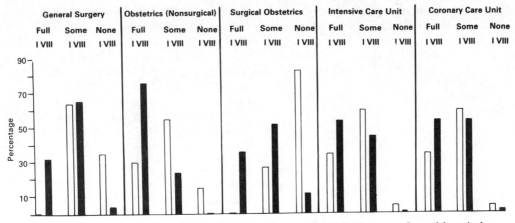

Fig. 3. Privileges granted to family physicians in specific clinical areas of rural hospitals.

the specific clinical areas for Regions I and VIII.

The conditions surrounding the granting of these specialized privileges are further reflected in Table 3, which shows the extent to which mandatory consultation is required for family physicians in order that they might be permitted to use hospital facilities in specific clinical areas. There was not as great a difference in required consultations in Region I and Region VIII as might be expected. However, in three of five specific clinical areas, more urban hospitals in Region I did require that family physicians obtain more consultation than in Region VIII. Rural hospitals in Region I also required more consultation in the area of surgical obstetrics.

In an effort to estimate trends for the future of family physicians in hospital practice, the administrators were asked to estimate the changes in the number of family physicians applying for hospital privileges over the past five years. There has been an increase in family physicians applying for privileges in the urban area of

Table 3. *Extent of Mandatory Consultation for Family Physicians in Specific Clinical Areas**

		Region I			Region VIII			
		All Cases	*Some Cases*	*Not Required*	*All Cases*	*Some Cases*	*Not Required*	**P Value†**
General surgery	Urban	37	61	2	16	59	25	.005‡
	Rural	26	49	25	11	59	30	NS
Nonsurgical obstetrics	Urban	6	76	18	11	53	36	NS
	Rural	2	41	57	3	41	56	NS
Surgical obstetrics	Urban	22	71	7	33	50	17	NS
	Rural	34	52	14	11	63	26	.03
Intensive care unit	Urban	35	51	14	20	48	32	.03
	Rural	20	47	33	10	54	36	NS
Coronary care unit	Urban	42	43	15	24	43	33	.03
	Rural	28	41	31	15	52	33	NS

* All figures in percentages.
† Difference between Regions I and VIII.
‡ P value <0.05 is statistically significant.
NS = Not significant.

both regions. In the rural area of Region I, there has been a significantly greater increase in application for privileges as compared to Region VIII (however, "rural" for New England is not the same as "rural" in the West) (Table 4).

In order to relate the degree to which privileges were made available to family physicians, an "average privilege score" was created by weighting the degree of privileges (full privileges = 3, some = 1, none = 0) and averaging across several clinical areas: general surgery, nonsurgical and surgical obstetrics, intensive care unit, and coronary care unit. (When a service was not available in a hospital, it was omitted.) The score deliberately gives a higher weight to full privileges. The range of scores was then divided into thirds.

Table 5 summarizes the differences in average privilege score according to various hospital characteristics. With the average privilege score, differences between Regions I and VIII were highly significant for the majority of hospital characteristics studied. Region I hospitals generally gave fewer privileges.

It is interesting to note that in those hospitals in both regions which had greater than a 25 percent proportion of family physicians on the staff, the regions were not statistically different when compared to their average privilege score. This suggests that in a hospital in either region with a large proportion of family physicians on the staff, differences in privileges granted

Table 4. *Change in the Number of Family Physicians Applying for Hospital Privileges in the Past Five Years**

	Region	Increase	Same	Decrease
Urban	I	45	39	16
	VIII	57	30	13
Rural†	I	64	26	10
	VIII	37	50	13

* All figures in percentages.
† Difference between Region I and VIII rural hospitals significant at P <.002.

between regions are not great. Also, if a hospital in either region had a clinical department of family or general practice, there was again no significant difference between regions, and *fewer* privileges were available to family physicians. However, a clinical department of family or general practice probably indicated a larger hospital with more specialists available in every category, and therefore more competition with family physicians.

Discussion

There are obvious limitations to this study design in that even with a geographic comparison adding a dimension to the initial study, this information cannot be extrapolated to reflect all parts of the United States. Areas of marked contrast were intentionally chosen, ie, the relatively rural Mountain states vs the much more densely populated New England states, with the understanding that differences between these areas are likely to be the greatest. The status of family physicians in other parts of the country probably falls between what has been reflected in this study.

Another limitation acknowledged in this paper is that the respondents, ie, the hospital administrators or their delegated personnel, were left to determine precisely what constituted full, some, or no privileges. These interpretations could differ considerably from hospital to hospital. For this reason, in determining the "average privilege score," the system was weighted in favor of giving emphasis to full privileges. A further problem is that information being derived from an administrative organization of the hospital may simply reflect by-laws rather than actual practice. Nonetheless, the significant difference in data obtained suggests some candor on the part of the respondents.

The information obtained raises several issues regarding the role of contemporary family physicians in hospitals. Perhaps most importantly, it documents that there

Table 5. *Average Privilege Score According to Hospital Characteristics**

	Region I			Region VIII			
	Low (0–1.00)	*Medium (1.01– 2.00)*	*High (2.01– 3.00)*	*Low (0–1.00)*	*Medium (1.01– 2.00)*	*High (2.01– 3.00)*	**P Value†**
Hospital location							
Urban	78	19	3	66	20	14	<.03‡
Rural	58	32	10	23	30	47	<.005
Number of beds							
≤99	60	30	10	20	26	54	<.005
≥100	74	23	3	53	27	20	<.005
Occupancy rate							
0–49%	60	30	10	24	28	48	NS
50–74%	67	26	7	36	24	40	<.005
75+%	73	24	3	54	29	17	<.005
Clinical department of family practice or general practice							
Yes	64	31	5	55	27	18	NS
No	72	22	6	30	26	44	<.005
Proportion of family physicians on staff $\left[\dfrac{FP + GP}{\text{active staff}}\right]$							
0–24	73	23	4	56	27	17	<.005
25–49	67	25	8	48	22	30	NS
50–74	44	37	19	18	41	41	NS
75+	29	57	14	29	23	48	NS

* All figures in percentages.
† Difference between Regions I and VIII.
‡ P value <0.05 is statistically significant.
NS = Not significant.

are significant regional differences in the United States. One frequently hears that family medicine varies considerably from one location to another, and whether this is a strength or weakness is left to individual interpretation. Rather than having a homogeneous mode of practice, the variation may reflect response to local needs and be a healthy difference.

The following issues are also raised by this study, although the data do not specifically address them:

1. *Physician satisfaction.* This had not been determined in the present study, in that physicians themselves were not contacted. In 1969, the American Academy

of General Practice (just prior to becoming the American Academy of Family Physicians) conducted an ambitious survey questioning all Academy members regarding their hospital practice and satisfaction with same.[10] The Academy received questionnaires from almost 20,000 physicians, and it determined that 89 percent had active staff privileges at one or more hospitals. Physicians were specifically asked if they were satisfied with their hospital privileges and 96 percent reported that they were, with only 4 percent stating that they were unduly restricted. These data are remarkable in view of the currently voiced concerns that family physicians are being severely limited in their opportunities to use hospital facilities.

It is interesting to speculate how many family physicians might be completely satisfied with their role even in the New England states where there are limitations. It may be that many physicians have voluntarily limited their hospital work in preference for ambulatory medicine, and that young physicians selecting careers as family physicians prefer not to care for or manage seriously ill patients in the hospital. At the conclusion of the initial survey of Region VIII, it was recommended that another study similar to the 1969 survey be conducted by the American Academy of Family Physicians. This study is presently being done; the results will reportedly be available within the coming year.

2. *Role of malpractice and malpractice insurance on limiting hospital work.* Many family physicians who previously had done obstetrics and surgery have reportedly limited their practice in these areas because of the great expense of malpractice insurance if these areas are included, and/or fear of a costly malpractice suit. This was a much publicized problem in the mid 1970s and, subsequent changes in the spectrum of family physicians' clinical work may now be reflected in the hospital privileges data obtained. If so, the stimulus for the "restrictions" would not have come solely from specialty colleagues forcing the generalist out of the hospital, but would represent considerably more complex issues. It is likely that both cost of malpractice insurance and fear of legal reprisals have had a significant impact on limiting the spectrum of a family physician's clinical work throughout the country over the past decade.

3. *Resistance from colleagues.* Hospital privileges are, in fact, determined by physicians, not administrators. There has certainly been marked resistance on the part of some of the specialty colleagues, as indicated above in the statement by the President of the American College of Surgeons in 1977. Other professional organizations have been very supportive and, in fact, have determined guidelines to assist in training family practice residents and in determining their future role. The best example of this is the jointly approved guidelines of the American Academy of Family Physicians and the American College of Obstetrics and Gynecology which addressed training of residents and appropriate hospital practice privileges in obstetrics and gynecology.[11] However, when family physicians are restricted from hospital facilities, either as a group or individually, one can certainly question the motivation of these actions. They are frequently couched in terms of "quality of care" for patients, while equally stringent documentation for competence and experience may not be required of other specialists to use the same facilities. Hence, the American Academy of Family Physicians has insisted that this be the sole basis for the granting of privileges. In fact, the Academy has provided free legal assistance to physicians who deem themselves unduly restricted and has provided considerable help for individuals with such problems. Such restrictions may come more from economic motivation, that is, concern for the consultant physician's income, than from genuine concern over patient care. Such factors influencing access to hospitals by family physicians must be considered highly unethical and illegal.

4. *Obstruction in addressing problems of health manpower and maldistribution.* The mandate is clear, from the public first, and secondarily from the government, for an increasing number of primary care physicians and for improved access to quality health care. In spite of the efforts of the Bureau of Health Manpower in providing considerable funds

to train primary care physicians, a great many students make career choices favoring subspecialty medicine. The extent to which this is influenced by fear of restricting the generalist in the hospital setting would be difficult to ascertain. But it is likely that regulations to ensure equitable granting of hospital privileges will have to be instituted nationwide if concerns over these problems are to be eliminated.

5. *Responsibility of the family physician.* Unfortunately, many of the current problems within the hospital, and some of the restrictions imposed, are the result of inappropriate use of hospital facilities by family physicians. As a specialist in breadth, the family physician must recognize his or her limitations and obtain consultation and referral when appropriate. When this has not been the case, criticism by colleagues in other specialties has been severe and warranted. This is particularly important regarding surgical and obstetrical procedures. If an individual's practice evolves so that he is not performing certain procedures frequently, and there are other specialists doing such procedures more frequently, limitation of one's clinical practice should be voluntary. Family physicians must have the intellectual honesty to periodically reevaluate their knowledge and skills. The spectrum and content of a family physician's practice is certain to evolve over time and his hospital work should reflect this accordingly.

Summary

The following conclusions can be drawn from this study: (1) Board certification of a family physician is more important in obtaining hospital privileges in New England; however, in the two areas studied, both a combination of documented medical experience and board certification have significant impact on likelihood of obtaining privileges; (2) there is significant restriction of family physicians in use of surgical and obstetrical facilities in the hospitals of New England, both in urban and rural settings; (3) there is remarkably little difference in access to intensive care units and coronary care units between family physicians in the urban Intermountain West and in New England; (4) the family physicians are required to have consultation more frequently in the New England States, both in urban and rural areas, than in the Intermountain West; (5) there has been a greater number of family physicians seeking privileges in rural hospitals in New England than in rural hospitals in the Intermountain West.

Authors' Update

The role of the family doctor in the modern hospital has interested me since my medical school days.

Over a decade ago, I was warned against becoming a general practitioner because I would not be able to work in a hospital. Although this concerned me, it was hardly sufficient to dissuade me from pursuing a career as a family physician. After completing a family practice residency, I had no problems obtaining hospital privileges for everything I wanted to do, which included general medical care for children and adults, and uncomplicated obstetrics. When I joined the faculty of a major medical school, I was surprised to find that students still expressed such grave concerns about hospital privileges, and that fear of being restricted was indeed a factor in career choice.

The research project presented here, and a previous study analyzing privileges for family physicians in the Intermountain states, were an attempt to determine if there really are significant limitations placed on family physicians. It is my impression that in most areas family physicians do have access to hospitals, and specific privileges are granted on an equitable basis, ie, documented experience and competence.

Unfortunately, there are many instances where family physicians and general practitioners have been unduly restricted from hospitals. I believe it is essential to continue to gather data related to these issues, and document trends which may lead to exclusion of the family doctor from the hospital.

In my opinion, the quality of health care of our patients and certainly the "health" of our discipline would suffer if we do not play a major role in the modern hospital.

REFERENCES

1. Petersdorf RG: The doctor's dilemma. N Engl J Med 229:628, 1978
2. ADFP takes action on hospital privileges: RE-Policy. AAFP Rep 3(3):1, 1976
3. Demonstrated ability should be keyed to hospital privileges. AAFP Rep 4(6):1, 1977
4. Hanlon CR: Address to American College of Surgeons Fellows, Clinical Congress, Dallas, Texas, November 1977. Bull Am Coll Surg 62(12):11, 1977
5. Keith DM: Family doctors' hospital privileges. Am Fam Physician 3(5):155, 1971
6. Hansen DV, Sundwall DN, Kane RL: Hospital privileges for family physicians. J Fam Pract 5:805, 1977
7. Warburton SW Jr, Sadler GR: Family physician hospital privileges in New Jersey. J Fam Pract 7:1019, 1978
8. AAFP board assists young FP in hospital privileges case. AAFP Rep 4(9)1, 1977
9. American Hospital Association Guide to the Health Care Field, annual edition. Chicago, American Hospital Association, 1979
10. American Academy of General Practice: Summary of Members' Practice Survey, Kansas City, Mo, American Academy of Family Physicians, 1969
11. ACOG-AAFP Recommended Core Curriculum and Hospital Practice Privileges in Obstetrics-Gynecology of Family Physicians, reprint no. 261. Developed by a joint ad hoc committee of the American Academy of Family Physicians, the American College of Obstetricians and Gynecologists, and the Council on Resident Education in Obstetrics and Gynecology, Kansas City, Mo, 1977

Importance of Obstetrics in a Comprehensive Family Practice*

Lewis E. Mehl, Calvin Bruce, John H. Renner

Four family practices in the San Francisco Bay Area, two of which did not include obstetrics and two of which did, were examined with reference to their patient populations and to the number of families for which they provided comprehensive, continuous family care. The groups practicing without obstetrics were found to do acute care primarily and, to a lesser extent, long-term care internal medicine, with very little pediatrics or gynecology. The groups practicing with obstetrics did significantly more minor surgery, gynecology, pediatrics, and psychotherapy. During the six-week study, the group practicing with obstetrics saw five times as many patients who were members of families receiving continuous, comprehensive care from the practice under observation. Psychotherapy done by the group including obstetrics was primarily family therapy; for the other group, individual therapy. If larger studies support these findings, then important implications are suggested for training programs in family practice and for the resident deciding to enter practice.

With the inception of training programs in family practice, many authors began to question the content of family practice. How much obstetrics, pediatrics, internal medicine, psychiatry, and surgery should the family practitioner know and practice? The range of opinion has varied from defining the family practitioner as a primary care internist to including the entire spectrum of medical practice within the family practitioner's domain, with the question of when to refer left to the discretion of the individual practitioner. Wilson[1] and Deisher[2] have seen the family physician as a synthesizer assisting the patient in integrating his personal health needs with his other needs and aspirations within his family and his community. Deisher calls for training in family practice to curb the tendency to teach ever more deeply in limited specialties and instead to promote the development of connecting insights which link one intensive discipline with another.

Haggerty[3] defines the family practitioner "as a medical specialist in the care of the family, doing little surgery and usually little or no obstetrics. They are primarily concerned with adult and child medical care . . . in ambulatory settings." McWhinney[4] describes the primary attribute of the family physician as commitment to the person rather than to a body of knowledge or a branch of technology. He states, "To a physician who achieves fulfillment from human relations it may not make much sense to say, 'I will commit myself to people provided they are over 14, or under 65, or under 14, or male, or female, or provided they are not pregnant.'"

In our opinion, the family physician's domain is the full range of health and emotional problems of the family and the relation of these problems to the family's cultural milieu. Whatever the family requires professional assistance or intervention for becomes the domain of the family physician—from delinquency to pregnancy, from well-child care to coronary care—with the family practitioner personally guiding the family through any further specialized care which may be required. This is a kind of family systems approach, synthesizing the general practice ethic of concern and commitment described by Balint[5] and the family systems approaches developed by Bowen,[6] Glick

* Reprinted by permission from *The Journal of Family Practice*, 3(4):385–389, 1976.

and Haley,[7] and Minuchin,[8] as well as many others.

We felt the need for a pilot study directed at determining how the inclusion or exclusion of obstetrics affected a developing family practice with regard to the configuration of patient problems encountered, the delivery of comprehensive, continuous family care, and the personal interest and satisfaction of the physician. We examined this in the context of several relatively new family practices in an area with easy access to specialists and a wide variety of health-care alternatives: the San Francisco Bay Area. It was felt that, as McWhinney[4] noted, trends in patient preference and selection procedures would be reflected in such a diverse area.

Methods

Four San Francisco Bay Area practices were chosen for this, two which offered obstetrical care and two which did not. The physicians' intentions upon entering practice and their training were otherwise similar. All had entered practice with plans to deliver comprehensive, continuous family health care. A brief interview with each group was obtained to document any differences between the groups in their philosophy toward health care, importance of obstetrics, the role of the obstetrician and the pediatrician, and their satisfaction with their practices.

All four practices included individuals with one or two years of post-medical school training. Practice 1 was composed of three physicians, ages 30, 34, and 38; practice 2, two physicians ages 28 and 32; practice 3, three physicians practicing as part of a multispecialty group, ages 34, 35, and 36; and practice 4, two physicians, ages 30 and 32. Practices 1 and 2 included obstetrics and are designated as group A; practices 3 and 4 did not and are designated as group B. Practice 1 had been in existence for five years, practice 2 for two years, practice 3 for eight years, and prac-

tice 4 for three years. A medical student was usually involved with practice 1. It is interesting to note, also, that practice 1 began with the intention of excluding obstetrics, but decided to include it during the first year of practice. Practices 3 and 4 were willing to provide prenatal care, but not delivery care. Given the availability of obstetricians, most patients did not elect this. All groups followed the recommendations of the American Academy of Pediatrics for well-child care.

Acute, episodic adult medicine visits for such ailments as sore throats and upper respiratory infections were defined as nonpersistent adult medical problems. Adult medicine visits were defined as including problems requiring long-term care. Pediatric sick and health maintenance problems were differentiated in the same manner. Diagnostic categories for other problems are self-evident. Orthopedic problems included bruises, falls, back pain, fractures, and other musculoskeletal problems. Lacerations were considered under episodic care. Minor surgery included such procedures as breast biopsy, needle aspiration and removal of sebaceous cysts. Procedures such as vacuum aspiration abortions, cervical cryocauterization, and intrauterine device insertions were defined as gynecological procedures. Skin biopsies were considered dermatological procedures.

For each practice, the reasons for patient visits over a six-week period were reviewed, and analyses of the frequency distributions of visits were carried out. The percent of patients seen who were members of families for which the group was providing continuous, comprehensive family care was calculated. Continuous, comprehensive family care was defined as care in which all members of the immediate family were seen for at least six months by the practice group. The communities in which the practices were located were similar in terms of ethnic and age composition and socioeconomic status.

Categories of office visits were defined

Table 1. *Attitudinal Differences between Family Practices Including and Excluding Obstetrics*

	Practice 1	Practice 2	Practice 3	Practice 4
Role of obstetrics in family practice	Integral; key to successful general practice of medicine	Very important; only way to provide total health care to a family	Not necessary for a successful family practice	Important, but obstetrician better trained to handle obstetrics
Relation of the obstetrician to family practitioner	Should be hospital based consultant	Should be hospital based consultant	Handles all obstetrics	Better able to handle obstetrics
Relation of pediatrician to family practitioner	Should be hospital based consultant	Special consultation only	Should handle some of pediatrics family practitioner not trained to handle	Better than family practitioner at handling pediatric problems
Satisfaction with practice	Very satisfied	Very satisfied	Mildly dissatisfied	Somewhat dissatisfied
Plans for the future	No change	No change	Considering more acute medicine and emergency medicine	Considering specialty training
Attitude toward obstetrics beginning practice	Not sure if wanted to be involved	Wanted to be very much involved	Wanted to be involved but practicalities made it difficult	Did not feel competent to be involved but would have like to
Role of family practitioner	Comprehensive family care	Comprehensive family care	Comprehensive family care	Comprehensive family care

so as to be mutually exclusive. Dermatological visits included skin problems in both geriatric, pediatric, and adult populations, with the exception of vulvovaginal problems which were included under gynecological visits. Orthopedic problems included those problems occurring in pediatric, geriatric, and adult populations, as did minor surgery and psychotherapy. Thus, pediatric, adult medical, and geriatric problems were defined as medical problems occurring in those specific age groups exclusive of dermatologic, orthopedic, minor surgical, psychiatric (meaning those problems to which therapy was applied), or gynecological problems.

Results

Table 1 illustrates attitudinal differences among the practices. Practices 1 and 2 were convinced of the importance of obstetrics in family practice, although practice 1 had excluded obstetrics at first. When questioned regarding this change, members of practice 1 stated that they had realized that "obstetrics was essential in the general practice of medicine." All practices felt that the role of the family practitioner was to provide continuous, comprehensive family care. Practices 1 and 2 were satisfied

with their practices and desired no major changes. Neither practice 3 nor practice 4 was satisfied with their practice. Practice 3 was considering changing their practice to encompass more acute and emergency medicine, while members of practice 4 were considering specialty training in internal medicine.

Table 2 presents the frequency distribution of various categories of office visits, and Table 3 and Figure 1 summarize the differences between groups including and excluding obstetrics. Certain differences are apparent. Practice group B saw fewer children than practice group A ($p < 0.001$), and saw many more adult medicine and acute, episodic problems ($p < 0.001$). Group A saw twice as many gynecological problems ($p < 0.001$), fewer geriatric problems ($p < 0.001$), more orthopedic problems ($p < 0.001$), an equivalent number of dermatological problems (not significant), more minor surgery ($p < 0.001$), and more psychotherapy ($p < 0.01$). Psychotherapy performed by group A was primarily marital and family counseling; that by group B was primarily individual counseling.

Table 4 and Figure 2 illustrate the percent of patients in each category of visit in which the patient seen was a member of a family receiving its comprehensive care

Table 2. *Frequency Distribution of Office Visits by Diagnostic Category*

	Practice 1 (Percent)	Practice 2 (Percent)	Practice 3 (Percent)	Practice 4 (Percent)
Pregnancy	21.6	18.3	0.3	0.2
Pediatric health maintenance	7.4	6.0	0.9	1.2
Pediatric sick visits	18.0	12.8	2.3	1.2
Gynecology visits	12.7	17.8	10.3	6.1
Geriatric visits	7.6	6.7	25.1	16.1
Adult medicine visits	7.2	12.7	22.0	23.2
Adult acute or episodic visits	13.5	16.5	29.4	50.8
Orthopedic visits	4.1	4.0	0.1	0.2
Dermatology visits	2.7	0.6	0.4	1.7
Minor surgery	3.0	2.5	0.1	0.2
Psychotherapy	2.2	2.1	0.2	1.3
Total	100.0	100.0	100.0	100.0

Table 3. *Intergroup Differences in Absolute Number of Patients Seen by Main Diagnostic Category of Visit*[1]

	Group A (Practices including OB)	Group B (Practices excluding OB)
Pregnancy	612	11
Pediatric health maintenance	216	26
Pediatric sick visits	500	45
Total pediatric visits[2]	716	71
Gynecology visits	500	187
Geriatric visits	225	524
Adult medicine visits	271	565
Adult acute or episodic visits	411	776
Orthopedic visits	122	6
Dermatology visits	37	26
Minor surgery	85	5
Psychotherapy	64	20
Total	3,058	2,199

[1] All differences are statistically significant to P < 0.001 except for psychotherapy where P < 0.01 and dermatology where P is NS.

[2] The sum of pediatric health maintenance and pediatric sick visits.

from the practice listed. From these tables it is seen that certain reasons for visit are much more likely in group A, including family therapy, minor surgery, pediatric care, and pediatric health maintenance. Table 5 illustrates the reason for visit of those patients who were members of families receiving their comprehensive care from the practice group. The table also illustrates the relative contribution of each diagnostic category to the total number of families seen. The number of entire families cared for by practice group A is approximately five times greater than for practice group B. The role of adult medicine visits in drawing families to the practice seemed to be the same for both group A and group B; the factor contributing to the greater number of families seen by practice group A seemed to be visits for pregnancy, pediatric health maintenance, pediatric sick visits, gynecology visits, and minor surgery visits.

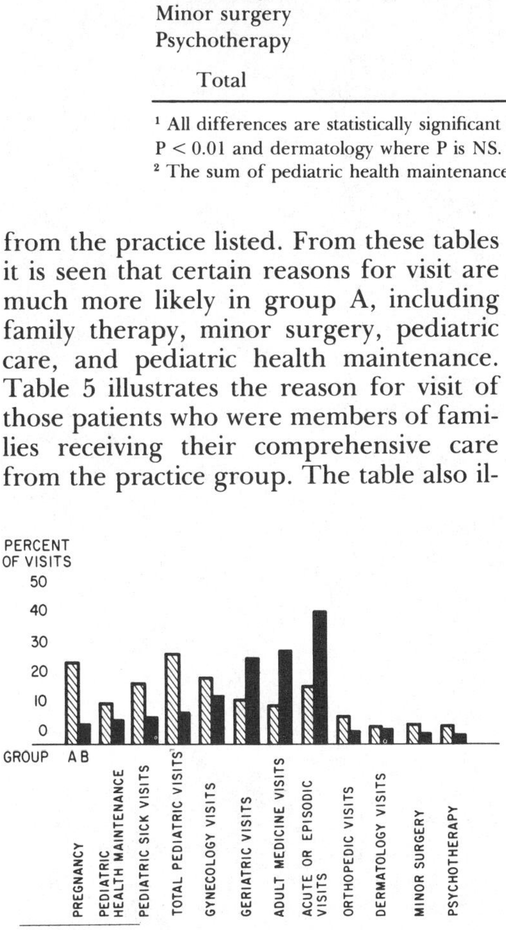

Discussion

From the data presented the hypothesis can be supported that obstetrics is of key importance in the establishment of a comprehensive family practice. Practice group B very much resembled the practice expected of a primary care internist, while practice group A better resembled the usual descriptions of a family practice, with a large pediatric population and see-

[1] Sum of pediatric health maintenance and pediatric sick visits.

Fig. 1. Bar graph of frequency of office visits by primary reasons.

Table 4. *Percentage of Times for Category of Visits in which the Patient Being Seen Was Part of an Entire Family Receiving Comprehensive Care*

	Practice 1 (Percent)	Practice 2 (Percent)	Practice 3 (Percent)	Practice 4 (Percent)
Pregnancy	84.1	79.5	12.11	51.31
Pediatric health maintenance	98.2	98.0	98.0	97.0
Pediatric sick visits	70.3	80.3	47.5	12.3
Gynecology visits	54.4	33.2	9.0	10.1
Geriatric visits	89.9	69.6	75.7	11.9
Non-acute adult medicine visits	57.6	45.2	14.5	12.2
Episodic adult visits	65.7	46.3	12.1	3.1
Orthopedic visits	80.3	49.6	22.5	5.0
Dermatology visits	81.1	75.0	14.9	10.1
Minor surgery	100.0	86.0	81.3	88.0
Psychotherapy	98.2	93.0	8.1	6.2

ing many problems other than internal medical problems. The data seem to support the hypothesis that without obstetrics a developing family practice becomes indistinguishable from the practice of a primary care internist. The study group was small, so that this hypothesis must be tested with a larger number of participants in a wider range of geographic areas. With only four practice groups, the attitudes of the practitioners may have had much to do with the characteristics of their practices. We think it is significant, however, that all

practice groups began with the same overall goal—providing comprehensive family medical care—and that three of the four began practice with plans to exclude obstetrics.

The dissatisfaction of members of practice group B may relate to the discrepancy between the type of practice they had anticipated and the characteristics of their existing practice. All had begun practice planning to treat entire families and to have a practice consisting of at least one-quarter pediatrics. The small numbers of families and children seen may have contributed to their dissatisfaction. This also relates to anthropological views of the function of the family and its clear relation to the begetting, bearing, and rearing of children. Variations of this basic theme are observed in primates as well as humans.[9] For the family practitioner not to be involved in this basic process may make him superfluous to the needs of the family.

We hope that this small pilot study will have some important results—namely that family practitioners will examine our conclusions in the light of their own personal experience and that directors of residency training programs will begin to explore the implications of this important factor. If larger studies support our hypothesis, then there are important implications for health-care planning and resident educa-

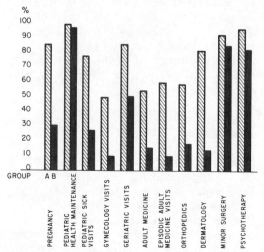

Fig. 2. Frequency of patient being a member of a family receiving comprehensive care.

Table 5. *Relative Contribution of Each Diagnostic Category for Visit to the Percentage of Families Receiving Comprehensive Care*

	Group A (Percent)	Group B (Percent)
Pregnancy	16.6	0.1
Pediatric health maintenance	6.9	1.0
Pediatric sick visit	12.3	0.5
Gynecology visit	7.7	0.8
Geriatric visit	6.2	1.0
Adult medicine visit	4.6	3.3
Episodic adult medicine visit	8.0	3.3
Orthopedic visit	0.2	0.04
Dermatology visit	0.1	0.1
Minor surgery	2.6	0.2
Psychotherapy	2.0	0.6
Total of Families Seen	57.0	11.14

tion in family practice. For the concept of comprehensive family care to remain viable, it would seem that obstetrics must remain an important part of family practice. For residents not planning to include obstetrics in their future practice, training needs will be different, and might best be met by a program resembling the primary care internal medicine training programs. For residents planning to include obstetrics in their future practices, then a broad-based training program is needed with much emphasis on obstetrics and gynecology, pediatrics, internal medicine, orthopedics, minor surgery, family psychotherapy, and other medical specialties. Future studies should utilize the independent physician profile or similar data for developing practices, and might also be able to ascertain the relation of geographical area of practice to the kind of resident education required.

REFERENCES

1. Deisher JB: What is so special about a family physician? West J Med 121:521–529, 1974
2. Wilson VE: Family practice—pioneer or slave to the past. Am Fam Physician 1(4):131–138, 1970
3. Haggerty RJ: Family medicine and pediatrics. Am J Dis Child 126:13–14, 1973
4. McWhinney IR: Family medicine in perspective. N Engl J Med 293:176–181, 1975
5. Balint M: The Doctor, His Patient, and the Illness. New York, International Universities Press, 1957
6. Bowen M: The use of family theory in clinical practice. Compr Psychiatry 7:345–374, 1966
7. Glick I, Haley J: Family Therapy and Research. New York, Grune & Stratton, 1972
8. Minuchin S: Families and Family Therapy. Cambridge, Mass, Harvard University Press, 1974
9. Morris D: Primate Ethology. New York, New American Library, 1969

What Do Family Physicians in a Prepaid Group Do in Their Offices?*

A. Sherwood Baker

Each family physician at the Permanente Group of San Diego was observed for one half-day. As with two earlier time studies, the time spent with each patient was tabulated to show the number of minutes used in each of the usual activity categories that are encompassed in a patient encounter.

Previously, similar studies had been carried out with rural practitioners in Missouri (1965) and rural and urban physicians in New Zealand (1975). The Missouri physicians practicing in pre-Medicaid days spent less time doing administrative work than their counterparts in this study, but appreciably more time in treatment and preventive activities. The time utilization of the physicians in prepaid groups was remarkably similar to that of the physicians in the fee-for-service system in New Zealand.

Medical practice in most industrialized societies is remarkably similar. Medical education is sufficiently general and reproducible, and natural patterns of illness in the human organism do not vary greatly. Age, culture, and weather play their parts in individual variations and incidence of sickness.

The practice of medicine may vary because of these illness factors, but it may be altered by the economics of the physician-patient transaction. How the individual physician answers the requests made of him/her, based on his/her own experience and skills, makes for interesting study. The educators would like to have a better feel for the appropriateness of their efforts. Payment agencies might be more realistic if they had more understanding of professional time needs.

It is not a straight-line function to correlate time usage of physicians to problem-solving. Illness presents in many stages and patients do not have identical powers to overcome them. Then too, therapeutic agents have varying effects.

Nonetheless, by simple observation of a physician at work, it is possible to identify threads of similarity or individual differ-

ence. In 1966, Parrish, Baker, and Bishop carried out a pilot study of time usage in the office practices of 25 rural Missouri general practitioners.[1,2] In that study, the data for each physician were provided by individual observers who were medical students assigned to the physicians. Because of the different observers used, uniformity in reporting can be questioned.

All the physicians were in private practice. The study antedated the introduction of Medicaid and Medicare, so the bulk of remuneration was still the responsibility of the patient on a fee-for-service basis.

In 1975, a time study was made of family physicians practicing in New Zealand. The form of remuneration was also fee-for-service, with the bulk of the fee paid to the physician by the government.

It appeared that there were many similarities between the Missouri and New Zealand practice patterns.[3] This suggested that another model for study would be worthwhile, specifically with a different form of remuneration.

Methods

The Southern California Permanente Group in San Diego is organized to make

* Reprinted by permission from *The Journal of Family Practice*, (2):335–340, 1978.

use of family physicians for a large component of its adult primary medical care. This time study covers half-day sessions for 22 of these physicians. Each half-day is scheduled to cover three and a half hours: patients are seen by appointment, with ten minutes being the usual allotted time. The physician may designate that he needs a 20-minute time period once during each session. Examples of such a need were for minor surgery, or to carry out an extensive examination.

In actual observations, the number of patients seen averaged 13.7 per physician per session, with a range between 11 and 16 patients. There was no obvious correlation between length of time that the physician had been with the group and the number of patients seen. As might be expected, those physicians who had been with the organization longest saw more "old" or "return" patients.

Thirteen of the physicians observed had been with Permanente two years or less. The other nine had been with Permanente for periods up to 12 years. The average time with Permanente was 3.9 years.

The average number of years of practice since medical school of the 22 physicians was 12, with the range between 2 and 31 years. Two of the physicians had just completed family practice residencies.

Results

Patient Profile

During the observation periods, 329 individual patients were seen (Table 1). Of this number, 163 were "new" to the practices of the physicians, but not necessarily to Permanente. Every effort is made to permit a patient to see the same physician, but prior scheduling or unavailability at times required some shifting.

At the time of the observation in January, a "slow-down" of Southern California physicians protesting the rise of liability insurance was threatening. The

Table 1. *Characteristics of 329 Patients Seen by Family Physicians in 24 Half-Day Sessions*

	Number	Percent
Age group		
Under 10 years	1	.3
10–20 years	28	8.5
20–60 years	266	80.1
60 and over	35	11.0
Time of patient in practice		
New patient	163	49.5
Old patient	166	50.5
Sex		
Male	157	47.9
Female	172	52.1
Race		
Caucasian	307	93.0
Non-Caucasian	22	7.0

Permanente Group had other malpractice insurance arrangements and did not contemplate such a work change. Consequently, in late 1975, several thousand new members joined the San Diego panel providing many of the "new" patients seen in January 1976, when these observations were made.

The ages of the patients were similar to those of the earlier study except for the very small number of children. This is understandable because the organization of the Permanente Group has provided pediatrician coverage for that age.

One child below the age of 10 and only 29 below the age of 20 were seen in the 329 patient contacts. Persons from ages 20 to 60 provided 266 patient contacts, and there were 35 patients over the age of 60.

More females (172) were seen than males (157). All but 22 of the 329 patients were Caucasian.

Problem Range

As with the New Zealand study, the problems were grouped into several major systems. Some patients had more than one problem, hence 329 patient visits elicited 358 complaints (Table 2).

Virtually no patients presented during the observation period with uncomplicated upper respiratory infection as the only reason for seeing the physician. At this time a "cold" clinic was in operation in the same building with care given by nurses and the family physicians in rotation. Hence the incidence of respiratory problems is slightly lower than might be expected in the study period.

Usage of Time

The author served as a detached time-keeper during each visit of a patient with a physician.[4] This minimizes the distractions to physician and patient. Should the physician be asked to record his/her own time, he may alter his rhythm or have a different judgment for classification than another physician also doing self-study. (An interesting apparatus for remote timing and self-observation audit has been described recently in England.[5]

The presence of a third party in the consulting room did not apparently modify the interaction of patient and physician. In those delicate interchanges where it did appear to be a deterrent, I stepped out and made an approximation of the time usage later. This actually happened on very few occasions and involved so little time that the overall results were not affected.

Time by Category (Table 3)

DIAGNOSIS. In the diagnostic category were included all the features of each patient visit involving history, physical examination, and all diagnostic procedures not involving submission of blood or urine samples. This use of time consumed 1,674 minutes of the total 5,661 minutes for the entire group. This gives each physician an average of 69 minutes for diagnosis per half-day, or 29 percent of his total time. This use of time was the largest for the group, but nine physicians spent more time in "other administration," two in "administration with the patient," and one used more time for "education and counseling."

TREATMENT. Treatment was defined as actual manual service of "laying on of hands." This involved accident management, dressing changes, gynecologic treatment, drainage of cyst and biopsy, minor surgery, joint injections, and removal of ear wax. Some of these procedures, such as ear washing, suture removal, and dressing

Table 2. *Classification of 329 Patients by Problems*

Problem	Total	Percent
Dermatologic	62	17.3
Musculoskeletal	59	16.5
Cardiovascular	52	14.5
Respiratory	48	13.4
Gastrointestinal	35	9.7
Urogenital	35	9.7
Neurologic and Psychiatric	32	9.0
Endocrinic and Metabolic	22	6.2
Hematolic	1	
Other	12	3.4
Total	358	100.0

Table 3. *Time Spent by Category**

	Minutes		Percent
	Total	Average	
Diagnosis	1,674	69	29
Treatment	193	8	3
Health Education and Counseling	795	33	13
Preventive Medicine	139	5.8	2
Personal with patient	16	−1	−1
Administrative with patient	963	40	16
Other administrative	1,213	50	21
Personal	264	11	4
Other	398	16.6	7
Total	5,661		

* Half-day office session.

changes were also done in a "nurses' clinic" and did not appear on the physician's time sheet.

The time used for treatment by the physicians in the 24 sessions totaled 193 minutes for an average of eight minutes per physician or three percent of the total minutes. Six of the physicians had no time allocated for this and one utilized 34 minutes for minor surgery.

HEALTH EDUCATION AND COUNSELING. The health education and counseling category might be construed in some instances as "treatment" since much therapy did take place. This, however, was used to include all the physician's instructions, advice, and counseling, including both dietary and activity modifications, which are part of the treatment activity of a verbal nature and given directly to each patient. The physicians used 795 minutes for this, averaging 33 minutes per session or 13 percent of the time spent with patients. The range was from 10 to 69 minutes.

PREVENTIVE MEDICINE. Preventive medicine included routine well-person physical examinations, pap smears and birth control measures, and immunizations and prenatal visits. In the case of the latter, this was not likely to be more than a diagnostic first visit as these physicians did not manage ongoing prenatal care or deliver babies. Also there were very few complete physical examinations because well persons or new subscribers had "health maintenance" examinations available at a different facility, but were seen for ongoing care by the physicians at La Mesa where the findings of these examinations could be corroborated or acted upon.

For preventive medical activities, the physicians used a total of 139 minutes, or 5.8 minutes per physician per half-day. This amounted to two percent of the time spent.

PERSONAL WITH PATIENT. The personal with patient category included discussion with the patient not related to the health problem presented. In the Missouri study this had occupied an appreciable amount of time, but in New Zealand amounted to only two percent of the total minutes. In this study it was even less, for a total of 16 minutes for all the physicians. Only five physicians were responsible for this total.

ADMINISTRATIVE WITH PATIENTS. This administrative category included all of the arrangements with patients for ongoing supervision and management, writing prescriptions, medical certificates, telephone calls, request for laboratory or x-ray determinations, or referrals to other physicians. Of the 329 patients seen, 30 were referred. Laboratory or x-ray assistance was requested for 124 patients. Time spent in making progress notes or in dictation in the presence of the patient was also included. A total of 963 minutes were consumed in this category, averaging 40 minutes per session and 16 percent of the total time. The variation was from 19 to 59 minutes. (The physician using 59 minutes dictated each of his progress notes in front of the patient and had the patient verify the notes.)

OTHER ADMINISTRATION. Other administration involved business phone calls, office matters, personnel relationships, and notes on charts of patients not present at that time. The total consumption of time for this was 1,213 minutes, averaging 50 minutes per half-day session or 21 percent of the time in the office. Nine of the physicians used more time for this than for diagnosis; 120 minutes was the greatest amount of time spent in this activity and three minutes was the least. (The low number was the time of the physician who did most of his dictation in the presence of the patient.)

PERSONAL. This personal category covered coffee breaks, snack time, reading mail, comfort stops, and telephone calls not related to work. The time spent purely with the author in discussion of the time study or medical matters was included here. Four percent of the working day was used this way, accounting for 11 minutes per physician and a total of 264 minutes. (One of the patients seen was himself an industrial engineer. He made the observation that most industries allow for a minimum of five percent of time usage for personal business and that 20 percent may be reasonable in certain occupations.) Eleven of the sessions showed no time at all used for personal needs.

OTHER. Other included activities related to medicine but not to the direct office contact with patients. This included reading medical literature, listening to tapes, or attending meetings. It also included a hospital visit by one of the physicians during the observation day. There were 398 minutes used this way, amounting to 17 minutes per physician per session, or seven percent of the total minutes.

Discussion

This study was designed to be a third inquiry into the time usage of family and general physicians (the first two were Missouri and New Zealand). A question existed regarding the validity of having a third party in the consultation room during the physician-patient encounter. As in

the studies of Missouri and New Zealand, this proved acceptable. The author elected to compare the three locations to demonstrate differences in time usage with different modes of remuneration (Table 4). Obviously, this could not be completely controlled. In the Permanente Group, a large organization makes certain uniform stipulations about office hours, work schedules, and accessibility to additional secondary and tertiary care, while the independent practitioners of New Zealand and Missouri were limited more by geography than personal choice.

The widest variation in time spent indicates that in 1965, Missouri physicians spent fewer minutes in administration than their counterparts in 1975 and 1976 in other settings. It must be remembered that 1965 antedated Medicare and Medicaid, so it might be appropriate to restudy a similar set of independent Missouri practices today.

Some modifications of the time utilization observed in this study may have derived from unusual circumstances. Half of the patients were seen by the physicians for the first time during this time study. Many were new to the practice as well as to the community. While many of the physicians were also new to the practice setting, no appreciable differences in use of time appeared, with the few exceptions already noted.

The Southern California group has

Table 4. *Percentage of Time Spent by Activity Category: Comparisons in Three Locations*

Activity Category	1965 Missouri	1975 New Zealand	1976 San Diego
Personal	2.6	1.3	4.0
Administrative (total)	6.5	29	37
Administrative with patient	—	19	16
Other administrative	—	10	21
Preventive medicine	13.5	8	2
Health information and counseling	19.3	12	13
Diagnosis	33.4	27	29
Treatment	27	7	3
Other	Not tabulated	7	7

gained efficiency by standardization of procedures, wide use of ancillary help, and easily available laboratory and x-ray facilities. Any attempt to grade the seriousness and urgency of the problems bringing patients to the physician in the three different settings would be futile. Personal habits and cultural norms would appear to have more to do with that than economic considerations.

This time study offers a further view of clinical practice that may be used in the preparation of family practice residents. Implications for the future form of practice may be drawn from the fact that these physicians spent more time with their records and less time in preventive activities than did the New Zealand and Missouri physicians. This may reflect part of the responsibility of belonging to a large group. But once again, as with the New Zealand study, it can be concluded that family physicians in English-speaking countries are more similar to each other than they are different.

Acknowledgment

The author wishes to thank Dr. Lauraine Kinney and the Family Practice Group of the Southern California Permanente Medical Group of La Mesa for their forbearance and help in this study. This study was supported by the Department of Family and Community Medicine of the University of Missouri—Columbia.

Author's Update

Currently, several thousand trainees are preparing to enter the field of family practice. Family practice residency programs have had to draw upon the traditional hospital-based programs of other specialities because other models are not readily available in many training sites. The skills of practice become modified in ambulatory settings.

This set of studies was conceived to demonstrate the use of time by the practitioner in each patient encounter. The variable factors of patient's problem, age, sex, and previous introduction to the physician were tabulated. There were notes made as to the ancillary use of laboratory and radiology services.

This study was conceived to see if prepayment made any difference in the method of office practice as measured previously in smaller office practices carried out by physicians in Missouri and New Zealand. The Missouri study was done at the time government programs were beginning, and the New Zealand form of remuneration is a mixture of government reimbusement and patient responsibility.

One conclusion is that practice habits are fairly similar in all settings and that training for those physicians had been fairly similar. There should be further studies to see if the physicians trained in the last decade have evolved different practice habits.

REFERENCES

1. Baker AS, Parrish HM, Bishop FM: What do rural general practitioners in Missouri really do in their offices? Mo Med 64:213, 1967
2. Parrish HM, Bishop FM, Baker AS: Time study of general practitioners' office hours. Arch Environ Health 14:892, 1967
3. Baker AS: What do New Zealand general practitioners do in their offices? NZ Med J 83:187, 1976
4. Cohart EM, Willard WR: A time study method for public health. Public Health Rep 70:570, 1955
5. Floyd CB, Livesay A: Self-observation in general practice: The bleep method. J R Coll Gen Pract 25:425, 1975

Results of a Needs Assessment Strategy in Developing a Family Practice Program in an Inner-City Community*

David Satcher, Jacqueline Kosecoff, Arlene Fink

The planners of an inner-city clinic and family practice residency program conducted a four-step needs assessment study to identify the importance, availability, and feasibility of local family practice services and objectives. Using mailout-mailback and supervised questionnaire data collection techniques, they contacted 1,020 consumers and providers. Those objectives rated most important and feasible and least available were given top priority for implementation, while the objectives rated important and unavailable but not currently feasible received research priorities.

This is a report of a needs assessment study conducted in 1975–1976 in the King-Drew service area of Los Angeles to assist in the planning of a family practice residency program and a family practice clinic or model unit. The King-Drew Medical Center consists primarily of the Martin Luther King, Jr. General Hospital and the Charles R. Drew Postgraduate Medical School. The center was developed to serve a community of about 350,000 persons of whom approximately 80 percent are Black, 15 percent have Spanish surnames, and 5 percent are white, Native American, or Asian. The community is well recognized as being medically underserved.

The major aim of this study was to determine the priority of family practice objectives in the King-Drew community by considering each potential service's importance, present availability, and feasibility. A secondary purpose of the study was to validate a needs assessment strategy not previously applied in a health setting.

Background: Family Practice in the Inner City

A comprehensive study conducted by the American Medical Association's Ad Hoc Committee on Education for Family Practice (Willard Report published in 1966) reported that the number of physicians engaged in family practice had declined dramatically between 1931 and 1966. Virtually no programs existed at the time for training physicians for family practice.[1] The committee therefore recommended that such training be made a national priority. Although significant progress has been made since the Willard Report, there is nevertheless cause for concern about the development of family practice in inner cities. The American Board of Family Practice has been established, together with over 364 family practice residency training programs with 6,531 residents,[2] but few family physicians practice in inner cities, and there has been a tendency among recent family practice graduates to practice in smaller communities as opposed to larger or more congested areas. Furthermore, very few minority physicians are involved in family practice residencies; in August 1979, only 705 of all residents in family practice (9.3 percent) were Black, had Spanish surnames, or were Native Americans (according to a telephone conversation with Ross R. Black, MD, Division of Education, American Academy of Family Physicians, August 1979).

Watts, where King-Drew's 400,000 Black and Spanish surname consumers are

* Reprinted by permission from *The Journal of Family Practice*, 10(5):871–879, 1980.

most concentrated, has a lower average income, a younger population, and a higher unemployment and death rate than Los Angeles County as a whole. Watts also has few available primary care services: many persons in the King-Drew service area depend on the hospital emergency services for their full range of medical care needs. As of 1972, when the King-Drew Medical Center opened, there was one physician per 609 persons in California, but in the King-Drew service area the figure was one physician per 2,200 persons.[3] In the entire Southeast Health Services Region, whose approximately 780,000 residents are served by the Medical Center, there are currently only 15 Board certified family physicians.[4] Only three of these family physicians practice in the Watts area. A recent survey of a random sample of 200 patients in the Walk-In Clinic at King-Drew Hospital revealed that while 75 percent preferred to have primary physicians caring for them, only 10 percent had physicians of any kind whom they could name.[5]

Given the comprehensive nature of family practice, the planners of the King-Drew Medical Center felt that a family practice program could well serve this community. In order to determine which of many potential family practice services were most relevant to local needs, and to make the most efficient use of available resources, the planners of this program undertook a survey to assess the needs of consumers and the priorities of providers in the community.

Needs Assessment Strategy Review

The evaluation literature was reviewed to identify needs assessment strategies appropriate for use at King-Drew. (The process of identifying needs and deciding upon priorities among them has been termed needs assessment.[6] A need is identified when observed conditions fall below what is considered to be an acceptable standard.) Several methods, most of which

were not formal needs assessment strategies, were identified as means of collecting information on health care needs and preferences of patient populations. They included the use of archival data, structured interviews, self-administered questionnaires, and open community forums.[4,7-10]

One needs assessment strategy, developed at UCLA for use in educational settings, was selected for use in the King-Drew study because it is community based and utilizes data from a variety of sources.[11] This strategy requires first developing a list of objectives that might potentially be transformed into program services. The relative importance of these objectives is weighed, and an assessment of existing programs determines discrepancies between important goals and currently available services. Finally, an analysis is conducted to identify the objectives considered by consumers and providers to be the most important, least available, and yet feasible to achieve.

Methodology

Identification of Objectives

Literature about the development of family practice programs was reviewed to identify potential objectives for a family practice program as defined by the medical community and to determine an appropriate survey method to ascertain community needs and preferences for medical services. In general, the literature focuses on issues of program administration, integration of the program in university teaching hospitals, and the content of family practice education in undergraduate and graduate programs.[12,13] While some of these studies describe the overall value of family practice per se,[7] they do not evaluate the relative importance of different family practice services in the surrounding community. In order to make such a comparison, the planners of the King-Drew program obtained additional statements of objectives from a review of 20 family practice residency programs throughout the country.[14] After listing the objectives, a group of two family physicians, one internist, an epidemiologist, two educational specialists, and two consumer representatives met to discuss and refine the statements of objectives. At this point, the list contained approximately 50 objectives. It was not modified until the needs assessment form was tested in a pilot study.

Sample Selection

The three groups identified for participation in the needs assessment study were consumers (actual or potential users of services), providers, and health care administrators. The total overall sample size was 1,022. A consumer sample of 350 households was systematically drawn from a probability sample of 1,000 households in the King-Drew service area representative of the racial, income, educational, housing, and employment characteristics of the service area. To ensure that former or current users of King-Drew Medical Center services were represented by the consumer sample, three additional subsets were included. These subsets consisted of participants in a monthly community forum (N = 100), consumers of outreach screening programs (N = 100), a sample of Walk-In Clinic patients (N = 150), and patients from a monthly Free Clinic (N = 24). The total size of the consumer sample was 724.

Sample providers included nurses, physicians, social workers, and medex students. Every third physician (N = 64) on the roster of the King Hospital and Drew Postgraduate Medical School faculty was selected so that all medical departments and professorial ranks were represented. Every fifth physician (N = 100) from a list of 500 community physicians was selected without regard to specialty. In addition, 20 social workers, 20 nurses, and 20 medex

students were systematically selected from the King-Drew Center. The total sample size of the provider group was 224.

Administrators (N = 74) were drawn from top and middle level positions at both King Hospital and Drew Postgraduate Medical School, and because of the limited number, all names were used.

Questionnaire Development

The survey's self-administered questionnaire listed the objectives and provided a modified Likert reference scale for rating the objectives in terms of importance, present availability, and feasibility. *Importance* was rated on a scale of 1 to 5 from "least important" to "most important." Respondents were instructed to assign at least two objectives to each of the five response categories (a Q-sort technique). *Availability* was rated on a scale of 1 to 3 from "not available" to "available but difficult to get" to "easily available." *Feasibility* was also rated on a three-point scale from "not feasible" to "feasible but difficult to get" to "easy to provide."

After a pilot test, 38 objectives were drafted into a final questionnaire which was prepared for administration in English and in Spanish. Because the pilot test indicated that many consumers had difficulty rating the feasibility of implementing family practice services, the feasibility scale was deleted from consumers' questionnaires. Only providers and administrators were instructed to rate the final 38 objectives in terms of feasibility as well as importance and availability.

Data Gathering

Two different data gathering methods were employed: the mailout-mailback technique and the supervised self-administered technique. All consumers in the Free

Clinic subsample, the Walk-In Clinic subsample, and 250 out of 350 persons in the household subsample were supervised as they completed their questionnaires. The remaining 100 consumers from the household survey, the Community Medicine Forum, the Outreach Screening Clinic, and the providers and administrators were sent questionnaires using a mailout-mailback method.

Plan of Analysis

Target objectives for the family practice center were selected based on a synthesis of the mean rating of objectives in terms of their importance, availability, and feasibility. By comparing perceived needs to the actual experiences of the family practice center in the year following the study, the planners evaluated the validity of the responses to the needs assessment study. The response rate (mailed vs supervised), the accuracy and completeness of data, and the estimated cost of mailing and supervising questionnaires served as determinants of the practicality of the needs assessment strategy.

Results

Response Rate

A large original sample size was selected on the assumption that it might be difficult to obtain responses from some of the subsamples and the mailout-mailback technique might yield poor return rates. The number of responses to the needs assessment survey confirmed this assumption (Table 1).

Of the 300 questionnaires mailed to consumers, 90 were returned due to incorrect addresses, and 54 were returned completed. Thus, the return rate was 18 percent for questionnaires mailed and 26 percent for those received.

Of the questionnaires mailed to community providers, 23 were returned with incorrect addresses, and 84, or 42 percent of the received total, were returned complete.

Of 424 attempts to obtain supervised self-administered responses, 20 failed due to incorrect addresses, 80 because respondents were not at home or refused to answer, and 94 because persons refused to participate (34 Walk-In Clinic patients, 2

Table 1. *Assignment of Participants to Data Gathering Methods and Return Rates*

Method Subsample	Assignments		Return Rate*	
	Frequency	*Percent*	*Frequency*	*Percent*
Supervised Self-Administration†				
Household	250	24.5	102	40.8
Walk-In Clinic	150	14.7	116	77.3
Free Clinic	24	2.3	22	91.7
Mailout-Mailback‡				
Community Medicine Forum	100	9.8	37	37.0
Household	100	9.8	5	5.0
Outreach Screening	100	9.8	12	12.0
Providers	224	21.9	84	37.5
Administrators	74	7.2	38	51.4
Total	1,022	100.0	416	40.7

* Frequency and percent of original assignments.
† Overall return rate for supervised self-administration was 57 percent.
‡ Overall return rate for mailout-mailback was 29 percent.

Free Clinic patients, and 58 in the household sample). Thus, 57 percent (240/424) of the original sample completed the questionnaires. Of the persons actually contacted, 74 percent (240/324) completed the questionnaire.

Largely due to the poor response rates for some of the subsamples participating in the mailout-mailback data gathering method, the overall response rate of 40.7 percent did not meet this study's target of 50 percent response. The number of returns was considered to be sufficiently large, however, for each group's needs to be reliably assessed. The proportions of consumers, providers, and administrators in the original and return samples were roughly equivalent, and there were few large differences in terms of sociodemographic and economic variables between the respondent and original planned samples.

Accuracy and Completeness

Among the respondents, 80 percent of the consumers followed the Q-sort direction to place at least two of the objectives in each rating category. Ninety percent of the providers and administrators responded as directed. Eighty-six percent of the questionnaires returned by consumers were complete, as were 90 percent of those from providers and administrators. Because none of the incomplete questionnaires represented more than four unanswered questions, missing data were ignored in the calculation of results.

Data Gathering Costs

Total cost for the mailout-mailback method was approximately $484. The cost of 424 attempted personal contacts was approximately $3,227, which included the cost of training questionnaire administrators. Thus, the cost per completed questionnaire in the mailout-mailback method

averaged to $8.89, and in the supervised self-administered method, $13.34.

Although the mailout-mailback survey had the advantage of being relatively inexpensive, the much higher return rate (74 percent compared to 26 percent) associated with the supervised questionnaire suggests that when community involvement is considered essential to a needs assessment in the inner-city, this more costly technique might prove worthwhile.

Selection of Target Objectives

In the overall sample, each objective was given mean ratings of importance, availability, and feasibility (Table 2).

The overall mean rating of importance for all objectives was 4.0 on a scale of 1 to 5. In addition, separate averages were computed and compared for each subgroup of consumers, providers, administrators, and provider/administrators (such as physicians who were also administrators, department chairpersons, or associate deans). For consumers the mean was 4.1, for providers 3.7, for administrators 3.8, and for provider/administrators 4.0. Consumers' ratings ranged from 3.5 to 4.6, providers from 2.75 to 4.45, and administrators from 2.26 to 4.63.

The objective perceived as most important in the total sample was Number 1, "to inform people about the kind of health services that are available to them" (Table 2). The objective perceived as being least important by the total sample was Number 24, "to care for persons of all ages and both sexes in the same clinic." Between consumers and providers, there were statistically significant differences in the rating in importance of 20 (52.6 percent) of the objectives; consumers and administrators differed significantly on 12 (32 percent), and provider/administrators and consumers differed significantly on 10 (29 percent) of the objectives. The most striking disagreement in the rating of consumers and administrators was on Number 11, "to conduct research to improve health care delivery." Consumers rated this 3.6 while administrators rated it 2.88, and providers 3.0. The greatest discrepancy between consumer and provider ratings appeared over Number 24, with an average rating of 2.75 for providers and 3.77 for consumers, and over Number 38, with consumers rating it 4.6 while providers rated it 3.21. Other objectives rated much higher by consumers than by providers included Number 4, cost control; Number 6, reduction of waiting time; Number 13, an-

nual physical examinations; and Number 20, the care of all members of the family by one physician. The only statements which providers rated higher than consumers were Numbers 8, 16, 17, 27, 28, and 32. These differences, however, were not significant. A striking finding in these results was the tendency for persons who were *both providers and administrators*—mostly department chairpersons and deans—to agree more closely with consumers than with providers or administrators in their ratings, particularly on Numbers 6, 11, 20,

Table 2. *Mean Ratings of Objectives*

Objectives	Importance* (Scale: 1–5)	Availability* (Scale: 1–3)	Feasibility† (Scale: 1–3)
1. Inform people about available health services	4.46	2.26	2.60
2. Teach families to identify dangers of common health problems	4.24	2.06	2.26
3. Help people get to a physician or hospital when needed	4.09‡	2.21	2.45
4. Reduce the costs of health care services in a clinic or doctor's office	4.05‡	1.69‡	1.63
5. Set up health care services in the community close to the people	4.15	1.98	2.04
6. Reduce the waiting time to see a doctor	4.02‡	1.78‡	1.95
7. Make clinic's hours fit community needs	3.86	1.89	2.10
8. Show people how to stay healthy by proper diet, exercise, etc.	3.83	2.03	2.31
9. Vaccinate against diseases like polio, measles, flu	4.26	2.49§	2.80
10. Screen for early stages of diseases like high blood pressure or diabetes	4.38§	2.26	2.53
11. Conduct research in health services delivery	3.47‡	1.77	2.15
12. Gather complete information about individuals' health and medical problems	3.90‡	2.08	2.15
13. Provide yearly physical examinations	3.82‡	2.03‡	1.92
14. Provide appropriate laboratory tests for diagnosis without waste	3.97§	2.13	2.33
15. Recognize and respond when people are in need of care	4.24	2.03	2.30
16. Provide the treatment that works and is safest for each patient	4.32	2.14	2.32
17. Allow patients to be responsible for some decisions about their health care	3.81	1.98	2.30
18. Closely follow people under treatment for an illness	4.28	2.12	2.30
19. Assist people in adjusting to life after a serious illness or injury	4.14‡	2.00	2.12
20. Provide health care to the whole family by the same doctor	3.77‡	1.84	1.85
21. Obtain patients' family history	3.65‡	2.05	2.38

(continued)

Table 2. *Mean Ratings of Objectives (continued)*

Objectives	Importance* (Scale: 1–5)	Availability* (Scale: 1–3)	Feasibility† (Scale: 1–3)
22. Identify and assist with family problems like child abuse and alcoholism	4.16‡	1.85	2.00
23. Involve other members of patient's family in maintaining health and treating disease	3.82‡	1.92	2.03
24. Care for persons of all ages and both sexes at the same clinic	3.45‡	2.02‡	2.04
25. Treat most common health problems in the same clinic	4.03‡	1.94§	2.17
26. Care for normal pregnancies and deliveries	3.88‡	2.44	2.63
27. Be sensitive to patients' feelings	4.19	2.13	2.60
28. Respect each patient as an individual	4.42	2.20	2.66
29. Seek patients' opinions about services offered in the family practice center	3.66‡	1.88	2.44
30. Have physicians recognize when they need help from other health care providers	4.13‡	2.14	2.40
31. Become aware of community health resources like family counselors and medical specialists	4.01	1.99§	2.50
32. Communicate clearly with other providers in making referrals and treating patients	4.00	2.07	2.41
33. Develop relationships which allow for long-term care of persons by the same providers	3.87	1.86	2.02
34. Ensure care of patients during a doctor's absence by accurate record keeping and informing other providers	4.48	2.08	2.45
35. Make the best use of the skills of each member of a family care team	4.15	2.01	2.34
36. Allow nurse practitioners and/or physician's assistants to provide care when possible	3.74	1.92	2.32
37. Become involved with community groups concerned with health, such as schools or churches	3.49‡	1.90‡	2.32
38. Make home visits when indicated	4.09‡	1.65	1.89

* N = 416.
† N = 122.
‡ Differences among groups at the .01 level.
§ Differences among providers, consumers, administrators, and provider/administrators at the .05 level.

22, 23, and 24. This similarity in rating patterns between consumers and provider/administrators in the King-Drew health care system may provide the basis for making the health care system more sensitive to community needs and concerns.

The scale for rating availability ranged from 1 to 3, and the overall mean was 2.1 with a range from 1.65 to 2.5. The objective that received the highest overall mean rating in availability (2.46) was Number 9, "immunizations against certain viral diseases." The lowest overall availability rating was given to Number 38, home visits. Ratings in availability by consumers, providers, and administrators tended to agree. Disagreement was significant at the .01 level for only four of the statements of objectives (Numbers 4, 13, 24, 37).

Only providers and administrators rated feasibility. The feasibility scale ranged from 1 to 3, and the overall mean feasibility rating was 2.1 with a range of 1.63 to

2.8. The highest feasibility rating was given to Number 9, "immunizations" (which also received the highest availability rating). The objective receiving the lowest feasibility rating was Number 4, "reducing the cost of health care." There were no statistically significant differences in the mean ratings between the provider and the administrators.

In order to assign a priority scale to the objectives, the rating results were synthesized by combining importance, availability, and feasibility ratings, as seen in Table 3. Top priority for *implementation* was given to those objectives rated high in importance and feasibility, and low in current availability. Four objectives were identified in this manner:

Number 5, To set up health services that are close to the people in the community
Number 22, To identify and assist with family problems that are threats to health
Number 25, To adequately treat the common or frequent health problems in the same clinic
Number 31, To make better use of community resources

Three of the objectives received top priority for family practice *research* because they were rated greater than 4.0 in importance but less than 2.0 for availability and feasibility:

Number 4, To reduce costs of health care
Number 6, To reduce the time a patient has to wait for health services
Number 38, To make home visits when indicated

Validity of the Needs Assessment Findings

The King-Drew needs assessment strategy resulted in identifying objectives that were important to the Watts community, not yet available to it, and feasible to translate into

Table 3. *Synthesis of Needs Assessment Results*

			Importance		
			2.5*–3.5	3.5–4.0	4.0–4.5
Availability 1.0–2.0	Feasibility 1.0–2.0			Objective: 20	Objectives: 4,6,38
	Feasibility 2.0–3.0		Objectives: 11,37	Objectives: 7,17,23,29, 19,33,36	Objectives: 5,31,22,25
Availability 2.0–3.0	Feasibility 1.0–2.0			Objective: 13	
	Feasibility 2.0–3.0		Objective: 24	Objectives: 8,12,14,21 26,31	Objectives: 1,2,3,9,10, 15,16,18,19, 27,28,30,32, 34,35

* No objective's average rating fell below 2.5 or above 4.5 in importance.

service through the family practice residency program. Seven objectives identified in the study have served to guide the center's development and research activities. In response to the Watts community's selection of the objective to provide health services that are close to the people, the model family practice center was organized, satellite activities were developed at two outlying clinics including the basement of a community church, and an evening clinic was established to meet the needs of persons whose daily work prevented them from visiting the clinic during regular hours. In response to the research objective, "to reduce the time a patient has to wait for services," one of the residents conducted a patient time flow study to determine the points of longest wait. The study resulted in a new approach to patient orientation and screening that has substantially reduced waiting time in the family practice center.

During the first year after the needs assessment, the family practice center's growth rate, patients' compliance with appointments, and the extent to which patients reported as family units demonstrated the validity of the study's findings. The family practice center grew at a rate of 100 new patients per month, and by the end of the eighth month approximately 450 patients were being seen per month. Whereas compliance with appointments had averaged between 50 and 60 percent for all of the outpatient clinics of the institution, by the sixth month of the center's operation its show rate was between 75 and 80 percent, and by the eighth month there were 150 patients, or 20 percent of the population, who were followed as family units.

Discussion

A review of the conditions surrounding the King-Drew needs assessment produces several possible explanations for the unexpectedly low response rate by consumers.

Although the respondent population resembled the entire consumer sample in age, family ties, and marital status, it appeared to have 1.5 to 2 years more education, which indicates that the less well-educated groups were less responsive, particularly to the mailed surveys, than others. (According to other studies conducted by Dr. John Ware of the Rand Corporation, response rates in community surveys range from 25 to 95 percent, and groups with lower socioeconomic status show poorer response rates.) Given the generally low educational level of consumers in the King-Drew service area, response rates might have been boosted had the questionnaire been shortened so that it took less than one half-hour to complete. Also, it was probably unrealistic to expect the majority of consumers in an area of such high mobility to be concerned about the family practice center's future. Among consumers who had otherwise become involved with King-Drew, eg, those who had participated in the Community Medicine Forums, the response rate was three times greater than it was among consumers in outreach screening programs, and six times greater than it was among people identified by probability sample of households. Even among providers, physicians working within King-Drew were about four times more responsive than practicing community physicians.

A review of the ratings reveals that while consumers and providers in the Watts area generally considered family practice objectives to be important, consumers tended to rate them higher than did providers. Consumers also attached great importance to improving access to health care, and to maintaining health and preventing disease. They gave a high rating (3.5) to the family unit objectives, but rated the access and preventive medicine objectives as more important. Perhaps this was because the community did not understand the concept of family unit medicine as well as it did other concepts in medicine, or perhaps the residents of Watts were primarily concerned with getting medical care, and considered the relatively sophisticated ideas, like treatment of families by medical teams, to be impractical priorities.

The strategy used in this needs assessment encouraged the kind of community input that is essential to the structuring of family practice units to improve health care delivery. The results from this study have been used at King-Drew in improving access to care and disease prevention, increasing compliance with medical care regimens, reducing waiting time and the cost of care, and in generally improving the design of the family practice center.

Acknowledgments

Preparation of this manuscript was assisted by a grant from the Robert Wood Johnson Foundation, Princeton, New Jersey. The authors wish to thank Dr. Robert H. Brook for his invaluable technical and editorial assistance in the preparation of this study and Ms. Sylvia Cox for the training of the surveyors.

Authors' Update

The purpose of the Needs Assessment Study conducted at the King-Drew Medical Center in 1975–1976, was to get useful input from the Watts community in the planning of the family practice center. This family practice center was to be the focus of the family practice residency program which would train family physicians to practice in Watts and similar inner-city communities. No such study had ever been done in the planning of a family practice program for an inner-city community in this country. The methodology was complex and strategy was itself an object of the study. In order to give useful input, a representative sample of residents in Watts had to give both time and thought to several statements of family practice objectives. A probability sample of 1022 persons

was selected to respond to a list of family practice objectives by rating them on a scale of 1 to 5 in terms of importance and availability. The provider component of the sample was also asked to rate the feasibility of each objective. Seventy-six percent of the sample responded to the house-to-house survey, but only twenty-six percent returned mailed questionnaires.

The results of the survey gave us useful information and raised some very difficult questions. First, we found that on a scale of 1 to 5 the community gave an average rating of 4.1 to statements of family practice objectives. In terms of ranking, they ranked health promotion activities, comprehensive care, and continuity of care above an emphasis on the family unit in terms of importance. Likewise, both consumers and providers rated cost reduction, reduction in waiting time and home visits as important, but questioned the feasibility of such objectives. We, therefore, selected these as issues for research while the other issues were objects of implementation.

The community has responded very positively to the family practice program and a second family practice center is now in operation and very busy. We have been successful at reducing waiting time by the use of time-flow studies; home visits have been organized around a team with the community worker as the primary visitor. Cost of the care continues to increase in an environment of uncontrolled inflation. Therefore, the Needs Assessment Study accurately prepared us for both the positive response which we have received from the community and for the areas of difficulty and concern with which we have had to work in implementing the program.

REFERENCES

1. Willard WR (chairman): Meeting the challenge of family practice. Report of the Ad Hoc Committee on Education for Family Practice of the Council on Medical Education. Chicago, American Medical Association, 1966

2. Annual survey of family practice residency programs, reprint No. 150. Kansas City, Mo, American Academy Family Physicians, 1979

3. Haynes MA: Health problems in the Martin Luther King, Jr. Hospital service area: Implications for community medicine programs. West J Med 4:118, 1973

4. Ashely M (ed): Health facilities: South East region, vol 1, series 3. Los Angeles, Department of Community Medicine, Drew Postgraduate Medical School-Martin Luther King, Jr. General Hospital, 1974

5. Satcher D: What inner-city residents expect from family practice. Urban Health 5(5):36, 1976

6. Anderson SB, Bale S, Murphy LT, et al: Encyclopedia of Educational Evaluation. San Francisco, Jossey-Bass, 1975

7. Wentz HS, Tindall HL, Zervanos NJ: Primary care research in a model family practice unit. J Fam Pract 1(1):52, 1974

8. Hochstim HR: A critical comparison of three strategies of collecting data from households. J Am Stat Assoc 62:976, 1967

9. Ware JE, Wright W, Snyder MK, et al: Consumer perception of health care services: Implications for the academic medical community. J Med Educ 50:839, 1975

10. Hulka BS, Zyzanski SJ, Cassel JC, et al: Scale for the measurement of attitudes toward physicians and primary medical care. Med Care 8:429, 1970

11. Klein SP, Burry G, Churchman DA: Evaluations workshop: Part 2: Needs assessment. Monterey, Calif, CTB McGraw-Hill, 1973

12. Belloff JS, Smoke PS, Weinerman ER: Yale studies in family health care: Part 2: Organizations of comprehensive pediatric care. JAMA 204:355, 1970

13. Stokes J: An experiment in the teaching of family medicine. J Med Educ 38:539, 1963

14. Special requirements for residency training in family practice. In American Medical Association: Essentials of Approved Residencies. Chicago, American Medical Association, 1973

Outreach by Primary-Care Physicians*

Matthew Henk, Jack Froom

Outreach can be accomplished by the primary-care physician if he institutes data systems that permit identification of cohorts of his patients by age, sex, diagnoses, and area of residence. These systems were used by the Rochester Family Medicine Program to identify and invite patients at risk to receive prophylactic influenza immunization, participate in an obesity treatment group, and receive screening tests for lead intoxication.

The primary physician's efforts to change the health status of his patients have generally been oriented toward individuals or families, rather than cohorts of patients or the community. The physician responds to patient-initiated encounters but rarely provides outreach services based on an analysis of the needs of his patient population. Outreach may be defined as medical intervention initiated by the health provider to meet the health needs that he perceives in his patient population; it requires that physicians take the initiative to contact their patients for the purpose of providing health services.

The addition of the role of community physician to that of personal-health provider requires some changes in physicians' attitudes and the acquisition of additional skills. The change in attitude involves taking responsibility for the health needs of the group in addition to those of the individual patient. The new skills required include the institution and use of data systems that permit identification of cohorts of patients by age, sex, diagnoses, and area of residence.

This article describes data systems that make outreach possible and gives details of three projects in which specific patient groups who were perceived to be at risk were identified and were invited to participate in procedures for their individual benefit.

Data Systems

The Rochester Family Medicine Program is a private, nonprofit teaching practice with a staff of five faculty and 30 family-medicine trainees. Medical care is provided for approximately 9,000 individuals. The age-sex register,[1] diagnostic index,[2,3] and file of patients' charts by geographic location,[4] are three parts of an integrated data system used by this practice.

Age-Sex Register

The age-sex register consists of a collection of 8 × 13-cm (3 × 5-inch) cards, one for each patient. The cards are color-coded, blue for males and pink for females, and they contain the following information: name, date of birth, marital status, census tract, identification of physician by code number, date of entry into the practice, and date of removal from the practice. Cards are filed by year of birth; males are grouped separately from females and cards are arranged alphabetically within each section. Cards are maintained for active patients only. Our definition of an "active patient" is one who belongs to a family from which one member visited the practice in the preceding two years.

* Reprinted by permission from the *Journal of the American Medical Association*, 233(3):256–259, July 21, 1975. Copyright 1975, American Medical Association.

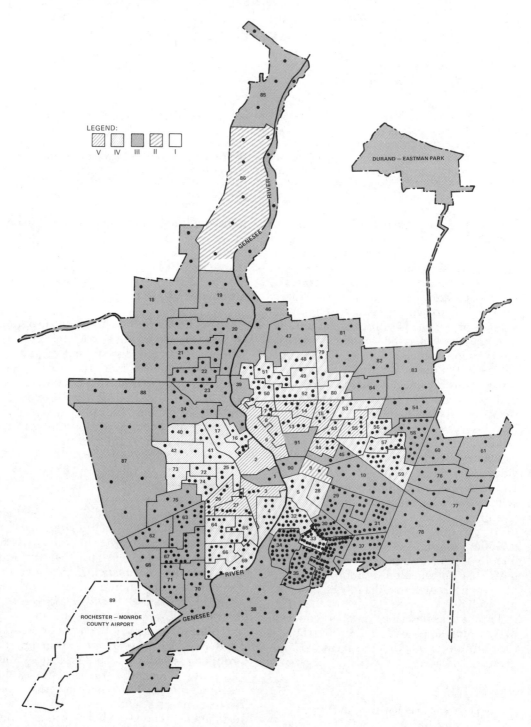

Fig. 1. Socioeconomic distribution of Rochester population by census tract. (For explanation of socioeconomic levels, see text.)

The Diagnostic Index-E Book

The diagnostic index-E Book is a loose-leaf binder containing 8 × 13-cm sheets of paper filed in an overlapping or "shingled" manner. There is one or more sheets for each diagnostic rubric or code number. The Royal College of General Practitioners Classification of Diseases, modified for use with problem-oriented records,[5] is used. The E Book sheets contain the following information: date of encounter, patient's name, type of episode (diagnoses newly made are recorded as "N" [new]; those that have been made by a previous physician and are still existent are recorded as "O" [old]), date of birth, a disposition code, and physician's name. If multiple diagnoses are made, the same information is recorded on the appropriate sheets for each diagnosis. Diagnoses of chronic conditions, such as diabetes mellitus or hypertension, are recorded only one time for each patient. Acute self-limited problems such as otitis media or pharyngitis are recorded as often as they occur.

Patients' charts are filed by the census tracts in which these patients reside. Census-tract directories, listing all of the addresses within a given census tract, and census maps are available from the Federal Bureau of Census.

Socioeconomic areas are delineated on the basis of a five-part composite index that consists of: median value of owned homes; median rental value; percentage of skilled, semiskilled, and unskilled workers; median years of education (of adults); and percentage of sound dwelling units. Five socioeconomic areas are delineated with V designated as the lowest. Cutting points between areas are based on a percentile distribution. Areas I and V each occupy 10% of the upper and lower limits of the distribution; areas II and IV, 20% each; and area III, 40%. A census-tract map illustrating the socioeconomic areas and our patient-population distribution in Rochester appears in Fig 1. and the distribution for Monroe County is shown in Fig 2.

Outreach Programs

Influenza Immunizations and Obesity Clinic

The age-sex register was used to define the population 65 years of age and older, and the diagnostic index was used to locate patients with the diagnoses of chronic obstructive lung disease, emphysema, chronic bronchitis, and ischemic heart disease. A single letter invited these patients to receive influenza inoculations. A total of 370 letters were sent, and 102 patients (28%) responded and received immunization for influenza.

An analysis of the socioeconomic status of the patients who were contacted and of those who responded is given in Fig 3 and 4. Our experience indicates that a single letter will produce a better response from the higher socioeconomic groups.

The diagnostic index was used to locate the 464 patients diagnosed as obese. This cohort of patients was invited by letter to participate in a Diet Workshop group. Of those contacted, 25 patients (5.4%) responded and enrolled in the group, which met weekly in our Family Medicine Unit.

Screening for Blood Lead Levels

A Directory of Street Addresses in High Risk Lead Belt Census Tracts was compiled by the University of Rochester School of Medicine and published by the Monroe County Department of Health. The census-tract filing system for patients' charts permitted the identification of those of our patients who resided in the area with a high-risk for lead intoxication. A single letter was sent to these families, inviting them to bring their children between the ages of 1 and 4 years to our clinic for determination of blood lead levels. Patients who did not respond after a one-month period were followed up with a single phone call. Identified as having an increased risk were 72 patients in the 1- to 4-year-old age group; 25 of these patients (35%) received a blood lead

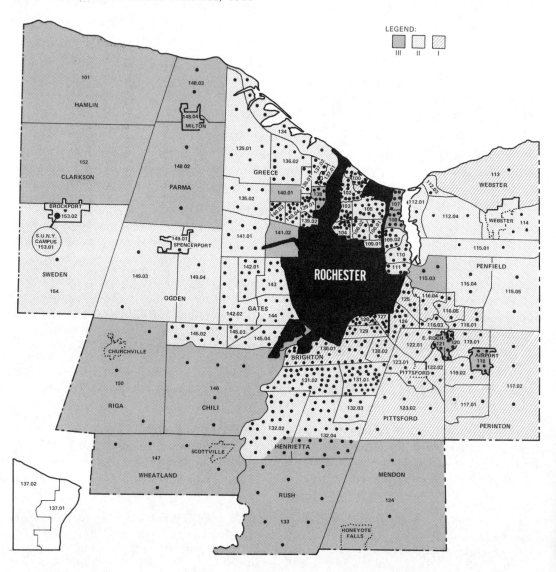

Fig. 2. Socioeconomic distribution of Monroe County population. (For explanation of socioeconomic levels, see text.)

level determination, and 9 patients (36%) had lead levels of more than 40μg/100 ml on initial screening.

Comment

Influenza causes excess morbidity and mortality in the aged and debilitated. The Public Health Service Advisory Committee on Immunization Practices recommends yearly influenza injections for these groups, although the immunization has only limited effectiveness. A mailing to the entire patient population would encourage excess utilization of these inoculations. The age-sex register and the diagnostic index can be used to identify the specific

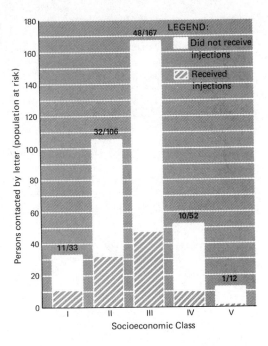

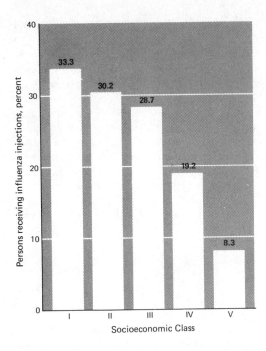

Fig. 3. Distribution of patients contacted for influenza injections by socioeconomic class. (For explanation of socioeconomic levels, see text.)

Fig. 4. Response to influenza outreach by socioeconomic class. (For explanation of socioeconomic levels, see text.)

cohort of patients who run the greatest risk if they contact influenza, and the outreach can be limited to this group.

Obesity is a difficult problem to treat, especially with traditional techniques. Group methods of treatment may give better results, although there are no long-term, rigidly conducted studies that prove this thesis. Nevertheless, if one wishes to start a group for any purpose, it is most efficient to recruit the entire group at the same time.

The diagnostic index permits identification of the entire cohort of obese patients (or any cohort of patients with a specific health problem) in the practice. This group can be contacted at one time and the feasibility of starting a treatment group evaluated.

The incidence of lead poisoning among children from inner-city areas as defined by blood lead levels in excess of 40 μg/100 ml appears to vary between 8.8% to

32.9%.[6] Other studies indicate that children in urban slums have higher mean blood levels than do suburban children.[7-9] The consequences of untreated lead poisoning could include serious central nervous system injury or renal damage.[10,11] Adults, except for those who have an occupational exposure, do not appear to be part of this high-risk group.[12] Eighty percent or more of acute toxic episodes occur during the summer months.[13]

It would therefore appear desirable to screen the population at greatest risk for lead poisoning. These are inner-city young children whose risk is greatest during the summer months. The technique of filing patients' charts by census tracts gives one the capability to screen this group with the greatest risk.

The primary-care physician can also use these data systems for research, audit or peer review, office management, and assessment of his continuing educational needs.[14,15] The pooling of data from many physician recorders could add to our knowledge of the natural history of diseases and may provide important clues to the epidemiology of diseases whose etiology is obscure.

The widespread use of outreach by primary physicians can have a considerable impact on the health of the general population. Improved access to patients with such problems as abuse of tobacco, anxiety, and hypertension, in addition to those described in this article, could contribute significantly to improved national health.

REFERENCES

1. Froom J: The age-sex register. J Fam Pract 1(1):45–46, 1974
2. Eimerl TS, Laidlow AJ: A Handbook for Research in General Practice. London, E&S Livingstone Ltd, 1969, pp 39–62
3. Froom J: Diagnostic index-E book. J Fam Pract 1(2):45–48, 1974
4. Farley E: Implications of filing charts by area of residence. J Fam Pract 1(3):43–47, 1974
5. Froom J: Classification of diseases. J Fam Pract 1(1):47–48, 1974
6. Gilsinn J: Estimates of the Nature and Extent of Lead Paint Poisoning in the United States, US Department of Commerce Publication No. NBS TN–746. Washington, DC, National Bureau of Standards, 1972
7. Lin-Fu J: Undue absorption of lead among children: A new look at an old problem. N Engl J Med 286:702–710, 1972
8. Seunee V: Lead poisoning. Am J Med 52:283–288, 1972
9. Blanksma L, Sachs HK, Murray EF, et al: Incidence of high blood lead levels in Chicago children. Pediatrics 44:661–667, 1969
10. Beyers RK, Jerd EE: Late effects of lead poisoning in mental development. Am J Dis Child 66:471–494, 1943
11. Chisolm JJ: Chronic lead intoxication in children. Dev Med Child Neurol 7:529–536, 1965
12. Lin-Fu JS: Vulnerability of children to lead exposure and toxicity. N Engl J Med 289:1229–1233, 1973
13. Chisolm JJ, Kaplan E: Lead poisoning in childhood: Comprehensive management and prevention. J Pediatr 73:942–950, 1968
14. Farley E, Treat D, Baker C, et al: An integrated system for the recording and retrieval of medical data in a primary care setting. J Fam Pract 1:44, 1974
15. Froom J, Rozzi C, Metcalfe D: Research comments: Computer analysis of morbidity reports in primary care. (Implications for a national morbidity survey). J Clin Comput 2:42–51, 1973

Establishing New Rural Family Practices: Some Lessons from a Federal Experience*

Roger A. Rosenblatt, Ira Moscovice

This study reports the experience of the National Health Service Corps in Washington, Oregon, and Idaho in establishing 20 new rural family practices over a six-year period. The practice structure, demography of the practice environment, and economic characteristics of the practices over time were analyzed in an attempt to isolate those factors which were associated with practice viability and physician retention. The outcome of each of the practices was examined in relation to the structure of the practice, training of the assigned physician, size of the town, and presence or absence of a group practice and supporting hospital.

The results indicate that it is possible for a new rural family practice to achieve financial equilibrium after approximately two years of operation. Forty-two percent of the physicians assigned to these practices elected to stay beyond their initial commitments; 17 percent of the sample made the transition into private practice. Factors associated with success included the presence of a hospital, group practice, and residency training. Impediments to success included service area population size below 4,000, lack of a hospital or group practice, and practices which mixed older and younger physicians. These data should be of use to physicians establishing new rural practices.

Rural areas have fewer physicians per capita than the rest of the United States.[1] These physicians are older, work longer hours, earn less money, and are more likely to be in solo practices than their urban counterparts.[2] Rural dwellers travel farther to obtain medical care, have relatively impaired health status, and use ambulatory health care services less than urban dwellers.[3] The relative disadvantage of rural areas has accelerated in the last two decades.[4]

There are a number of potent forces which promote maldistribution of physicians. They can be divided into six major areas: economic incentives; social and professional environment; specialty orientation; organizational frameworks; professional liability; and ancillary services. In each of these areas current conditions favor physicians who choose to practice in urban areas.

First, the current incentive system differentially rewards the urban practitioner. He is able to earn more and work less.[2] Secondly, the urban physician has increased access to professional peer relationships, coverage arrangements, and continuing medical education. Physicians traditionally come from white, middle class, urban families. Medical schools and residencies are preponderantly located in the cities and suburbs. Thus, physicians and their families seek to replicate the environments in which they are most comfortable when they choose a practice location.[1]

The proliferation of narrowly based specialists is a third factor which has had a deleterious effect on the provision of rural medical services. Specialists require a large population base to generate an adequate case load. The sparse population densities found in rural areas are not sufficient to support specialists. In the last two decades, medical schools have produced a cohort of physicians who are unable to practice medicine in rural America without abandoning the bulk of their training. The lack of organized structures for the delivery of med-

* Reprinted by permission from *The Journal of Family Practice*, 7(4):755–763, 1978.

ical care in rural areas has exacerbated the problem of maldistribution. As services have become less available, rural dwellers have developed patterns of health-care seeking behavior that circumvent local resources. Years of poor or nonexistent services have caused people to seek their care through distant or nontraditional practitioners. These habits are very difficult to modify, particularly for the new, young physician attempting to establish himself in a small rural community.

Added to the difficulty of establishing new organizational modes for the delivery of rural health care is the dearth of established group practices in these areas. The current mode of practice increasingly relies on the provision of medical care by a group of providers, physicians and supporting personnel.[5] Areas that have these organizational matrixes are much more likely to attract new physicians.[6] Resident training increasingly emphasizes the coordinated team approach to the provision of medical services in all settings, by generalists as well as specialists.[7] The absence of even rudimentary group structures in rural areas imposes another major obstacle to the establishment of new practices. Rather than merely adding one physician to an operational unit—an addition that results in only marginal additional costs to the stable practice—one must establish de novo several physicians in order to create the appropriate group structure. This is more complex, more costly, and tends to increase initial operational deficits. In addition, small scale delivery systems are inherently more unstable than larger aggregations of providers. The loss of one physician or a simple personality conflict can fatally disrupt small practices.

The increasingly volatile professional liability problem has had a disproportionate impact on the rural physician. Because the nature of such a practice requires a broad range of medical services, the physician is usually forced into the higher liability categories. Yet the relatively small numbers of obstetrical and surgical procedures performed often are insufficient to cover the premium costs. Thus, rural generalists are in a dilemma. If they abandon part of their professional repertoire, their patients must travel to obtain certain basic services. If they retain these procedures as part of their practice, their financial viability is threatened.[8]

The last major impediment is the erosion of other medical services in rural areas. Rural hospitals, in particular, have disproportionately felt the impact of the increasingly complex and costly regulation of the hospital industry. In general, the same standards are applied indiscriminately to rural and urban hospitals.[9] In addition, the rural hospitals built under the aegis of the Hill-Burton Act have been seriously undercapitalized in recent years. This has led to a relative lack of modern equipment and facilities to support rural physicians in hospital settings. The lack of rural physicians, the increasing regulatory burden, and the creeping obsolescence have threatened the financial and professional equilibrium of many smaller hospitals. Recent work has documented the symbiotic relationship that exists between rural primary care practices and rural hospitals.[10] In addition to hospital services, the whole gamut of public health, social, and supportive services taken for granted in urban areas are often missing in rural areas.

Two major movements over the last decade have been designed largely to redistribute physicians. The first has been the creation of the specialty of family medicine. One major impetus for the revival of this discipline was the perception that the solution of the rural manpower problem required the training of a more broadly based, self-sufficient physician. A large number of medical school and residency programs have been launched with federal and state support in an attempt to solve the maldistribution problem.[11] The hypothesis has been that the emerging family medicine resident will possess skills that match the medical, organizational, and social characteristics and needs of rural settings. The hope is that graduates of such programs are more likely to settle and remain in underserved areas.

A second major effort has been undertaken by governmental agencies and foundations which underwrite the creation of new rural delivery systems. The largest program of this type has been the National Health Service Corps (NHSC) which by 1977 had grown to a field strength of 725 health care providers, the majority in rural settings.[12] In addition, a number of grant programs have been sponsored by the federal government and by private foundations designed to increase the amount and range of health services in rural areas.[13]

Rural areas have an acute need for young, well-trained physicians. A growing number of family practice programs are creating such physicians. Governmental and private programs are assisting in the establishment of new rural practices. Yet, many of the structural constraints mentioned above create major barriers to the establishment of viable rural practices.

This paper is an examination of the experience of the NHSC in the northwestern United States in establishing new rural practices. The experience garnered during six years of initiating new family practices in areas critically deficient in physicians should be of considerable use to young physicians who desire to locate in rural areas. Certain recurrent patterns emerge from an examination of these practices that may be of use in identifying and overcoming the major impediments, and predicting which areas and which organizational modes predispose to success. As increasing resources are directed at the problem—and as large numbers of family practice graduates complete residencies and are interested in rural practice—it becomes crucial to base future efforts on the lessons of past experience.

Background

Since its inception in 1971, the NHSC has established 25 new physician practices in the states of Washington, Oregon, and Idaho; 20 of these practices are now more than two years old. During the period of this study, the NHSC offered assistance only to communities in which the physician to population ratio fell below 1 to 4,000 people within the relevant medical service area. By definition, these were areas where traditional health care delivery systems had largely deteriorated, often due to the death or retirement of aging general practitioners. Although in most cases a fragmentary health care system persisted, it was inadequate to meet the bulk of the medical care needs of the populace. Due to a lack of local physicians, a large proportion of the affected population received its ambulatory and inpatient services outside of the community. Often, other medical care institutions, such as hospitals, were moribund or had succumbed.

Working in conjunction with a community-based nonprofit sponsor, the NHSC initiated efforts to rebuild and staff a comprehensive health care delivery system. The major emphasis was on bringing physicians as rapidly as possible to the applicant community. Using a national recruiting system, the NHSC was successful in almost every case in placing physicians on a voluntary basis in each approved community.

Each community selected for NHSC assistance received extensive and uniform technical assistance before and during operation. Physician assignees, members of the sponsoring nonprofit boards, and members of the practice supporting staff were assisted by federal staff and members of an experienced practice management firm. Practices were closely monitored as they developed, and regular site visits were made during the study period.

Methodology

In this paper, the performance of the NHSC practices is analyzed in two different ways. In the first analysis, the practices are stratified according to their relative success in attaining their primary goal: the establishment of independent primary care practices in underserved areas. In the second analysis, a subset of the practices is examined for their economic growth and development. These analyses are designed to identify those characteristics of newly developed rural practices which predispose to success and to highlight areas where intervention may improve the outcome.

The definition of success in new practices is perplexing and challenging. The ultimate test of success in the present system of care is the establishment of a viable, independent, sustained private practice of medicine. Yet rigid application of such an endpoint tends to distort the situation. Many rural practice situations, and especially those served by the National Health Service Corps, represent settings in which normal market situations have proven unsuccessful. From the consumers' standpoint, the continuous provision of medical services represents a substantial improvement in the delivery system.

For the analysis, four distinct and quantifiable stages of success were defined. The first is the situation in which the physician, after subsidy by the NHSC, elects to remain in his setting independent of continued direct federal support. In the second category are those who elect to remain in their communities beyond their initial two-year commitment; although they extend their tour of duty in the communities to which they have been assigned, they do not leave the relative security of a salaried Public Health Service berth. The third category comprises those communities in which the physician initially assigned leaves at the conclusion of his commitment, but in which the practice as an institution persists. Replacement personnel are recruited without a hiatus in the delivery of medical service. In the fourth category the practice fails, and the assignee either leaves or is withdrawn. Failure may result from strife at the community level, a severely under-utilized practice, or inability to recruit a replacement physician.

Another measure of success is financial self-sufficiency: that point at which a practice is collecting enough money from fees for services rendered to pay for the expenses of the practice and the salaries of the providers. For the second analysis, nine sites were selected in order to focus on the aspects of practice development on which financial self-sufficiency depends. The nine sites selected for intensive analysis were those with the most complete and accurate financial records; they did not differ significantly from the 20 practices in the sample universe with respect to age of site, number of physicians, size of service area, or practice outcome.

The 20 practices which comprise the study universe were not uniform. They varied in the size of the town in which they were set, the configuration of the medical care team assembled in these towns, and the relative access to other medical care services, such as hospitals. Although clearly there was a spectrum of practices, they did tend to cluster around three fairly well-defined configurations.[14] The first (System 1) included those settings with a medical service area of greater than 10,000 people, a minimum of three physicians,* and a small, full-service hospital. The second (System 2) had a medical service area of 5,000–10,000 people, a minimum of two physicians, and was served by a hospital with a limited range of traditional services. The third setting (System 3) lacked inpatient facilities; generally, the medical service area of these towns was between 3,000–5,000 people and at least one physician was required.

It would be misleading to suggest that there is a complete overlap between the size of the service area, the number of physicians, and the range of available inpatient services. Yet, in general, these three factors were closely linked.

Of the nine sites selected for the second

---

* The number of physicians noted in each system means all practicing physicians in the service area, whether or not they were members of the NHSC.

analysis, there were three sites in each of the three types of designated configurations. The practices' economic data were obtained through the use of the existing monitoring system, in which each site submitted a detailed monthly statement of operations (MSO) which included the important economic data about the site.

For this study, the data were normalized for number of provider full-time equivalents (FTE) to ensure the comparability of data across sites, and then plotted against time. A fuller description of the technique can be found in a recent publication.[10] This allowed the examination of the growth and development of the key indicators of practice performance-productivity as measured by gross charges and receipts, and number of patients seen; managerial efficiency as reflected in overhead expenses and collection; and relative success as measured by the practices' ability to attain economic self-sufficiency.

Using these two approaches, it is possible to examine the outcome of a group of new rural practices, and focus on the economic experience of a set of these practices.

Results

Practice Success and Community Characteristics

Table 1 shows selected characteristics of 20 communities in the Northwest in which NHSC practices have operated for two years or longer. These communities are distributed evenly among the four possible outcomes for a practice, as defined earlier. Those communities in which the practice failed are strikingly different from the other communities. Most of the practices that failed were solo, and all of the towns lacked hospitals. In none of the sites that failed were any of the physicians residency-trained. One noticeable difference is the small size of the medical care service area, suggesting that there is a minimum size service area below which physician practices cannot be expected to survive.

The differences among the other three groups are not as clear. One suggestive variable is that four of the five communities in which the physicians "went private" had hospitals. One possible explanation for this factor emerges from the financial

Table 1. *Rural Practice Outcome and Community Characteristics*

Practice Outcome	Sample Size	Average Size Medical Service Area †	Number of Group Practices‡	Type of Group Practice* NHSC Only	Hybrid	Number with Hospitals in Community	Percent of MDs Residency Trained§
Made transition to independence	5	9,600	4	3	1	4	18
Extended commitment	5	6,800	3	3	0	2	58
Replaced initial assignee	5	8,400	3	2	1	2	30
Practice stopped operating	5	3,200	2	0	2	0	0

* A hybrid practice is one in which the NHSC assignee(s) practices in conjunction with a community physician who was in practice at the time of application. A NHSC Only practice indicates that all the physicians initially were members of the NHSC.
† Medical service area is calculated from the estimates of the local health planning unit at the time of application to the NHSC.
‡ A group practice is defined as an organized cooperative medical practice with at least two physicians working conjointly.
§ This percentage applies to all NHSC physicians ever assigned to the community who have completed residencies in family medicine, internal medicine, or pediatrics.

data to be presented. Yet from the marked overlap in groups 1 to 3, it is apparent that there are no unequivocal elements which can be isolated as the sine qua non of success.

Group practice situations also appear to enhance success. In this study, a group practice was defined as two or more physicians working conjointly in a shared medical practice. It was readily apparent that the solo physician in a community without other physicians was not a viable model in these settings; each of the three practices in which the assignee was the only provider in town failed.

One initial hypothesis was that placing a newly graduated physician with an existing practitioner would be worthwhile because the less experienced physician would be given a source of counsel and support. The converse appeared true. In three of the four cases in which a hybrid practice was established, either the practice failed or the group arrangement was dissolved. Generational difference, expressed largely in differences in professional approach, caused conflict in many cases. In addition, the disparate financial arrangement experienced by a private physician and his government-salaried partner was a constant irritant.

Table 2 summarizes the status of the 55 physicians placed in the Northwest since 1971. Thirty-five percent of all assignees ever placed are still in their initial two-year

period of commitment. The majority of this group has been residency trained in family medicine, reflecting the increased supply of family physicians, the interest of the group in rural practice, and the conscious attempt to recruit residency-trained family physicians whenever possible.

Of the 36 assignees who completed their two-year commitment, 15 (42 percent) stayed in their community beyond their initial commitment. The majority elected to remain within the relative security of the Public Health Service; six made the transition to independence. Of those who did choose to remain beyond their initial commitments, 40 percent were residency trained, as opposed to 20 percent of those who left at the completion of their initial obligation. This suggests that there is a higher likelihood of residency-trained individuals remaining in small rural practices.

Economic Growth of Practices

Figures 1 through 5* present five critical indicators of practice performance compared among the three major types of practice configurations described earlier. After the starting period there were no

* Figures 1 through 5 are adapted from figures and data presented in Reference 10 and are presented with the permission of the Lippincott Company.

Table 2. *Status of NHSC Physician Assignees in Pacific Northwest—1971–1977*

| | | Residency Training Status | | | |
Status	Assignees (%)	Family Practice	Internal Medicine	Pediatrics	None
Currently in initial two years of assignment	19 (35)	11	3	0	5
Extended assignment in NHSC	9 (16)	4	0	0	5
Made transition into private practice	6 (11)	1	1	0	4
Left their community at conclusion of assignment	20 (36)	1	2	1	16
Died	1 (2)	0	0	0	1
Totals	55 (100)	17	6	1	31

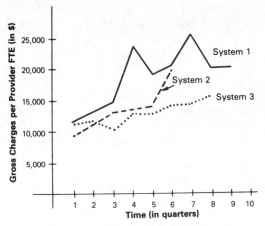

Fig. 1. Gross charges per provider FTE. System 1—Service area >10,000; ≥3 physicians; full service rural hospitals. System 2—Service area 5,000 to 10,000; ≥2 physicians; limited service hospital. System 3—Service area 3,000 to 5,000; ≥1 physician; no hospital.

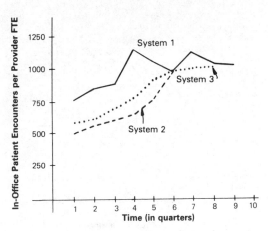

Fig. 3. In-office patient encounters per provider FTE.

major differences among the three systems in practice collection ratio and number of encounters. All three types of practice settings attained a plateau of about 1,000 encounters per quarter—16 patients per working day—after approximately two years of operation. In the same time period, the collection ratio stabilized at about 80 percent. It is of interest to note that in System 3, gross charges were considerably lower than in Systems 1 and 2. The lack of a hospital practice decreased the ability of

physicians to charge for the traditional services performed in the hospital and this in turn appeared to impair the financial viability of their primary care practices.

Figures 4 and 5 support this supposition. All three systems show a decrease over time in the practice expense ratio. The expense ratio is the total expenses incurred by the practice, excluding provider salaries, divided by gross charges, and is a measure of practice overhead. System 3, however, is unable to reduce its overhead to the 50 percent level the others are able to attain. The explanation parallels that

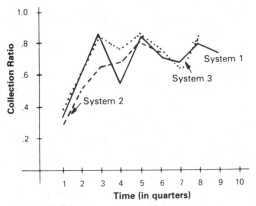

Fig. 2. Practice collection ratio.

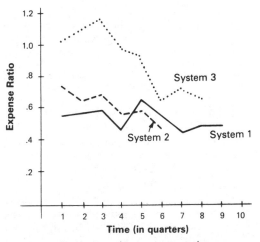

Fig. 4. Practice expense ratio.

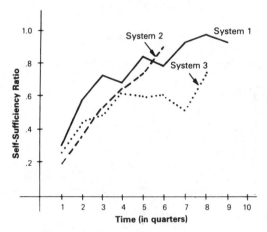

Fig. 5. Practice self-sufficiency ratio.

given above. Since practices in System 3 do not have ready access to a hospital, they are deprived of the revenue generated from that source. The hospital is basically a free workshop for the physician, and it is logical to assume that a practice without access to a hospital would have commensurately larger overhead.

One crucial test of a new rural health-care practice is the degree to which it is able to reach financial equilibrium. The self-sufficiency ratio compares the practices' ability to collect revenues with their expenses—overhead plus provider salaries. System 1 practices reached 95 percent of self-sufficiency at two years; System 2 practices reached 89 percent of self-sufficiency at 1½ years; and System 3 practices reached 71 percent of self-sufficiency at two years.

Again, the data suggest that the rural practice without access to a hospital has a more difficult struggle to become self-supporting. When this economic impediment is added to the professional liabilities of being at a distance from a hospital, the ultimate viability of this model without external subsidy may be questionable.

On the other hand, after two years of operation, the six practices with local hospital access were largely independent of external governmental support. Patient revenues were able to defray most of the overhead and the bulk of the physicians' salaries.

Discussion

The establishment of new independent family practices in small rural areas is a difficult proposition. The data presented here demonstrate that even with a coordinated, cohesive, and well-funded effort by the federal government, only 17 percent of all the physicians placed in a six-year period successfully made the transition to independent practice. On the other hand, the program does demonstrate that in the Northwest new practices can be started in areas where traditional medical care systems have largely disappeared, and the majority of them will increase their productivity and their financial stability with time, achieving a large measure of self-sufficiency within two years of initiation.

The data presented here emerge from a fairly homogeneous area of the United States, the Pacific Northwest. There are regional variations in the structure of rural health care delivery. Yet a number of provocative suggestions emerge which may be of use to young physicians planning to set up practices in rural areas, to planners and administrators designing rural health care systems, and to communities seeking physicians.

First, it is highly unlikely, in the present structure of medical care, that new rural practices will be able to begin without external support, both administrative and financial. Facilities and equipment require large capital expenditures; to this must be added the operational subsidy to cover the deficit experienced during the first two years of operation by the new practices. The resultant financial risk—even without considering the attendant professional and organizational difficulties—greatly diminish the likelihood that new physicians will establish such practices without assistance.

The evidence also suggests that there are certain elements whose absence greatly reduces the likelihood of financial success. There may be a minimum service area size in which a contemporary family practice can exist. The cutoff point in this study appeared to be about 4,000 people; no practice started in towns with medical service areas smaller than 4,000 was able to retain physicians. Size of service area is highly correlated with two other variables: the presence of hospital facilities and the establishment of a group practice. Ready access to hospital facilities is essential to the recently trained physician, be he specialist or generalist. In this study, towns with hospitals were more likely to retain physicians. A hospital practice allows the physician to broaden his scope of services, both in the variety and complexity of services supplied, without a concomitant increase in overhead cost. Thus the absence of a hospital in a rural community frustrates the physician's ability to fully use his skill and deprives him of a source of income that may be critical to his financial success.

These data may appear to run counter to the current argument that small, rural hospitals are often inefficient, under-utilized, and may provide care at a questionable level of quality.[15] Although this paper does not focus on the problems of the rural hospital, it does emphasize the symbiotic relationship between the rural hospital and the rural physician. Governmental and educational strategies, which on the one hand increase the supply of broadly trained physicians to rural areas and on the other hand undermine the viability of the hospitals in which they work, compound the problem of developing viable rural health care strategies.

Group practice is increasingly the desired model among young physicians. It takes a certain minimum population to generate enough encounters to support a group of physicians. In this small sample, the most successful sites tended to be group practices, in particular group practices composed of peers. Towns smaller

than 4,000 have difficulty supporting even two physicians, and may be unable to retain any. In this study, the only places where solo NHSC practices persisted were in communities of greater than 10,000 people which had other physicians with whom the NHSC assignees shared coverage.

Physician training also appears to be an important factor in determining the capacity of the rural physician to adapt to and master his environment. In this study, there was greater likelihood that a physician who had finished a residency would remain in the community after his initial commitment. In talking and working with the physicians assigned, it became evident that the majority of those who had not completed a residency felt overwhelmed by the professional demands of their situation. Conversely, those who had completed a residency, although challenged, were exhilarated by the opportunity to translate their academic preparation into the reality of practice.

The residency trained group displayed greater managerial aptitude and interest and involved themselves more completely in the organizational and community aspects of the practices. The experience of working in a model family practice in a family medicine residency appeared to be an important factor in increasing the flexibility of the assigned physicians. Establishing record systems, choosing appointment schedules, defining collection policies, and carrying out personnel management are an important part of every new rural practice. Physicians who had completed family medicine residencies were familiar at a working level with the concept of practice management, and were able to successfully structure their practice environment without unnecessary conflict or stress.

There are many rural areas in this country in which there is a critical need for the establishment of well-organized health care systems. The recruitment and retention of young physicians is an essential component of this process. Certainly, the establishment of a new primary care practice presents the young physician with the opportunity to create a practice environment that will fully use his talents and mesh with his interests. The information presented here should be helpful in meeting that challenge.

Acknowledgments

The authors wish to acknowledge the support of the Center for Health Services Research at the University of Washington (Grant #HS 01978), and the cooperation of the Region X Office of the National Health Service Corps.

REFERENCES

1. Factors Influencing Practice Location of Professional Health Manpower: Review of the Literature. In Health Resources Administration (Hyattsville, Md): DHEW publication No. 75-3. Government Printing Office, 1974
2. 1975 Net Income and Work Patterns of Physicians in Five Medical Specialties. In Department of Health, Education and Welfare, Social Security Administration (Washington, DC): Research and Statistics Note No. 13. Government Printing Office, 1977
3. Davis K, Marshall R: Primary health care services for medically underserved populations. In Health Resources Administration (Hyattsville, Md): Papers on the National Health Guidelines: The Priorities of Section 1502. DHEW publication No. (HRA) 77-641, Government Printing Office, 1977
4. American Medical Association: Profile of Medical Practice. Chicago, American Medical Association, 1972
5. Madison D: Recruiting physicians for rural practice. Health Serv Rep 8:758, 1973
6. Evashwick C: The role of group practice in the distribution of physicians in nonmetropolitan areas. Med Care 14:808, 1976
7. Scherger JE, Eaton MH, Flaherty S, et al: A nurse practitioner in a family medicine residency: Role description and impact of continuity on the practitioner-patient relationship. J Fam Pract 5:791, 1977
8. Reynolds JA: Tips from the big groups on heading off malpractice problems. Med Econ 54(1):173, 1977
9. Popko K: How regulation affected two community hospitals. Hosp Progr 58:80, 1977
10. Rosenblatt R, Moscovice I: The growth and evolution of rural primary care practice: The National Health Service Corps Experience in the Northwest. Med Care 16(10):21, 1978
11. American Academy of Family Physicians: Data Summary, 1977, mimeograph, Kansas City, Mo, AAFP, 1977
12. Department of Health, Education and Welfare, Health Services Administration: National Health Service Corps Notes. Rockville, Md, Public Health Service, April 1978, p 2
13. Martin E: The federal initiative in rural health. Pub Health Rep 90:291, 1975
14. Blackman A, Moscovice I: Highlights of the second working conference on state government's role in improving rural health service. Seattle, Wash, Center for Health Services Research, University of Washington, 1977
15. Spitzer W: The small general hospital: Problems and solutions. Milbank Mem Fund Q 48:413, 1970

Changes in Hospital Emergency Department Use Associated with Increased Family Physician Availability*

John R. Hilditch

This study explores the effect of an increase in the family physician to population ratio on use of the hospital Emergency Department in a community. Two household surveys were conducted, the first before a community health center was established in an underserviced community, the second survey three years later. During this period there was a fivefold increase in the family physician-population ratio. Use of hospital Emergency Departments decreased. Respondents were more likely to have called their physician before going to the Emergency Department. If they did not call, the reason for not doing so was less likely related to physician unavailability. A decrease in the level of perceived illness in the community was also found.

This study was undertaken to determine the effects of establishing a community health center on selected aspects of the health care behavior of the residents of a medically underserviced community. This report presents some of the findings of the study, with particular emphasis on hospital Emergency Department use.

The study was undertaken to determine if an increase in the ratio of family physicians to population would lead to an altered pattern of hospital Emergency Department use. Would the utilization rate decrease? Would the type of problems taken to the Emergency Department be more likely acute? Would care from family physicians more often be sought prior to the Emergency Department visit? When respondents attended the Emergency Department without first trying to contact their physician, would the reasons be less often related to physician unavailability?

The Community

In October 1972, a community health center was established in an urban neighbor-

hood in metropolitan Toronto. This community had a population of about 10,000 people living in rented apartments and townhouses. About 15 percent of the dwellings were publicly subsidized housing units. Medical care provided within the community was confined to one family physician.

A building development in 1972 and 1973 added more apartments and townhouses, most of which were condominiums. In 1975, the community health center had been active for three years, with four family physicians, nurse practitioners, a social worker, a nutritionist, a laboratory, a pharmacy, an x-ray unit, and a physiotherapy department. In addition, two private family physicians established practice in the community in 1973. A major physician-staff turnover occurred during the first six months of 1975. At this time three physicians left the health center and also set up practice in the community. The net result was a change from a physician to population ratio of 1:10,000 in 1972 to 1:1,800 in 1975.

The policy of the community health center, and also to a great extent the other medical groups in the community, was to provide extended hours of operation (70

* Reprinted by permission from *The Journal of Family Practice*, 11(1):91–96, 1980.

Table 1. *Household Characteristics*

Characteristic	Phase 1	Phase 2	Statistical Test
Mean number of persons per household	3.3	2.8	$\chi^2 = 1.62$, $df = 1$, $0.25 > P > 0.1$
Male:female ratio	49:51	45:55	$\chi^2 = 1.61$, $df = 1$, $0.25 > P > 0.1$
Age (years) % ≤17	33.0	35.0	
% 18–45	58.0	52.4	$\chi^2 = 4.29$, $df = 2$, $0.25 > P > 0.1$
% ≥46	9.0	12.6	
Marital status of adults % single	18.4	22.6	
% married	72.9	67.1	$\chi^2 = 2.47$, $df = 2$, $0.5 > P > 0.25$
% separated, widowed, divorced	8.6	10.3	

hours per week), plus 24-hour physician coverage. A small emergency treatment room in the health center was provided with the aim of treating minor emergencies, thereby avoiding the necessity for some visits to local hospital Emergency Departments.

Methods

Two household surveys were conducted in the community. The first one, conducted in the summer of 1972, was completed just before the community health center opened. This is referred to as Phase 1 of the study.[1] The second was conducted three years later in the summer of 1975, and is referred to as Phase 2 (Tables 1 and 2).

Phase 1 was a household survey of a randomized sample of addresses in the community. The interview schedule was administered by trained interviewers, in the respondents' homes. Out of a population of about 10,000 people, the sample consisted of 141 households, comprising 467 people. The representativeness of the sample was verified by comparison with 1971 census data.

The Phase 2 survey involved the same community but because of the large building development the population was estimated to be 18,000. The addresses selected for the sample in Phase 1 were used to make up the sample for one stratum in Phase 2, with the intention of obtaining a "before and after" measure of a subsample of respondents who had lived in the community at the same address from 1972 to 1975. A second stratum consisted of a random sample of the addresses in the new development. The first stratum consisted of 176 households, 494 individuals. This report presents data from Phase 1, and only the first stratum from Phase 2, so that

Table 2. *Sociodemographic Characteristics*

Characteristic	Phase 1	Phase 2	Statistical Test
Percentage with post-secondary school education	23.4	33.0	$\chi^2 = .106$, $df = 1$, $.9 > P > .75$
Median family income	$9,932*	$11,454†	See *, †
Percentage in technical, professional, or managerial jobs	18.1	27.7	$\chi^2 = 7.7$, $df = 1$, $P < .01$
Percentage Canadian born	55.4	45.1	$\chi^2 = 10.2$, $df = 1$, $P < .01$
Percentage who have lived in community less than 1 year	35.1	35.9	$\chi^2 = .04$, $df = 1$, $P > .9$

* 95% confidence interval ($7,615–$11,266).
† 95% confidence interval ($10,363–$12,545).

comparisons are made using samples from the same addresses.

In order to view the findings regarding Emergency Department use in light of use in the broader community, data on total annual hospital Emergency Department visits were obtained from the Ontario Ministry of Health for the years 1972 and 1975.

Results

Sample Characteristics

A comparison of household sociodemographic characteristics in Phases 1 and 2, presented in Tables 1 and 2, show few changes. There is an increase in the proportion of foreign born persons. More people are employed in the professional, technical, and managerial occupations. The median family income was lower than that for the whole of metropolitan Toronto ($11,454) in Phase 1 but was proportionately even lower in Phase 2 (metropolitan Toronto median family income, $18,050).[2] The population continues to be mobile. Another indication of this is that the repeat sample in Phase 2 revealed only 5 out of the original 167 families in Phase 1.

Emergency Department Use

A marked difference was found in Emergency Department visiting rates. In Phase 1, 22.1 percent of respondents had visited a hospital Emergency Department at least once in the preceding one year; in Phase 2, 13.8 percent had visited ($\chi^2 = 12.53$, P < .01). Calculated on the basis of visits per 1,000 persons per year, in Phase 1 there were 280/1,000 persons per year; in Phase 2 there were 174/1,000 persons per year (Table 3).

There was essentially no difference between Phase 1 and Phase 2 regarding the acuteness of the problem for which the respondents visited the Emergency Depart-

Table 3. *Use of Emergency Departments*

	Number of Visits					
	0	*1*	*2*	*3*	*4 or More*	**Total**
Phase 1	363	82	13	5	3	466
Phase 2	426	54	11	2	1	494

$\chi^2 = 12.53$, *df* = 4, *P* < 0.01.

ment. The problem was reported to have begun within the previous 24 hours by 81.9 percent in Phase 1 and by 83.1 percent in Phase 2 ($\chi^2 = .04$, P > .9).

During the two weeks before the Emergency Department visit, 13.5 percent of the visitors in Phase 1 consulted their physician about the same problem. In Phase 2, 19.4 percent had done so ($\chi^2 = 1.1$, .5 > P > .25).

In Phase 1, 81.6 percent went directly to the Emergency Department; 18.4 percent attempted to contact their physician, then went to the Emergency Department. In Phase 2, 35.8 percent attempted to contact their physician; 64.2 percent went to the Emergency Department directly ($\chi^2 = 65.4$, P < .001). Those who went directly to the Emergency Department were asked why they did not first try to contact their physicians. The replies are displayed in Table 4.

Reasons were then classified by those relating to physician unavailability (indicated by an * in Table 4), and other reasons. In Phase 1, 54.9 percent of reasons were related to physician unavailability, compared to 39.5 percent in Phase 2. Although specific reasons (ie, "I have no doctor" and "Doctor too far away") show differences from Phase 1 to Phase 2, the general comparison is of only borderline statistical significance ($\chi^2 = 3.63$, .10 > P > .05).

Other reasons for these changes in patterns of Emergency Department use were examined. Perhaps the decreased visiting rate was part of an overall change in Toronto. More than half of the visits from this neighborhood were made to the three closest hospitals (58 percent in Phase 1 and

Table 4. *Reasons Given for Going Directly to Emergency Department*

Reason	Phase 1 (N)	Phase 2 (N)
It is the best place for the problem	30	4
* My doctor is unavailable/ could not see me	22	12
* I have no doctor	13	3
* My doctor is too far away	9	1
My problem was a real emergency	6	18
* My doctor is ill/away	1	1
Other	1	4
Total	**82**	**43**

$\chi^2 = 22.8$, $df = 6$, $P < .001$.

* Reason related to physician unavailability.

60 percent in Phase 2). In the three years between Phases 1 and 2, there was a 5 percent increase in the population of the municipalities in which these hospitals are located. During the same time period, there was, on the average, a 16 percent increase in the Emergency Department visits in these hospitals (range from 1 to 33 percent). This strongly suggests that, while visiting rate decreased in the study community, in the broader community the rate of Emergency Department use was increasing.

Could the changes be attributed to a change in the composition of the community? Only three of the sociodemographic variables, place of birth, occupation, and income changed from Phase 1 to Phase 2.

Emergency Department use was unrelated to any of these variables.

Another possible reason for the decrease in Emergency Department utilization could be a difference in the amount of perceived illness between Phase 1 and Phase 2. Respondents were asked to report if they had felt ill during the two weeks preceding the interview. In Phase 1, 25.3 percent of respondents reported feeling ill compared to 14.2 percent in Phase 2 (P < .001) (Table 5).

This difference in perceived illness could easily account for much of the difference in rates of Emergency Department visiting.

In both phases, 60 percent of the "sick people" did not see a physician for their problem because it was not important enough (Table 6).

However, when other reasons were given, in Phase 2 these were less often related to physician unavailability than in Phase 1.

Strengths

This study gives the opportunity to study sociodemographic characteristics, perceived health problems, and health care behavior over time. Of particular interest are the changes in health care behavior associated with an increase in family physician availability. It also gives an opportunity to examine population based Emergency Department utilization rates rather than utilization rates reported from hospital statistics.

Table 5. *Illness in Past Two Weeks*

	Phase 1		Phase 2	
	(Number)	*(Percent)*	*(Number)*	*(Percent)*
Felt sick	118	25.3	70	14.2
Did not feel sick	349	74.7	424	85.8
Total	467	100.0	494	100.0

$\chi^2 = 18.8$, $df = 1$, $P < .001$.

Table 6. *Reasons for Not Visiting Physician*

Reason	Not Important	Physician Not Available	Other	Totals
Phase 1	22	12	3	37
Phase 2	6	2	6	14

$\chi^2 = 8.7$, $df = 2$, $P < .025$.

Weaknesses

This study has the "weaknesses" of any survey research in that the data are derived from the subjects' opinions and recall and may not be entirely accurate. Since this research consisted of two surveys, three years apart, considerable attention was given to keeping the interview schedule and the research methods as nearly alike as possible. However, with change in research personnel and other unforeseen problems some differences occurred leading to areas of incomparability. Finally, although the study was originally designed to examine the effect on the community of the introduction of the community health center, many changes occurred in this community in the three years, including a near doubling of the population, and the addition of other physicians as well as those in the health center. Thus, there was great difficulty in separating the effects of the health center from other important factors.

Discussion

The ratio of family physicians to the population in the community increased from 1:10,000 to 1:1,800 with the addition of the community health center and of other family physicians to the community. This ratio is close to the overall Ontario ratio for 1961 to 1971 reported by Spaulding and Spitzer.[3] Clearly, the community in this study was medically underserviced in 1972, in Phase 1 of the study. Associated with this increase in family physician avail-

ability, per capita hospital Emergency Department visiting rate decreased by 40 percent. During the same period of time Emergency Department visiting rate increased in the broader community. This is similar to the findings of other investigators. Moore et al, who studied the effect of a neighborhood health center on Emergency Room visiting rates, observed that the rates remained constant over two years in the study community, but the overall community rate rose during that time.[4] Hochheiser et al reported a 38 percent decrease in Emergency Room use by children in the community served by a neighborhood health center.[5]

An unexplained and confounding finding in the present study is a decreased illness reporting rate, which could account for all or part of the decreased visiting rate. The higher level of illness reported in Phase 1 could be accounted for by either "significant" illness or "trivial" illness. In both surveys the perception of the importance of the problems was the same. In Phase 1, however, respondents were more likely to use "physician unavailability" as a reason for not seeking medical care for their problems. It appears reasonable to suggest that family physician availability had an effect on the "seeking care" behavior in general of the study community.

Other findings, in any case, suggest that increased family physician availability had effects on health care behavior. There was an increase in the proportion of persons who contacted their physician immediately before the Emergency Department visit. This suggests that the family physician is more often playing a role in providing care for conditions perceived as urgent. Also seen is a difference in the reasons given by those who attended the Emergency Department without first contacting their physician. Reasons related to physicians' unavailability are less often stated. Emergency Department use was not related to measured sociodemographic factors, so changes in these could not account for the observed findings.

There are several likely reasons for the use of the hospital Emergency Department as an alternative to care in the family physician's office for urgent problems.[6,7]

First, hospitals have better developed and organized their Emergency Departments in the last 10 to 15 years. This is possibly a reaction to the increased demand, but at the same time has made the Emergency Department a more effective place to deliver a large volume of acute care. Secondly, supportive services, such as radiology, laboratory, consulting services, and hospital admission, if necessary, are easily accessible, certainly more so than in most family physicians' offices. Thirdly, even when a family physician takes calls in the "off-hours," the patient may not wish to bother the physician, or may fear the problem will be considered trivial. Immediate 24-hour availability can be offered in the Emergency Department, with no questions asked regarding the appropriateness of the visit. Fourthly, with virtually 100 percent of Canadians covered by health insurance, there is no financial deterrent to this rather expensive form of health care. Finally, some family physicians encourage the use of the hospital Emergency Department for urgent care of their patients' problems, not only during off-hours, but during the day, when close scheduling of patients may make it difficult to also deal with "unscheduled" problems.

Many family physicians, however, do offer care to their patients in "off-hours" and would prefer to look after all aspects of their patients' care, including urgent problems.[8] This study demonstrates that family physician availability does have an effect on the use patients make of local hospital Emergency Departments.

Acknowledgments

Much of the data analysis and preparation of this manuscript was undertaken while the author was Visiting Associate Professor with the Department of Family Medicine, University of Washington, Seattle, Washington. He wishes to acknowledge the support and encouragement of Dr. Theodore Phillips and Dr. John Geyman of that department. He wishes also to thank Dr. James Logerfo and Dr. William Richardson of the School of Public Health and Community Medicine, University of Washington, for their helpful comments and criticism during the preparation of this manuscript. This report is based on data collected as part of a project funded by the Ontario Ministry of Health, DM-199, and a project funded by Sunnybrook Hospital 71-27.

REFERENCES

1. Hilditch JR, Demanuele F, Neumann B: Flemingdon Park Health Survey, Phase One. Toronto, Ontario, Sunnybrook Hospital, 1973
2. Statistics Canada: Consumer Income and Expenditure Division: Income Distribution by Size in Canada. Ottawa, Information Canada, 1976
3. Spaulding WB, Spitzer WO: Implications of medical manpower trends in Ontario 1961–1971. Ontario Med Rev 39:527, 1972
4. Moore GT, Bernstein R, Bonanno R: Effect of a neighborhood health center on hospital emergency use. Med Care 10(3):240, 1972
5. Hochheiser LI, Woodward K, Charney E: Effect of the neighborhood health center on the use of pediatric emergency departments in Rochester, New York. N Engl J Med 285:148, 1971
6. Chaiton A: Trends in emergency department utilization. Can Fam Physician 21(1):115, 1975
7. Torrens PR, Yedvab DG: Variations among emergency room populations: A comparison of four hospitals in New York City. Med Care 8(1):60, 1970
8. Bass M: A profile of family practice in London, Ontario. Can Fam Physician 21(9):113, 1975

Attitudes and Patterns of Practice: A Comparison of Graduates of a Residency Program in Family Medicine and Controls*

Michael Brennan, Moira Stewart

Two groups of graduates of the University of Western Ontario Faculty of Medicine were compared. The study group had satisfactorily completed a two-year residency program in family medicine at the University, commencing at graduation from medical school; the controls had completed a one-year internship after graduation, but had not pursued specific residency training in family medicine. Both groups were engaged in family practice in Ontario at the time of the study. As predicted, the groups differed in their attitudes; the graduates were more satisfied with practice than the controls and placed more importance on emotional factors in illness. Anticipated differences in patterns of care provided were also found. Family medicine graduates conducted proportionately more noninstitutional care. The findings were not generalized beyond the one program. The advantages and limitations of program evaluation through studies of graduates are discussed.

Most evaluations of residents in family medicine programs have used data collected while the resident was actually in the program.[1-3] "Before" and "after" comparisons have been made frequently. The present study attempted to extend information about the impact of programs on residents in family medicine. Its goal was to compare the graduates of one program, the Department of Family Medicine, University of Western Ontario (UWO), London, Ontario, with a group of controls who had not taken specific residency training in family medicine. All physicians in the study had graduated from the UWO Faculty of Medicine and taken their graduate training in London, Ontario.

The Program, the Hypotheses and Assumptions

The residency in family medicine from which the study group was drawn is a two-year program commencing at graduation

* Reprinted by permission from *The Journal of Family Practice*, 7(4):741–748, 1978.

from medical school and has the following characteristics designed to influence the behavior of its graduates: (1) the three medical centers in which the residents were trained are geographically removed from hospitals by distances of three fourths to 15 miles; (2) the duration of block training in the centers is 12 months for almost all the program graduates; and (3) the teaching faculty are entirely practice-experienced family physicians.

The curriculum has been designed to provide a total, intensive learning experience which is heavily oriented toward comprehensive, continuous, community and preventive health care. The program's duration, content, and structure have been changed over the past ten years. However, given the overall objectives of the program, it seemed reasonable to expect measurable differences in attitudes and behavior between the graduates and the more traditionally trained physicians. Indeed, a previous study by Brock supports this expectation.[4] She found three differences between family medicine residents and other general physicians in their patterns of referral: (1) the family medicine trained physicians referred less frequently to medical specialists; (2) they referred more frequently to nonmedical community resource people; and (3) they more often sent a letter to the consultant when making the referral.

Underlying the predictions concerning attitudes and patterns of practice, which are stated under Results, were value assumptions which corresponded, as closely as possible, to the goals of the UWO program. For example, we predicted that the graduates would have a stronger belief in the importance of emotional factors in specific illnesses, reflecting the philosophy expressed in the departmental publication.[5] Although some judgments underlying the predictions may not be widely accepted, most are generally acceptable. In any case, the results of the present study will not be generalized beyond the UWO program.

Methods

Selection of Participants

The goal of the study was to compare family medicine graduates with controls who had similar undergraduate education and hospital rotations. Therefore, the study group was restricted to those graduates of UWO medical school who had also taken their residency training in family medicine in London. Further, the control group included only those graduates of UWO medical school who remained in London for their internship year. The procedure for selection is shown in Figure 1. The study and control groups consisted of all physicians who met the criteria.

The undergraduate performances of all physicians in the study were examined and no important differences were found be-

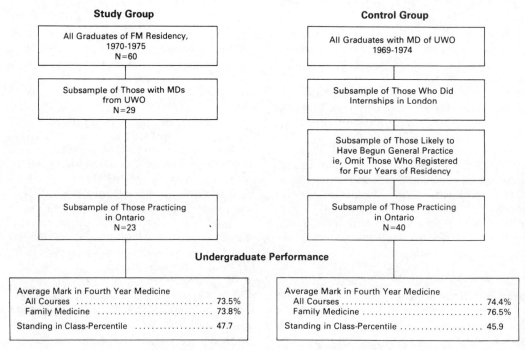

Fig. 1. Criteria for selection. Both groups beginning practice 1970–1975 inclusive. (For undergraduate performance, there was no statistically significant difference between the groups; $t < 1.4$ on 60 df, $P > .05$.)

tween the two groups in their marks for all four years of medical school education. Figure 1 shows the average fourth-year marks to illustrate this finding.

Sources of Data

Questionnaire

A 33-item questionnaire was developed for the study. Questions dealing with physician satisfaction were based on the work of Becker, Drachman, and Kirscht[6] and focused on physician satisfaction with patient relationships and with the quality of care. The items concerning the physicians' attitudes toward the importance of emotional factors were derived from recent work of one of the authors (Stewart MA: Development of a questionnaire to assess attitudes of family physicians, unpublished). The remaining items, regarding background information, staff, medical records, and workload were devised for this study. The whole questionnaire was pretested for clarity on five residents.

Ontario Health Insurance Plan Data

Data on billings for certain kinds of services were made available through the Ontario Ministry of Health, Data Development and Evaluation Branch, Information Systems Division, for a three-month period from September to November 1975 and were identified by groups of physicians rather than by individuals to maintain confidentiality.

Results

The Participants

Of the 63 (23 + 40) questionnaires mailed, 21 (91.3 percent) and 35 (87.5 percent), or the family medicine and control

groups respectively, were completed and returned after two follow-up letters. The respondents had been in practice from a minimum of one year to a maximum of six years.

The control group, chosen because its members' training differed from that of the family medicine graduates, showed some internal variation in training. Of the 35 controls who completed the questionnaire, 27 began general practice immediately after internship; the other eight had from 4 to 12 months additional hospital training, mostly in anesthesia and internal medicine.

It should be noted that the study and control groups did not contain equal proportions of physicians newly in practice. In fact, 42.1 percent of the graduates began practice in the summer of 1975 compared to 15.7 percent of the controls. These physicians would therefore have been in practice at the longest for three months before the Ontario Health Insurance Plan billings. Because the length of time in practice might reasonably be expected to affect other variables, the study and control groups were compared within these four subgroups: practice begun in (a) 1975, (b) 1973–1974, (c) 1972, and (d) 1970–1971. Unless otherwise stated, the differences found between the study and control groups as a whole were maintained when subgroups who had been in practice similar lengths of time were compared.

Professional Satisfaction

It was predicted that the family medicine graduates would express a greater degree of professional satisfaction than the controls. Of the ten items regarding satisfaction, three showed a 30 percent difference between the groups, differences which attained at least a 0.10 level of statistical significance. The family medicine graduates presented more positive attitudes than the controls (Table 1).

Table 1. *Physician Satisfaction: Percentage of Physicians Who Agreed with the Statement*

Statement	Family Medicine Graduates (N = 21)	Control Group (N = 35)
I find my work satisfying	90.4	95.3
My medical practice corresponds to my expectations prior to beginning practice*	90.5	60.0
My practice provides an opportunity for me to perform at my optimal level*	76.1	45.7
I think the time I have to spend with each patient is too limited†	19.0	54.3
Relationships with patients are usually satisfying	100.0	97.1
Most of my patients are "good patients"	89.5	87.8
I find I can practice good quality patient care.	90.5	82.4
Additional relevant questions:		
Closed practice (answer = yes)	33.3	14.7
Enough time for recreation (answer = yes)	71.4	74.3
Time spent on continuing medical education (answer = >7 days per year)	38.9	38.2

* Stratified $\chi^2 > 2.7$ on 1 df, $P < .10$.
† Stratified $\chi^2 > 5.4$ on 1 df, $P < .02$.

Medical Records

As anticipated, the family medicine graduates used Problem-Oriented Medical Records more than the controls (Table 2). They also implemented a data retrieval system more frequently. Approximately the same percentage of both groups used family folders.

Access to Allied Health Care Professionals

Program graduates were predicted to have greater access to allied health care professionals than controls. The findings revealed slightly more access to registered nurses in the study group and approximately the same frequency of access to social workers. The most striking difference concerned the public health nurse attachment which was more common for the family medicine graduates than the control group (71.4 and 48.3 percent, respectively).

Association with College of Family Physicians in Canada

The program graduates, as predicted, were more likely than controls to be associated with the College of Family Physicians. Of the family medicine graduates, all were active members and 81.0 percent were certified members. Of the controls, 29.2 percent were active members and only 2.4 percent were certified.

Table 2. *Medical Record Keeping: Percentage of Physicians Who Used the Following Systems*

Systems	Family Medicine Graduates (N = 21)	Control Group (N = 35)
Problem-oriented medical record*	76.2	44.1
Family folders	66.7	60.0
A method of data retrieval	23.8	3.0

* Stratified $\chi^2 = 2.5$ on 1 df, $P \approx .10$.

Teaching Involvement

Questionnaire responses indicated that the program graduates were engaged in part-time teaching approximately twice as often as controls (38.1 compared to 17.6 percent).

Choice of Group or Solo Practice

The prediction that program graduates would more likely choose some form of group practice was based on the fact that the family medicine teaching centers are all group practices. This prediction was not supported and the data indicate that slightly more than 50 percent of both family medicine graduates and controls were in group practice as opposed to solo practice.

Choice of Practice Site by Size of Population

The prediction that study and control groups would not differ greatly in terms of the population of their practice sites was not supported by the data. In fact, the family medicine graduates were more likely to practice in areas of fewer than 50,000 people, whereas the controls were

more likely to live in cities of 50,000 or more (Table 3).

Patient Contact

As predicted, almost one half of the controls said they saw 40 or more patients per day compared to one in five family medicine graduates. The residency graduates spent more time with their patients (Table 4).

Kinds of Services Provided in a Three-Month Period

The average number of services, as determined from Ontario Health Insurance Plan (OHIP) billing data, was 166.61 for family medicine graduates and 176.61 for the control group per week.

The OHIP data were used to test certain hypotheses of interest concerning the style of practice of the family medicine graduates and controls.* The first of these stated that family medicine graduates, whose training stressed noninstitutional patient care, would carry out proportionately fewer services in active-treatment hospitals and more services in offices or outpatient settings than controls. The differences, al-

Table 3. *Percentage of Physicians by Population of Practice Sites*

Population	Family Medicine Graduates (N = 21)	Control Group (N = 35)
0– 1,499	19.0	2.9
1,500– 2,999	4.8	2.9
3,000– 9,999	23.8	17.1
10,000– 49,999	19.0	11.4
50,000– 99,999	14.3	20.0
100,000–499,999	19.0	42.9
500,000+	0.0	2.9
Total	100.0%	100.0%

* Tests of the statistical significance of differences in the proportions shown in Tables 5 to 8 were conducted in two ways: (1) χ^2 on contingency tables with N's of 41,152 and 87,195. All results were significant (P < .001), indicating that the differences revealed in the OHIP billings were true differences and not due to chance in sampling that particular three-month period; and (2) analysis of covariance was done with the physician as the unit of analysis, and the dependent variable being the proportion in question; the independent variable, the group (family medicine or control); the covariate, the number of years in practice; and the total degrees of freedom, the number of participants (57 minus 1). None of the analyses of covariance revealed statistically significant differences: any differences noted between the groups are merely suggestive, requiring further study with larger groups of physicians.

Table 4. *Percentage of Physicians by Number of Patient Contacts*

Patient Contacts	Family Medicine Graduates (N = 21)	Control Group (N = 34)
Patients per day		
Under 40 patients	76.2	60.0
40 or more patients	23.8	40.0
Total	100.0%	100.0%
Length of time spent with each patient*		
0–10 Minutes	23.8	52.9
11–15	61.9	44.1
16–30	14.3	2.9
Total	100.0%	100.0%

* Stratified $\chi^2 > 2.7$ on 1 *df*, $P < .10$.
(The variable was dichotomized: 0 to 10 minutes, >10 minutes).

though not statistically significant, support the hypothesis and, it can be argued, have implications for the cost of care (Table 5). The difference in the proportion of hospital services cannot be explained by different proportions of surgical services, which were 8.26 percent and 8.40 percent for the family medicine and control groups, respectively. The second prediction stated that family medicine graduates, whose training focused on community-oriented medicine, could be expected to visit patients at home more frequently than controls. The figures in the third row of Table 5 show a small difference in the direction predicted.

Preventive Care

It was predicted that family medicine graduates, whose discipline stresses continuous and preventive care, would generate a higher frequency of preventive billings than controls. The first row of Table 6 shows that the differences were negligible. Also relevant to preventive care, the family medicine graduates were expected to carry out more well-baby visits per newborn than the controls. The second row of Table 6 shows virtually no difference between the two groups.

Attitudes Toward and Management of Emotional Factors

Of the six questionnaire items dealing with emotional factors, four showed a 20 percent difference between the two groups, one of these was statistically significant and another was close to significance (Table 7). These differences were as predicted. Table 8 shows that family medicine graduates, whose program had stressed the recognition and management of psychological problems, conduct proportionately more psychotherapy than do the physicians in the control group.

Table 5. *Hospital, Office, and Home Services Provided in a Three-Month Period (OHIP data)*

Place Service Provided	Family Medicine Graduates (N = 19)	Control Group (N = 38)	Ratio FM/C
Hospital	17.8	25.9	0.69
Office–out-patient	79.7	71.4	1.12
Home	1.9	1.4	1.36
Other*	0.6	1.3	0.46
Total	100.0%	100.0%	
Total number of services	41,152	87,195	

* Included such services as x-ray, pulmonary function, care in a nursing home.

Table 6. *Preventive Care Provided in a Three-Month Period (OHIP data)*

	Family Medicine Graduates (N = 19)	Control Group (N = 38)	Ratio FM/C
Percentage of all billed preventive services*	7.4% (41,152)	7.9% (87,195)	0.94
Number of well-baby care billings per newborn care billings†	7.8 (101)	7.7 (280)	1.01

* OHIP billing codes: General Assessment (A003), General Reassessment (A004), Well-Baby Care (A002), Well-Child Care (K014), Primary School Examination (K015), Secondary School Examination (K016), Annual Health Examination (K009).
† OHIP billing codes: Well-Baby Care (A002)/Newborn-Baby Care (H001).

Continuity and Comprehensiveness of Care

The family medicine graduates whose training stressed total and continuous care were predicted to have a higher proportion of newborns for whom care was also given to the mother. The Ontario Health Insurance Plan data allowed calculation of the following indicator of continuity:

$$\frac{\text{Number of billed services for total care, delivery, or attendance at labor and delivery*}}{\text{Number of newborn care billed services}} \times 100 \text{ percent}$$

The indicator was 96.0 percent of 101 for family medicine graduates and 83.9 percent of 280 for controls. Although these data seem to support the hypothesis, the authors recommend that better indicators of continuity be tested before any firm conclusions are drawn.

Discussion

The study has shown that the attitudes of family medicine graduates of UWO were

* "Attendance at labor and delivery" is an OHIP billing category that covers situations where the patient has been transferred to the care of a specialist for the delivery but the family physician is present.

different, on the whole, from those held by the control group. Specifically, the graduates were more likely to respond positively to questions relating to greater professional satisfaction, and to stress the importance of emotional factors in illness. The differences in patterns of practice between the two groups, in spite of being small in absolute terms, supported all the hypotheses except the one regarding billed preventive services.

Despite the consistency of the findings, the authors recommend caution in their interpretation. First, one must recognize that the observed differences cannot be interpreted as solely the effect of the family medicine program. Rather, the findings may represent the combined effect of: (1) selection into the program, whether self-selection on the part of the medical student or faculty selection; (2) unmatched characteristics of the physicians and practices making up the two comparison groups; and (3) the family medicine program itself.

To assess part of the influence of faculty selection in creating differences in the two groups, the undergraduate marks were compared. No statistically significant differences could be found (Figure 1). Self-selection, of course, must be recognized as important even though no direct measurement of it could be made. In a more definitive study, data on attitudes measured during medical school could be included, in order to assess the role of self-selection.

Table 7. *Percentages of Physicians Who Found Psychological Problems Important in Most Cases (questionnaire response)*

	Family Medicine Graduates (N = 21)	Control Group (N = 35)
Asthma*	66.7†	40.0
Peptic ulcer	95.2	97.1
Vomiting of pregnancy‡	65.0	40.0
Essential hypertension	57.2	48.6
Rheumatoid arthritis	40.0	22.9
Patient-visits in general	66.7§	45.7

* Stratified $\chi^2 = 2.5$ on 1 df, $P \approx .10$.
† Represents three categories combined 'all, most, many cases' as opposed to 'some, few, no cases.'
‡ Stratified $\chi^2 > 2.7$ on 1 df, $P < .10$.
§ Represents 50 percent or more patient visits.

To eliminate potential bias due to unmatched characteristics of physicians in the comparison groups, questionnaire data were reanalyzed on a set of 13 pairs matched for the year of entering practice and the population of practice site. Essentially the same differences as those reported earlier were found. Unfortunately, because the OHIP data was group data, they could not be analyzed in pairs. Although it would be desirable for future studies to attempt to match graduates and controls as closely as possible, there was no evidence in the present study that unmatched characteristics created exaggerated differences between the groups.

A second limitation of the study was that it did not directly measure two very important variables, quality and cost of care. The indirect measurements used can be said to have implications for quality and cost, but one is reticent to draw even tentative conclusions until more direct assessments can be made. The authors recognize the importance of such variables as use of laboratories, investigative procedures, x-rays, and prescribing habits, and although they were unable to gather valid data for the present study, they are currently engaged in a search for methods to examine more directly the questions of quality and cost of health care services.

The limitations described above were somewhat offset by the advantage of assessing a program through data from its graduates. As Corley said, "the validation of an education program lies in the professional practices of its graduates."[7] Now that the number of graduates from any one program is approaching an adequate sample size and because, through projects such as the one reported here, the problems of assessing graduates are being recognized and overcome, such studies might well evolve as an integral component of family medicine program evaluation.

Table 8. *Billed Services for Psychotherapy (OHIP data)*

	Family Medicine Graduates (N = 19)	Control Group (N = 38)	Ratio FM/C
Percentage of all billed services which were for psychotherapy	5.15 (41,152)	2.66 (87,195)	1.92

Acknowledgments

The authors wish to thank the family medicine graduates and controls for their participation in this research. The authors acknowledge with gratitude the encouragement of Dr. Ian R. McWhinney, Chairman of the Department of Family Medicine, University of Western Ontario and his department for its financial support. They wish to thank Dr. Leifur Dungal for his helpful suggestions during the development of the project and Maureen Beamish, Helen Simpson, and Donna Greer for their research assistance. Drs. Carol Buck and Martin Bass provided valuable comments on the manuscript.

The authors gratefully acknowledge the assistance of Mr. Ron Quan, Assistant Head, Allocation, Data Development and Evaluation Branch, Information Systems Division, Ontario Ministry of Health, in obtaining the OHIP data.

Dr. Moira Stewart is supported by a National Health Research Scholarship from Health and Welfare Canada.

REFERENCES

1. Kane RL, Leigh EH, Feigal DW, et al: A method for evaluating patient care and auditing skills of family practice residents. J Fam Pract 2:205, 1975
2. Snope FC, Sadler GR, Currie BF: Quality assurance in community-based education for family practice in New Jersey. J Fam Pract 3:333, 1976
3. Molineux J, Hennen BK, McWhinney IR: In-training performance assessment in family practice. J Fam Pract 3:405, 1976
4. Brock C: Consultation and referral patterns of family physicians. J Fam Pract 4:1129, 1977
5. Department of Family Medicine: A Handbook. London, Ontario, The University of Western Ontario, 1975
6. Becker MH, Drachman RH, Kirscht JP: A field experiment to evaluate various outcomes of continuity of physician care. Am J Public Health 64:1062, 1974
7. Corley JB: In-training residency evaluation. J Fam Pract 3:499, 1976

Changes in Patient Perceptions toward a Family Practice: A Case Study*

Paula L. Stamps

This paper presents the results of an evaluation of a family practice that focuses on changes in patient perceptions over five years. The evaluation includes an analysis of patient attitudes as well as behavior. Patient attitudes are measured by means of a personal interview and behavior is analyzed by creation of a Family Utilization Index. Significant changes are noted in the areas of both reported and actual utilization, with fewer changes in the areas relating to patients' perceptions of health and illness or in attitudes toward either the model of family practice or the specific site of obtaining care. This is not a definitive model for evaluation of family practice, but it is one of the few empirical studies available and suggests the need for more documentation of the effectiveness of family practice as a model for delivering primary care services.

Since the establishment of the American Board of Family Practice in 1969, the growth of family practice programs has been impressive. By the end of 1969 there were 30 accredited residency programs in family practice and by 1974, 206 residency programs were approved, with more than half of all medical schools having a Department of Family Medicine.[1-3]

Most of the literature that surrounds this rapidly growing field is philosophical and definitional, rather than empirical. This includes defining the various roles of a family physician and the type of training needed, as well as describing the differences between family practice and other generalist-oriented models of delivering primary care.[1-9]

The major concept underlying the model of family practice is that of one provider with a generalist orientation who will provide a patient with comprehensive, continuous health services in a family setting and who will maintain responsibility for the patient's total health needs throughout all interactions with the entire health care delivery system.[5,10,11]

To date, there has been no empirical analysis of either the implementation of these functions or the response of patients, analysis that is requisite to an evaluation of the impact of family practice as one method by which primary medical care can be delivered. The following three criteria are suggested as tools in such an analysis:

Criterion I: Perceptions of Health and Utilization of a Family Physician

The perception of health and illness is a central value in determining patient utilization of any provider. The patient's perception of health, if closely allied to the view set up by the family practice model, would encompass a concrete view of health, larger than merely organic complaints and including personal and occupational stresses. Health concerns should involve all aspects of a family's life as a social unit and as a part of the larger social organization, the community. Use of a family physician should include all members of the family for both routine preventive care and care for acute and chronic conditions.

* Reprinted by permission from the *Journal of Community Health*, 4(3):232–241, 1979. Copyright 1979 by Human Sciences Press, New York, NY.

Criterion II: Patient's Perceptions of the Role of the Family Physician

The family physician should be viewed as providing entry into the health care system—a point of first contact. In this role, he/she should be perceived as the physician to whom the entire family goes and who serves as the central source of health information as well as health care.

Criterion III: Utilization of Other Health Resources

If the patient complies with the model of family practice, he/she will consult the family physician on all issues of health care, including referrals. The patient should maintain a continuing relationship with the primary physician as he/she is involved with any other health resources. The information and communication system should be centered around the family physician.

All of these criteria focus on the expected patient response to the model of family practice in order to allow measurement of the impact of family practice on the patients. The underlying assumption is that consumers must be receptive to the values and goals of family practice before the model can provide them with appropriate care. This paper presents one empirical case study of an evaluation of the family practice model based on the measurement of these three criteria.

Methods

Even though the major concepts of family practice—continuity, comprehensiveness, and family-oriented care by one provider—may be carried out in another setting, it is imperative to measure the achievement of these objectives in a family practice setting. Therefore, this study involves a family practice residency program that is associated with a medical school having full-time physicians, teaching faculty members, and residents.

Data were collected on two samples of patients seeking care at the Family Medicine Clinic: The first group consisted of 150 patients interviewed in May 1970 and the second group comprised 135 patients on whom data were collected in June 1975. In neither case was it a true probability sample. The respondents are those who kept their appointments, not the total population of people making appointments. Moreover, although the patients were selected randomly, one systematic bias was introduced: if a patient (either adult or an adult bringing a child in for care) was in acute pain he/she was eliminated from the sample. This involved only a very small number of patients with urgent and serious illnesses who had made same-day appointments. Finally, new patients were not included in either study.

The first source of data was an interview comprising 30 open-ended and structured questions verbally administered to the patient by a personal interviewer. Since the interview process was incorporated into the customary patient flow procedures there was no reticence on the part of the patients to respond to the interview. Although it was not possible for the interviewer to be present at all times the clinic was open, an interviewing schedule was set up so that all clinic hours were represented.

The second source of data was an analysis of the medical records of the family units made the same day the interview was given. These data included the total number of persons in the family unit as well as a description of those who were active patients, the length of time the family had utilized the clinic, and the total number of visits made by the family unit. The medical record was also used to corroborate responses in the interview to demographic questions (age, number of children, marital status, occupation, and education) as well as to questions on reported utilization of other health resources.

Results

The results will be presented separately for each of the three evaluation criteria. In order that the changes be presented in a proper perspective and because it was not possible to conduct a prospective study a demographic description of the two samples is included.

Demographic Variables

There are few significant demographic differences in the two samples over the five-year period. Both samples are composed of about 20% men and 80% women and both are two-thirds nonwhite, primarily Black. The age range in both samples is similar, with 60% between the ages of 15 and 29. According to Hollingshead's social class index, which provides a weighted score for education and occupation,[12] almost 60% of both samples are categorized in the lower two social class categories.

The only significant difference in demographic characteristics of the two patient samples is marital status. There are significantly greater numbers of unmarried patients in the 1975 sample (67%) compared with the 1970 sample (50%). This increase is due to more divorces rather than to increasing age or widowhood.

The implication of the demographic stability of the two patient samples is that any changes discovered in the analysis of attitudes and utilization patterns are not caused by demographic shifts in the patient samples themselves.

One other factor that might affect utilization patterns is the length of time a person had been a patient at the clinic. In both 1970 and 1975 about 35% of the families had been patients at the clinic for the full 35 months of the study period, and 15% had been patients for less than 12 months.

Criterion I

As seen in Table 1, a majority of the sample identify bad health as resulting primarily from medical problems, with about half of both groups indicating that problems at home can affect a person's health. There are differences, however, regarding the types of information a physician needs to know in order to take good care of a patient. In 1970, 70% of the sample indicated the doctor needs only medical information; in 1975, the majority recognize a need for both personal and medical information on a patient.

Table 1. *Comparison of 1970 and 1975 Responses on Selected Interview Items for Criterion I*

Interview Items for Patient Perceptions of Health/Illness	Year of Study			
	1970		1975	
	(number)	*(percent)*	*(number)*	*(percent)*
Causes of bad health				
Medical only	105	70	97	72
Medical plus others	45	30	38	28
Problems at home affect health				
Yes	67	45	70	52
No	83	55	65	48
Information needed by family physician*				
Medical only	105	70	52	39
Personal and medical	45	30	83	61
Physical examination				
Yes	78	52	82	61
No	72	48	53	39

* Statistically significant by chi square at the 0.05 level of significance.

One way to measure the relationship of perception of health and health behavior is to examine utilization of preventive health services. The gauge in this study was the number of patients having a complete physical examination. Although the percentage rose between 1970 and 1975, this increase is not statistically significant. What is important is that the increase is not spread evenly over the sample: Those who are classified into the lowest social classes have had the greatest increase in physical examinations. For example, only 21% of the lowest social class had a physical examination in 1970 and in 1975 this had risen to 45%.

It is intriguing to note that both items indicating behavioral responses (i.e., having a physical and types of information needed by a physician) demonstrate changes over the five-year period, even though responses to items about causes of bad health and value of preventive medicine have remained the same. Although these two samples do not verbally acknowledge the relationship between physical and emotional health, they seem to have changed their behavior in this direction. The analysis of actual utilization patterns in the medical record further explores this question.

A Family Utilization Index with the following components was created in order to summarize utilization patterns of an entire family unit:

1. The number of persons in the total family who are patients at the clinic compared with the total number of persons in the family.
2. A description of the individuals within the family who are active patients (i.e., mother only, mother and children, etc.)
3. Length of time the family has utilized the clinic.
4. The total number of visits made by the entire family.

Separate proportional scores were devised for each of these four components and the weighted total score is referred to as the Family Utilization Index.[13] It does not take into account the objective medical needs of a family, nor is it applicable to a one-member family. Despite these limitations, however, it does provide a crude way of quantifying a behavior pattern that is central to the value structure of the family practice model.

Table 2 shows that there have been remarkable and significant utilization changes as measured by the Family Utilization Index. The shifts of scores are due primarily to the increased total number of

Table 2. *Distribution of 1970 and 1975 Respondents by Category of the Family Utilization Index*

Utilization Index Category*	1970 Study		1975 Study	
	(number)	*(percent)*	*(number)*	*(percent)*
A.	33	22	36	27
B.	13	9	20	15
C.	26	17	12	9
D.	22	14	28	21
E.	37	25	11	8
Single member family†	19	13	28	20
Totals	150	100	135	100

$\chi^2 = 22.57$; 5df; $P < 0.005$.
* Categories are highest utilization to lowest, with A being the highest utilization.
† Those who were classified as single-member households were exempt from calculations involving the Family Utilization Index. These increased between 1970 and 1975, primarily due to the increased number of unmarried patients.

visits of a family unit, which is caused by the increased proportion of family members coming to the clinic (component 1 of the Family Utilization Index). Whereas 40% of the later sample fall into the top two categories of utilization, 30% of the 1970 sample are accounted for within these two categories. Thirty-eight percent of the first sample and only 28% of the 1975 sample fall into the two lowest categories. It should be noted that these differences are understated: because the shift in scores upward was so great, the range of scores for 1975 was revised upward in order to retain the lowest category for comparison.

In five years, the patients of this Family Medicine Clinic have changed their utilization patterns to become more consistent with the criteria of the family practice model. That the changes noted in the interview responses are less than expected is probably related to the fact that these are values that change slowly and require a more sophisticated means of measurement than this interview schedule.

Criterion II

Six of the seven items on the questionnaire that measure opinions about patient definition of a family doctor show significant changes, all in a positive direction toward the model of family practice. Many more patients stated they had what they would consider a family doctor; more patients in every utilization category stated that they had a stronger and more continuing relationship with one physician (Table 3). Although this change is true for all utilization categories, it is most dramatic among those patients with lower utilization indices. In 1970, the percentage of patients identifying a family physician was 69% in categories A, B, and C and 42% in categories D and E; in 1975, 78% of those in categories A, B, and C identified a family physician, and almost 70% of those in the two lower categories identified with a family physician.

Moreover, there was a significant shift in identifying the Family Medicine Clinic itself as the source of family-oriented care. In 1970, only 54% of the patients cited the clinic as where their family doctor is or noted that the clinic is their "family place," in comparison with 74% in 1975. This shift is also most dramatic among those in the lower utilization classes. Reinforcing this is the increased ability of a patient to name the specific physician with whom he/she has an appointment: In 1970, 24% could not name their physician, but in 1975 it had dropped to 2%. This is not necessarily related to more patients seeing the same

Table 3. *Comparison of 1970 and 1975 Responses on Selected Interview Items for Criterion II*

Interview Items for Patient Perception of Role of Family Physician	Year of Study			
	1970		1975	
	(number)	*(percent)*	*(number)*	*(percent)*
Identification with a family physician*				
Yes	82	55	100	75
No	68	45	35	25
Arrange appointment with consultant				
Yes	129	86	122	90
No	21	14	13	10
Family physician contact patient*				
Yes	96	64	70	51
No	54	36	65	49

* Statistically significant by chi square at the 0.05 level of significance.

physician, since that remained at 60% in both samples. Rather, it seems to be related to a stronger identification with the clinic as a place to receive family-oriented medical care services.

The respondents were asked two questions with respect to their expectations about the function of a family physician: one related to the role of the family physician in making referrals to a consultant and the other to the family physician's taking the initiative in contacting the family about health matters. More than 80% of both samples want the family physician to make arrangements for their seeing a consultant but significantly fewer patients want their family physician to contact them about health-related matters such as immunization or appointment reminders or test results. The latter figure, which has decreased from 64% to 51%, is not related to the utilization category and indicates that most people are seeing their physicians on a more regular basis, are able to have enough contact with their physician, and therefore have access to this information.

Criterion III

Theoretically, the patients in these two samples should have no significant sources of health care other than those referred by a Family Medicine Clinic provider. In one interview item that simply asks for "other

places" of care, there are no significant differences noted over time in the percentage reporting use of other health resources (Table 4). There has been, however, a change in the type of resource utilized: In 1970 it was most likely a primary care physician, but in 1975 it was usually a free immunization clinic. In 1970 there was no relationship between the Utilization Index and reported utilization of these other resources. In 1975, however, those persons in the higher utilization categories were more likely to have no other sources of care. Those in the lower utilization categories in both samples are more likely to have other physicians.

The most significant change in utilization of other resources is in emergency care. There was a strong and significant increase in the percentage of those contacting the clinic for emergency care in 1975 over 1970. This increase is directly related to a higher Family Utilization Index. Once again, the greatest change has been in the two lowest utilization categories: in 1970, 38% of these two groups (D and E) noted that they would call the clinic in an emergency and in 1975 this had increased to 58%. This trend was strongly encouraged and supported by the clinic physicians.

Discussion

The most striking changes that have been documented in this study are those related

Table 4. *Comparison of 1970 and 1975 Responses on Selected Interview Items for Criterion III*

Interview Items for Use of Other Health Resources	Year of Study			
	1970		1975	
	(number)	(percent)	(number)	(percent)
All other sources of care				
None	113	75	107	79
Other	37	25	28	21
Source of emergency care*				
Consult clinic	69	46	87	64
Other source	81	54	48	36

* Statistically significant by chi square at the 0.05 level of significance.

to actual utilization patterns, as quantified by the Family Utilization Index. Those items measuring general concepts or definitions of health and illness and those dealing with the theoretical model of family practice show the least change, while those items relating to specific situations involving the clinic or behavior-worded items show the greatest change.

The patients interviewed in 1975 have evidenced fairly dramatic changes in the utilization of the Family Medicine Clinic, in many of their attitudes toward family practice, and especially in their opinions toward the clinic itself. In many cases, those most responsible for the significant changes are those in the lower utilization categories, although the changes are prevalent throughout the entire 1975 sample. It may be said that at the end of this five-year period the patients have significantly changed their utilization patterns and their attitudes so that they are much closer to the model of family practice than were the 1970 patients interviewed.

It is difficult, however, to place these changes in a proper perspective for two basic reasons. Methodology is the first limitation, i.e., interviewing two separate samples of patients instead of conducting a five-year follow-up of the same group of patients. Since this is not a prospective study, it is possible that the 1975 sample is composed of those patients who may be termed "survivors," those who were more predisposed to the clinic. Although the second group interviewed have not been patients for a longer period of time than the first group, there may be other factors biasing the results. It is therefore imperative to state that no causality is implied in this study; without conducting a prospective study it is impossible to state that the clinic is responsible for the changes noted in the 1975 sample. Furthermore, although the demographic changes in the patient population are minimal, the results cannot be generalized to the community. It is more appropriately viewed as a case study of one family medicine clinic.

The second limitation is the Family Utilization Index itself. There are several scoring and computation-related decisions that are arbitrary. Although a dramatic change is obvious, in some cases there is no relationship between being classified in a high utilization category and a specific behavior or attitude obtained from the interview. Those in the higher utilization categories, for example, are no more likely to have a closer identification with a family physician, nor are they more likely to feel the need to relay personal and biographical information to their physician. In both of these cases, the entire sample demonstrates significant changes that are unrelated to the Family Utilization Index itself. However, in many cases, especially those items measuring utilization of other resources, the Family Utilization Index is significantly related to the variables in the expected direction. Those patients classified in the higher utilization categories are, for example, more likely to contact the clinic in an emergency and are less likely to have other sources of primary care.

The Family Utilization Index is an attempt to document the relationship of behavior (i.e., utilization) and attitudes toward family practice as a model with one specific family practice as a provider site. Although it has been treated here as an independent variable, realistically the relationship between utilization and attitudes is much more complex and multidimensional. Utilization patterns no doubt cause changes in attitudes but are also certainly influenced by the attitudes of the person as he/she interacts with a provider in a specific environment. This method of analyzing utilization patterns in a family context is suggested as one means of documenting changes in behavior when it may not be possible to detect the more subtle shifts in values and attitudes that may be represented in an interview. Moreover, creating an index provides criteria against which to evaluate provision of ambulatory care services.

Any such model, however, is only valid if

those responsible for its implementation actually carry out the suggested behaviors. No effort, other than observational and anecdotal, was made to document whether the providers (residents and full-time family physicians) were encouraging patients to alter their behavior and attitudes to be more congruent with the model of family practice. Insofar as this is a residency program it is probably valid to use the described model as the behavior of the providers. Therefore, the use of the Family Utilization Index is one place to start in the effort to examine empirically the implementation of the model of family practice. While this study can provide no definitive results, it does expand the possibilities for evaluation strategies.

The Family Utilization Index itself is not suggested as a final evaluation technique; rather, it is intended to open up ways of analyzing family practices. More research is required, not only on the Family Utilization Index but also on family practice as a method of delivering primary care. The index itself should be validated in other family practice sites, with special attention paid to the weighting of the components and the computation of the index. The actual behavior of the providers should be compared with the model of family practice in order to validate the criteria used in the Family Utilization Index. More importantly, a prospective study is crucial in being able to reach stronger conclusions about the impact of family practice on a family's utilization patterns. This would make comparative studies with other methods of primary care possible and thereby facilitate more accurate assessment of the impact of the family practice model on our health care delivery system.

REFERENCES

1. Pellegrino ED: Expectations for family medicine. J Med Educ 74:356–367, 1972
2. Petersdorf RG: Internal medicine and family practice. N Engl J Med 293:326–332, 1973
3. Stein MF, Maniscalo AE: General internists and family practitioner. Ann Intern Med 81:713–714, 1974
4. Janeway C: Family medicine—fad or for real? N Engl J Med 291:337–343, 1974
5. McWhinney IR: Family medicine in perspective. N Engl J Med 293:176–181, 1975
6. Ransom DC, Vandervoort HE: The development of family medicine. JAMA 225:1098–1102, 1973
7. McFarlane AH, Norman GR, Spitzer WO: Family medicine: The dilemma of defining the discipline. Can Med Assoc J 105:397–398, 1971
8. Reynolds RE: Primary care, ambulatory care, and family medicine: Overlapping but not synonymous. J Med Educ 50:893–895, 1975
9. Menke W: Divided labor: The doctor as specialist. Ann Intern Med 72:940–943, 1970
10. Willard W: Meeting of Challenge of Family Practice: Report of the Ad Hoc Committee on Education for Family Practice of the Council on Medical Education. Chicago, American Medical Association, 1966
11. McWhinney LR: Continuity of care in family practice: Part 2—implications of continuity. J Fam Pract 2:373–374, 1975
12. Hollingshead A, Redlich A: Social Class and Mental Illness. New York, John Wiley and Sons, 1958
13. Stamps PL: Toward evaluation of family practice: Development of a family utilization index. J Fam Pract 7:767–779, 1978

ABSTRACTS

Marsland DW, Wood M, Mayo F: A data bank for patient care, curriculum, and research in family practice: 526,196 patient problems. J Fam Pract 3(1):3–6, 1976

The health care problems that 88,000 patients presented to 118 family physicians over two years were evaluated. From July 1, 1973 to August 1, 1975, 82 family practice residents and 36 practicing family physicians recorded all patient problems evaluated during each 24-hour period onto a daily work sheet. The daily work sheet was basically an appointment list turned into a data input sheet for keypunching, the information then being stored and correlated in a computer. The secretary in the practice would record the patient's name, date of birth, and sex on the work sheet. After evaluating the patient, the physician would record the problem or problems that were addressed. The secretary would then code the problems recorded on the daily work sheet using the USA Modification of the Coded Classification of Disease of the British Royal College of General Practitioners.

Recorded during this 25-month interval 526,196 primary health care problems for all age groups were combined, from one week of age on. The problems were arranged into 22 major diagnostic categories. Teaching and nonteaching practices were compared. The profiles were remarkably similar. The suburban, urban, and rural practices were compared. These profiles were also remarkably similar, except for a greater frequency of trauma and problems of the respiratory system in rural practices.

The data bank is arranged into two formats. The first is diagnoses ranked by frequency to the 99th percentile. The second part is diagnoses ranked by frequency in each of the 22 major disease categories. Within each major disease category the data are further subdivided into the age groups of 1 week (0) to 4, 5 to 9, 10 to 14, 15 to 24, 25 to 34, 35 to 44, 45 to 54, 55 to 64, and 65+ years. The age groups are further divided into male and female. The 50th percentile of all 526,196 problems was contained in 23 descriptive diagnoses; the 70th percentile was contained in 63 descriptive diagnoses; the 80th percentile was contained in 102 descriptive diagnoses; and the 95th percentile was contained in 234 descriptive diagnoses.

A 4 percent recording error was noted between the patient's record problem list, the daily work sheet, and information stored in the computer.

A major criticism of any descriptive study is that the description only reflects the individual experience of the recorder. It is also accepted that any system such as this can be criticized as being too restrictive in scope, as being concerned only with that which is recognized and understood and not with the ill-defined and unknown areas of the natural history of patient disease as it exists in community practice. This is the most exciting and potentially productive area of future investigation in family medicine, and the work-sheet methodology used in this study was developed for the express purpose of such investigation.

This methodology for indexing the problem-oriented record allows the physician to know the patients by diagnosis within his practice. This individual practice information could serve as a focal point for longitudinal audit, board recertification, and continuing education within the discipline of family practice. The larger comprehensive profile of family practice contained within the data bank could serve as a reference point for future prospective studies that would lead to the development of curriculum and patient care systems and new understanding of the natural presentation of disease in the community.

Knopke HJ, McDonald E, Sivertson SE: A study of family practice in Wisconsin. J Fam Pract 8(1):151–156, 1979

Selected Wisconsin family physicians have studied their practices with the help of the Department of Continuing Medical Education of the University of Wisconsin Medical School. Detailed descriptions of family practice were obtained by studying 100 Wisconsin family practices over a three-year period through Individual Physician Profile (IPP). IPP is aimed at helping family physicians identify their individual educational needs. In the first step, data are collected from the physician about every patient contact (a contact is defined as any interaction between physician and patient requiring the physician's medical judgment) for one different day a week for four weeks. A pocket-size tape recorder is lent to the physician for this purpose. The patient problems indicated by the physician are coded into the Eighth Revision International Classification of Diseases, Adapted (ICDA) and these data are then computerized. The computer generates a practice profile.

The physicians participating in this study were described as using five practice types: 22 were in solo practices, 35 were in single specialty practices with five or fewer physicians, and 8 were in single specialty practices with more than five physicians. The remaining 35 physicians practiced in multispecialty groups, 13 of these in groups with five or fewer physicians, 22 in groups with more than five physicians.

The 100 self-enrolled physicians were located in towns ranging in population from less than 2,500 to over 50,000. During the sampling period, these 100 family physicians had 17,416 patient contacts (average 43.5 per day), and reported a total of 28,803 diagnoses, averaging 1.7 diagnoses per patient contact.

The distribution by type or location of patient contacts included 61.7 percent in physician offices, 20 percent in hospitals, and 14.9 percent by telephone. The remaining 3.3 percent were divided among hospital Emergency Rooms (1.5 percent), nursing homes (0.3 percent), and house calls (0.8 percent).

The relationship of diagnosis to patient age is further demonstrated by comparing the ten specific diagnoses occurring most frequently for each age group (Figure 1). For all six age groups, the ten most frequently occurring specific problems accounted for a large portion of all diagnoses recorded for that age group. The range was from 28 percent of all diagnoses in the 35- to 49-year age group to 47 percent of all problems in the 0- to 14-year age group.

When compared to other published studies with data on epidemiology of patient problems, regional differences can be anticipated, not only between major categories but also between more specific patient problems within a single category. For example, the combined incidence of hyperthyroidism and hypothyroidism was 0.71 per 1000 patient contacts in the Wisconsin study and 1.78 for 1000 patient contacts in Virginia, i.e., more than two times greater than the incidence in Wisconsin. Such data prompt the questions:

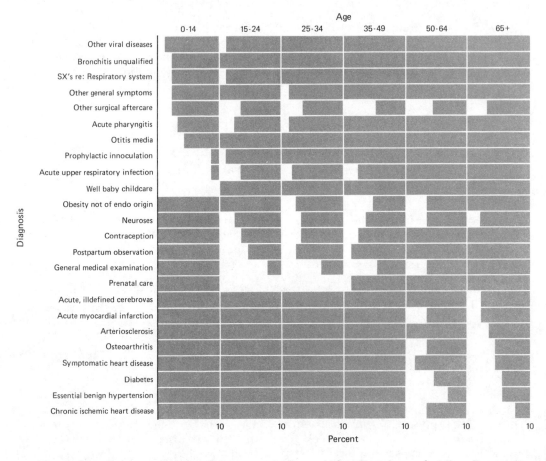

Fig. 1. Most frequent diagnoses by percent and age. (After Knopke et al: J Fam Pract, 8(1):151, 1979.)

Are thyroid metabolic disturbances more common in Virginia than in Wisconsin? If so, why? Or, are the differences due to the varying language used by physicians and the coding systems employed between the two studies? More detailed studies of practice profiles between states and regions might provide answers to these types of questions.

D'Elia G, Folse R, Robertson R: Family practice in nonmetropolitan Illinois. J Fam Pract 8(4):799–805, 1979

A description of the activities of a sample of family physicians in southern Illinois resulted from a field study of nonmetropolitan medical manpower and practice conducted by the Southern Illinois University School of Medicine. Descriptions of the medical practices of 19 family physicians in a nonmetropolitan area are based on a sample of one third of the family physicians in a 16-county area. Data were obtained from office patient records, hospital operating room logbooks, an interview with the physician, a questionnaire completed by the physician, and a questionnaire completed by the office nurse-receptionist.

Family physicians spent an average of 33 hours per week in office practice, and 25 hours per week in hospital practice, including patient rounds, Emergency Room, and operating room activities. They managed an average of 123 office patients per week. The family physicians reported seeing an average of 11 patients per day (range of 4 to 17 patients) as they made hospital rounds.

Each patient record sampled was categorized in terms of the reason for the visit, and the results are presented in Table 1.

While an analysis of diagnoses indicates that 40 to 50 frequently identified problems constitute the majority of the patient volume, an assessment of the range of diagnoses encountered suggests that the family physician manages problems cover-

Table 1. *Percentage Distribution of Reasons for Visit*

Reason for Visit	Percent
Nonoperative (acute) problems	40
Long-term follow-up	22
Preventive, well-maintenance	20
Office procedures	12
Postoperative evaluation	3
Preoperative evaluation	2
Other	1
All reasons	100

Reprinted by permission from D'Elia et al: J Fam Pract, 8(4):799, 1979.

ing all the organ systems and all the stages of human growth and development. The family physicians are providing pediatric, obstetric, general medical-surgical, and geriatric care. They provide care in office, operating room, Emergency Room, hospital ward, and other settings. As part of the surgical manpower pool, the family physicians perform surgery, assist surgeons, and refer patients to surgeons in the community or in larger centers.

***

Frey JJ, Rice CA: Family practice in Massachusetts: A comparison of residency trained family physicians with the general practitioner experience of 1967–1968. J Fam Pract 10(4):663–671, 1980

An analysis of data collected from a one-year survey of the activities of seven residency trained family physicians practicing in Massachusetts was carried out. These data were compared to a study of activities of Massachusetts general practitioners done in 1967–1968. Both hospital and health center encounters were analyzed.

In April 1977, the Department of Family and Community Medicine of the University of Massachusetts Medical School began monitoring the clinical experiences of family physicians and family practice residents in four affiliated community

based centers. Three of these four health centers have one or more residency trained family physicians on their staff. Of these physicians, three practice at an urban neighborhood health center, one at a rural health center which serves an eight-town area in north central Massachusetts, and three are members of a group practice in a town of 75,000. Data for this report were accumulated over a year's time from July 1977 through June 1978, from the practices of these seven residency trained family physicians. By the end of the study year, the physicians involved had averaged 2.7

Table 1. *Sites of Patient Encounters in Practices of Residency Trained Physicians and General Practitioners*

Site of Visit	Residency Trained Physicians		General Practitioners	
	*Number**	*Percent†*	*Number**	*Percent†*
Office	19,867	81.5	9,190	71.6
Home	41	0.2	719	5.6
Hospital (inpatient)	4,332	17.8	2,772	21.6
ER‡/Extended Care/Other	126	0.5	154	1.2
Total Encounters	24,366	100.0	12,835	100.0

Reprinted by permission from Frey, Rice: J Fam Pract, 10(4):663, 1980.
* Number = Number of encounters.
† Percent = Percent of total encounters.
‡ ER = Emergency Room.

years in practice, ranging from 1 to 6 years. Of the seven physicians, five had been doing obstetrics.

Table 1 shows the number of encounters that occurred at each site, including office (health center), home, hospital inpatient, and extended care facility/emergency room/other. A comparison of the distribution of the sites of visit for residency graduates and the 15 Massachusetts general practitioners shows that encounters with residency graduates were more often office based (82 percent, vs. 72 percent for general practitioners).

The age distribution of the practices paralleled that of the general practitioners, particularly the younger general practitioners. The sex distribution was also comparable. However, over one third of all health problems recorded during the

study were for preventive or nonillness visits. This represented a significant percentage increase over the general practitioners.

In 1967, a group of general practitioners in Massachusetts set out to look at their practices and find reasons why patients sought help from their physicians. Ten years later, this study has found that, in many areas, what they did and what graduates of a training system (which did not even exist at the time they did their work) do, are not that dissimilar. Both groups deliver preventive, acute, and chronic health care to individuals of all ages and both sexes over a broad range of medical problems. Both studies were descriptive in nature and said nothing about the quality of the care that was given and little about the manner in which it was delivered.

Dixon AS: Survey of a rural practice: Rainy River 1975. Can Fam Physician 22:693–703, 1976

A study of family practice in a small rural community in northwestern Ontario was conducted over a one year period from January 1, 1975–December 31, 1975. An attempt was made to define the population at risk and, in addition to recording morbidity in terms of illness episodes, study

was made of referral patterns in the practice and the use of a small hospital staffed solely by a family physician.

Rainy River is a small town in northwestern Ontario with a population of 1200. Patients are drawn from 30 miles to the north and 15 miles to the east—comprising some

450 square miles. The two major employers in the town are the Canadian National Railway and a factory which makes snowmobile clothing. The outlying population is mainly involved in farming, tree cutting and, in the summer, running tourist camps. There are two Indian Reserves 30 miles north of the town. The majority of the practice population falls into the middle and lower income groups. Medical services are provided by the Rainy River Clinic, which is situated in the basement of a small Red Cross outpost hospital. It is staffed by one or two physicians. For eight months of the year under investigation a second physician also worked in the clinic. Fort Frances, 60 miles to the east, is the closest town of any size (population 10,000), and its clinic provides referral services in general surgery, orthopedics, internal medicine, obstetrics, and gynecology. Otherwise, the nearest referral center is Winnipeg, some 150 miles to the west.

An age/sex register was constructed to define the practice population, and hence the population at risk. A record was kept in the register of those patients who attended the clinic during the study year, thus defining the "attending population." Illness episodes were recorded in an "E" Book. The Canuck Classification was used, and entries were made only for patients who appeared in the age/sex register—casual attenders were not included.

There were 2404 people in the practice ("population at risk") of whom 1167 (48.5 percent) were male, and 1237 (51.5 percent) were female. Of the population at risk, 1646 (68.5 percent) attended on at least one occasion during the year. Attendance was defined as a direct patient/doctor contact. Any indirect contact, e.g., by telephone, was not included. Of the 1646 attending patients, 780 (47.4 percent) were male, and 866 (52.6 percent) were female. There were 3523 recorded episodes of illness during the year, of which 369 were episodes classified as "miscellaneous," and included routine medical examinations, Pap smears, antenatal attendances, and prophylactic procedures.

In the absence of comparable Canadian figures, comparison was made with the results of the first (May 1955–April 1956) and second (Nov. 1970–Oct. 1971) United Kingdom National Morbidity Surveys. The number of patients consulting per 100 population at risk was higher in Rainy River for males (66.8 per 100), and also for the combination of males and females (68.5 per 100), (Table 1).

On a total of 217 occasions, 207 patients were referred for specialist opinion. Table 2 shows the distribution of referrals ac-

Table 1. *Comparison of First and Second U.K. National Morbidity Surveys and Rainy River Survey*

	U.K. 1st National Morbidity Survey May 1955–April 1956	U.K. 2nd National Morbidity Survey Nov. 1970–Oct. 1971	Rainy River Survey
Patients consulting/100 population at risk	m 63.5 f 70.2 p 67.0	m 63.1 f 70.9 p 67.2	m 66.8 f 70.0 p 68.5
Episodes/person at risk*	m 1.21 f 1.44 p 1.33	m 1.42 f 1.80 p 1.62	m 1.20 f 1.41 p 1.31
Episodes/patient consulting*	m 1.9 f 2.1 p 2.0	m 2.3 f 2.7 p 2.5	m 1.79 f 2.02 p 1.92

Reprinted by permission from Dixon: Survey of a rural practice: Rainy River 1975. Can Fam Physician 22:693–703, 1976.
* These figures exclude prophylactic procedures and antenatal episodes.

cording to specialist opinion sought. Of all referrals, 78.7 percent were to general surgery, orthopedics, obstetrics and gynecology, or internal medicine. As a result of referral, 124 hospital admissions resulted (57.1 percent of all referrals). There were 173 referrals to surgical specialties; 79 (45.7 percent) of these referrals resulted in the performance of some kind of surgical procedure.

Figures from the Rainy River survey indicate that 16.7 patients per 100 population at risk were in a hospital on at least one occasion during the year. This included patients admitted to the Rainy River Hospital and to other hospitals as the result of referral. The presence of Indian patients in the practice presented special problems, and a higher proportion of the Indian population at risk were admitted to hospital. The admission rate for non-Indian patients was 13.3 patients per 100 at risk.

Table 2. *Distribution of Referrals According to Specialty*

	Number of Referrals	Percent of Total
General surgery	78	35.9
Orthopedics	36	16.6
Obs./gyn.	30	13.8
Internal medicine	27	12.4
ENT	13	6.0
Urology	11	5.1
Dermatology	5	2.3
Psychiatry	5	2.3
Pediatrics	4	1.8
Ophthalmology	4	1.8
Neurology	3	1.4
Plastic surgery	1	0.5
Total	217	100.0

Reprinted by permission from Dixon AS: Survey of a rural practice: Rainy River 1975. Can Fam Physician 22:693–703, 1976.

Mechanic D: The organization of medical practice and practice orientations among physicians in prepaid and nonprepaid primary care settings. Med Care 13(3):189–204, 1975

This is an extensive study based on a survey of a national sample of primary care physicians in office-based practice conducted in 1970 and 1971. The characteristics of respondents and nonrespondents, in terms of social and demographic variables, were comparable with the population from which they were sampled although older physicians, those in fee-for-service practice, and physicians who neither had specialty boards nor belonged to a specialty society responded somewhat less. In this study, data are reported for 710 general practitioners and 179 pediatricians included in the sample.

Data are presented on office-based general practitioners and pediatricians working in varying practice settings. Fee-for-service physicians were found to spend more time in direct patient care activities than those in prepaid practice, and to devote more time to each patient. The data suggest that the patient load characteristic of general practice in prepaid groups encourages a more assembly line practice which is less responsive to patients than the pattern characteristic of fee-for-service practice. Prepaid physicians work during scheduled hours and may deal with increased load by processing patients more rapidly. Fee-for-service physicians tend to respond to increased demand by working longer hours. The responsiveness of primary care physicians to patient problems

Table 1. *Comparisons of Various Aspects of Work**

Aspects of Work	Group		Nongroup		Prepaid Group	
	General Practitioners (N = 113) (%)	Pediatricians (N = 43) (%)	General Practitioners (N = 606) (%)	Pediatricians (N = 136) (%)	General Practitioners (N = 108) (%)	Pediatricians (N = 154) (%)
Use of diagnostic procedures during previous two weeks						
5 or less	8	35	10	29	1	29
6–7	3	19	9	26	7	28
8–9	12	19	21	24	19	29
10–12	64	21	51	20	63	12
13	13	7	10	1	10	1
$\bar{X}$	10	7	9	7	10	7
SD	3	3	3	3	2	3
Reports use of following procedures on occasion or more frequently						
"Tape" sprains	88	72	86	78	65	53
Excise simple cysts	89	23	94	29	69	10
Open abscesses	96	74	99	92	88	75
Suture lacerations	96	81	98	85	86	51
Do proctoscopic or sigmoidoscopic exam	86	42	83	43	64	23
Take and interpret your own electrocardiograms	81	44	70	25	84	47
Do vaginal exam with a speculum	98	42	99	32	95	38
Use a laryngoscope	62	72	49	60	36	62
Do uncomplicated obstetrics	58	5	59	7	15	1
Do well-baby care	81	100	91	97	49	99
Do simply psychotherapy	98	95	96	93	94	94
Do pap smears	93	9	98	10	84	12
Set simple fractures	80	35	81	50	50	10
Do major general surgery	35	0	34	5	3	0
Take and interpret selected x-rays in your office	88	65	58	32	86	66

Reprinted by permission from Mechanic: Med Care, 13(3):189, 1975.
* Figures represent percentage of N.

seems to reflect primarily their social orientations to medical practice and the time pressures they face.

The physicians were presented with 14 diagnostic procedures and were asked to indicate which procedures they used in the previous two weeks. Table 1 presents the distribution of the number of procedures used. On the average, general practitioners in nongroup practice use fewer procedures, whereas among pediatricians, those in prepaid practice report the lowest average number of procedures used. Differences among practice settings were found to be relatively small. A different picture emerges in responses to a list of 15 relatively commonly used procedures shown in Table 1. On the average, both general practitioners and pediatricians in prepaid practice are less likely to report using these procedures. For example, physicians in prepaid practice are less likely to report that they tape sprains, excise simple cysts, suture lacerations, do proctoscopic or sigmoidoscopic examinations, do uncomplicated obstetrics, or set simple fractures. Among general practitioners, those in prepaid practice are less likely to report using each of the 15 procedures except for the interpretation of electrocardiograms.

Data are also presented on sociodemographic and professional characteristics of primary care physicians in varying settings, workload, use of diagnostic and laboratory procedures, social orientations to medical practice, satisfactions and dissatisfactions, and attitudes toward sociopolitical aspects of medical care. Suggestions are offered for improving the responsiveness of prepaid practice.

Galazka SS, Lundeen PB: An approach to locating a family practice office in a metropolitan area.
J Fam Pract 8(2):333–336, 1979

The problem of locating a family practice within an urban area is faced by many physicians each year. The ultimate decision will affect the health care services for many of an area's population and requires the mobilization of significant financial resources. The purpose of this paper is to present a simple and economically feasible approach to locating a family practice office within a metropolitan area.

The Grand Rapids area of Michigan serves as the population base for this investigation. An Office Location-Population Profile was determined from census tract population data and known physician office distribution. Based on this information, a subsegment of the total area was delineated as a possible neighborhood for an office location and a physician-population ratio for this subsegment was determined. This was compared with recommended ratios. A statistical profile of the population within the area considered as a possible site location was developed using information available through census bureau statistics. Finally, a direct survey of a random sample of households within the selected area was performed.

Of those people surveyed, approximately 68 percent obtained their health care outside of the immediate geographic area and more than 50 percent stated that they did not presently have a family physician. Over half the people surveyed stated that they would use the services of a new family physician located so as to provide ready access to their immediate area.

The use of a statistical profile and neighborhood health care survey provide a perspective on the population from which one can anticipate health care needs. The census tracts which were studied were composed of young families with children and a low-to-middle income. Only half had family physicians, and over half would use the services of a new family physician located within their neighborhood. The health care needs of this population would be quite different from those of a population with a significant proportion of people in a geriatric age group. Services to be provided should emphasize prenatal and obstetric care and developmental pediatric care, as well as general medical care provided within the context of the family unit. Lower income families might require greater access to nutritional services, and blue-collar workers might require access to services with evening rather than daytime hours. These objective data are helpful in health care planning as well as site location.

Wanderer MJ, Suyehira JG: Obstetrical care in a prepaid cooperative: A comparison between family practice residents, family practitioners, and obstetricians. J Fam Pract 11(4):601–606, 1980

The American Academy of Family Physicians and the American College of Obstetrics and Gynecology have jointly studied Obstetrics as practiced in this country and have recognized the necessity of family physicians providing a large portion of this nation's obstetrical care. The committee has developed guidelines to be used for the training of these physicians. In addition, they have agreed that hospital privileges for the physicians providing this care should be based on documented training and proven competence rather than arbitrary criteria developed in various localities. However, the practice of obstetrics and the granting of hospital privileges to family physicians continues to be controversial. Unfortunately there is a paucity of objective data on which to base discussion. This study is intended to add to the fund of knowledge regarding process and outcome and quality of obstetrical care provided by different physician groups.

Group Health Cooperative of Puget Sound is a prepaid, consumer-owned health care program located in the Seattle metropolitan area. At the time of the study, the patient population was approximately 200,000 persons served by 200 physicians, of whom 90 were family practitioners/general practitioners, 11 of whom practice obstetrics, and 20 obstetricians.

The Family Practice Residency consists of 12 family practice residents who supply comprehensive and family oriented care to approximately 4000 patients. There are three groups of physicians who provide obstetrical services: family practice residents (FPR), family physicians (FP), and obstetricians (OB). Ninety percent of deliveries were performed by the OB group.

Deliveries between July, 1975 and July, 1977 were tabulated and 200 deliveries each of the FP and FPR groups were reviewed, as were a randomly selected group of 200 OB deliveries. All hospital charts were reviewed for 81 variables.

FPR had more patients who were poor, single, and nulliparous. They presented later in pregnancy, were more often anemic, and had an increased incidence of venereal disease. The FPR and FP groups documented major psychological problems and depression more frequently. The OBs used caudal and epidural anesthesia twice as often as FPR and FP groups, who used more local, pudendal, or no anesthetics. Except for an increased incidence of third-degree lacerations in the FP group, total maternal and fetal complications were few and equally divided among the groups. FPR and FP delivered 78 percent and OB's 38 percent of their own patients.

The documentation of process and outcome of obstetrical care in this audit and in other studies show that the family physicians, family practice residents, and obstetricians provide a comparable quality of care. There are areas of divergence that require further study and more sensitive indicators of process/outcome need development.

Ranson PJ: Changing trends in family practice obstetrics. Can Fam Physician 24:222–231, 1978

In 1973, Canadian family physicians delivered two thirds of the total number of babies born. Since trends in some countries show less involvement of the family physician in obstetrics and even more reliance on the obstetrician/gynecologist as the primary care physician for women, this study was designed to find out if obstetrics could be adequately practiced in a small rural hospital by family physicians with occasional surgical help. Also, a questionnaire was sent to 200 family physicians, 100 in Ottawa and 100 in Vancouver, to ascertain their present involvement in obstetrics.

Obstetric cases for a five year period were audited in a 72 bed, active, fully accredited hospital with approximately 10 obstetrical beds, one labor room, and a reasonably equipped delivery room. A fetal stethoscope is the only monitoring equipment. The obstetrics is done by eight family physicians with two general surgeons doing the cesarian sections. Any cases needing referral go to Ottawa (40 miles). The audit included the quantity of obstetrics done as well as the proportion of complicated dliveries, number of consultations (own colleagues and referrals away), C-section rate, and finally fetal outcome. The complicated deliveries included abnormal presentations, prolonged labor, postpartum hemorrhage, rectal tears, etc.

A questionnaire was sent to 100 randomly picked family physicians in Ottawa and 100 in Vancouver asking several questions:

1. Whether total obstetrical care was practiced or just antenatal care.
2. Number of babies delivered each year and percentage referred to obstetricians.
3. Whether the family physician felt competent practicing obstetrics, found it financially rewarding and enjoyed it, or considered obstetrics a necessary duty.

The survey of obstetrics done by family physicians in Vancouver and Ottawa shows that the majority of family physicians still practice obstetrics, although in Ottawa 33 percent were not involved in obstetrics and 16 percent were involved in antenatal care only. Those who did not practice obstetrics cited the main reasons as "too time-consuming" and "not financially rewarding." Table 1 summarizes the findings of the surveys of Vancouver and Ottawa family physicians.

The audit of obstetrics in the rural hospital, although small, suggests that family physicians are providing adequate obstetrical care in this setting with occasional surgical help. Very few referrals were made to obstetricians. The C-section rate and perinatal mortality rate are near the national average.

As a result of this study, the following conclusions are drawn:

1. Obstetrics is central to the practice of family medicine. Practicing just antenatal care is a poor alternative and not a developing trend.

Table 1. *Survey of Obstetrics Done by Vancouver and Ottawa Family Physicians*

	Ottawa		Vancouver		Total	
	Number	*Percent*	*Number*	*Percent*	*Number*	*Percent*
No. responding	80	80	76	76	156	78
No. in total obstetrical care	41	51	70	92	111	71
<20 deliveries/yr	7		11		18	
20–30 del./yr.	11		18		29	
30–40 del./yr.	11		21		32	
40–50 del./yr.	5		9		14	
50 > del./yr.	7		11		18	
Antenatal care only	13	16	2	3	15	10
No obstetrics practiced	26	33	4	5	30	19
Not financially rewarding	43	83	47	62	90	73
No. who felt competent in obstetrics	44	85	70	99	114	92
No. who felt obstetrics a duty only	14	14	10	14	24	14
No. who enjoyed obstetrics	45	86	62	88	107	87

Reprinted by permission from Ranson: Can Fam Physician, 24:222, 1978.

2. Obstetrics has become a sophisticated specialty requiring more knowledge and expertise.
3. New family physicians practicing obstetrics should have more mandatory obstetrical training, i.e., six months in an approved teaching hospital.
4. More postgraduate obstetrical courses should be offered to family physicians currently practicing obstetrics.
5. Obstetrics can be practiced adequately in small rural hospitals without an obstetrician but these areas can reduce their perinatal mortality by early diagnosis of high risk pregnancy and early referral in utero.
6. A significant number of city family physicians do not practice obstetrics and this may be mainly on the basis of poor financial reward.

Geyman JP, Gordon MJ: Orthopedic problems in family practice: Incidence, distribution, and curricular implications. J Fam Pract 8(4):759–765, 1979

The spectrum of orthopedic problems encountered by family physicians in everyday practice has received little study in the past. This paper presents and analyzes the incidence and distribution of orthopedic problems in general/family practice based on four sources of secondary data. These sources include the National Ambulatory Medical Care Survey (NAMCS), a Family Practice Service in a large military teaching hospital, a state-wide study in Virginia, and two community-based family practice settings in Washington State.

The NAMCS data involve a probability sample of approximately 15,000 patient problems seen by general/family physicians during 1976. The Madigan data involve a total of approximately 5000 patient visits for musculoskeletal problems over a 16-month period from September 1, 1975 to December 31, 1976. The Family Practice service of Madigan Army Medical

Table 1. *Overall Distribution of Orthopedic Problems*

	Madigan (%)	NAMCS (%)	Washington (%)	Virginia (%)
Chronic musculoskeletal problems	57	57	56	54
Sprains and strains	24	32	27	28
Fractures	6	10	14	14
Other	13	1	3	4
Totals	100	100	100	100

Reprinted by permission from Geyman, Gordon: J. Fam Pract, 8(4):759, 1979.

Center is staffed by 23 family practice residents under the supervision of the program's eight faculty members. The residents and faculty provide comprehensive care for a known population comparable in age and sex composition to civilian communities. The Virginia data involve analysis of over 500,000 patient problems presented to 118 family physicians in rural, suburban, and urban settings in Virginia over a two-year period. The individual practice data include all visits for musculoskeletal problems in two selected family practices in Davenport (population 1,471) and Spokane, Washington (population 174,500) for 12-month periods during 1977–1978.

The overall incidence of orthopedic problems comprised about 10 percent of all office visits in the NAMCS and Madigan studies and 8.6 percent in the Virginia Study. Table 1 displays the breakdown for chronic musculoskeletal problems, sprains and strains, and fractures for the NAMCS, Madigan, Washington, and Virginia studies.

All four available secondary sources of data provide interesting comparisons of the rank order by frequency of specific fractures and nontraumatic orthopedic problems. The seven locations of fractures shown in Table 2 account for about 90 percent or more of all fractures in each of the four studies, and show a high level of agreement in terms of comparative frequency of the most common kinds of fractures. Table 3 shows the comparative rank order of frequency among the four available studies for specific nontraumatic musculoskeletal problems, and again, a high level of comparability is evident. A notable exception is the reversal in ranks between low back pain and bursitis, tenosynovitis, and synovitis. Together these six problems accounted for well over 50 percent of non-

Table 2. *Comparative Rank Order of Fractures*

	Madigan	NAMCS	Washington	Virginia
Carpal, metacarpal, tarsal, and metatarsal bones	1	1	1	1
Phalanges of foot or hand	2	2	3	2
Radius, ulna	3	3	2	5
Tibia, fibula	4	5	5	3
Clavicle	5	6	7	6
Ribs	6	4	4	4
Humerus	7	6	6	—

Reprinted by permission from Geyman, Gordon: J Fam Pract, 8(4):759, 1979.

Table 3. *Comparative Rank of Non-Traumatic Musculoskeletal Problems*

	Madigan	NAMCS	Washington	Virginia
Low back pain	1	1	3	1
Osteoarthritis	2	2	2	2
Pain in joint (arthralgia)	3	5	5	5
Bursitis, tenosynovitis, synovitis	4	3	1	3
Syndromes related to cervical spine	5	—	—	6
Rheumatoid arthritis	6	4	4	4

Reprinted by permission from Geyman, Gordon: J Fam Pract, 8(4):759, 1979.

traumatic musculoskeletal problems in each of the four studies.

The studies that have been discussed represent a wide range of patient populations in different parts of the country. Although the commonalities of these studies are striking, there may be considerable variation in the spectrum of orthopedic problems seen and managed by individual family physicians in different practice settings.

Perry BC, Chrisinger EW, Gordon MJ, Henze WA: A practice based study of trauma in a rural community. J Fam Pract 10(6):1039–1043, 1980

Tonasket, Washington, an agricultural town with a population of 900, is situated 125 miles from the nearest referral center. The clinic in Tonasket serves a sparsely settled agricultural area containing several small communities with a population base of approximately 8000. The economy of the area is based on apples, cattle, and lumber. The family physicians in Tonasket became concerned at the volume and severity of the injuries treated in their practice. They came to believe that trauma had a significant detrimental effect on the community and that injuries comprised a remarkably large portion of their practice.

The study population comprised all patients who sought care from the Tonasket clinic providers in either the clinic or the Emergency Room. The study period extended from August 15, 1978 through November 15, 1978. During the three-month study period, the clinic personnel recorded 4734 visits for all causes. Of all visits to providers, 818, or 17.3 percent, were for injuries. Males were involved in 68.2 percent of injury episodes; 29.9 percent of all episodes of injury occurred on the job. Teenagers and young adults were the most frequently injured, with 55.7 percent of all injuries occurring in the 10- to 29-year age group.

Falls were the most common cause of treated injuries in this study, followed by being "struck by an object" and "tool injuries." Other causes of injury are tabulated in Table 1. A majority totaling 64.3 percent of all episodes involved injury to an extremity. Eye injuries comprised an additional 9.1 percent of episodes. Table 2 shows that the predominant types of injuries were contusions, lacerations, strains and sprains, and fractures. These four

Table 1. *Major Reasons for Cause of Injury Stated by Patient or the Family*

Cause of Injury	Number of Cases	Percent of Cases
Fall	139	28.7
Struck by object	55	11.3
Tool injury	52	10.7
Automobile	34	7.0
School athletics	30	6.2
Struck stationary object	28	5.8
Chainsaw	15	3.1
Motorcycle	14	2.9
Altercation	14	2.9
Sport not otherwise specified	13	2.7
Insect sting	11	2.3
Ingestion	10	2.1
Burn	10	2.1
Horse related	7	1.4
Other	53	10.9
Total	485	100.0

Reprinted by permission from Perry et al: J Fam Pract, 10(6): 1039, 1980.

Table 2. *Types of Injuries Treated by Providers* *

Type of Injury	Number of Episodes	Percent of Episodes
Contusion	107	22.1
Laceration	102	21.0
Sprain and strain	96	19.8
Fracture	65	13.4
Corneal abrasion	30	6.2
Puncture	30	6.2
Foreign body (eye)	23	4.1
Closed head trauma	16	3.3
Burn	14	2.9
Foreign body (tissue)	12	2.5
Insect sting	11	2.2
Secondary infection	9	1.9
Dislocation	6	1.2
Ingestion	4	.8
Internal ligamentous injury (knee)	4	.8
Blunt trauma (abdomen)	3	.6
Traumatic iritis	3	.6
A-C separation	2	.4
Lacerated liver	2	.4
Rust ring (cornea)	2	.4
Finger amputation	2	.4
Blunt trauma (chest)	1	.2
Amputation of leg	1	.2
Bracheal plexus strain	1	.2
Other	41	8.5

Reprinted by permission from Perry et al: J Fam Pract, 10(6): 1039, 1980.
* May include more than one type of injury per episode so that percent total is greater than 100.

types of injuries accounted for 76.3 percent of all injury episodes. The categories of closed head trauma, blunt abdominal trauma, blunt chest trauma, fracture, and dislocation were combined to form a category of "serious injury." Serious injuries accounted for 20 percent of all treated injuries. Motorcycle, automobile, and horse-related accidents accounted for most of the serious injuries.

The most frequently performed procedures were for laceration and orthopedic care. Consultation was obtained in 9.9 percent of patients treated for trauma. Four percent of trauma patients required admission either at the local hospital or at the referral hospital.

Practice-based studies may be effective in identifying preventable patterns of injury. Specific mechanisms of injury may be prevalent in the community and not be noticed by health or occupational workers.

For example, in this study eye injuries occurred in 9.1 percent of all encounters due to trauma. Further investigation revealed that most agricultural workers did not wear eye protection in the field or shop. After the results of this study became known, public education about eye protection was begun.

The role of the rural family physician is central to the treatment of the injured patient. It is hoped that mechanisms will be identified through which the family physician may also markedly reduce the incidence and sequelae of injury.

Huygen FJA: Primary health care for the elderly. In selected papers from the Eighth World Conference on Family Medicine. Occasional Paper 10, J R Coll Gen Pract, May, 1980

This paper is written by a solo family physician who has practiced for 35 years in a large semirural practice in the Netherlands. He is also a part-time Professor of Family Medicine and Director with a multidisciplinary staff. At this Institute, information is obtained from a computer-based "continuous morbidity registration system" which records the morbidity presented to family physicians in four practices: two urban and two rural. Based on this information, the characteristics of the morbidity pattern of the elderly are described and their implications for primary health care are discussed.

In the Netherlands about 11 percent of the population are over 65, but they form about 15 percent of the workload of general practitioners. General practitioners care for about 90 percent of the aged population.

This study is based on records for five years from a population of about 12,000. Table 1 lists the prevalence of the "top 20" diagnoses made by the general practitioners in more than 3,000 patient-years observed in people of 65 and over. There are marked sex differences: obesity, arthritis, hypertension, nervous disorders, varicose veins, diabetes, and urinary infections are more prevalent in women, while bronchitis, earwax, and coronary infarctions are more prevalent in men.

The "top 20" diagnoses of Table 1 cover more than 60 percent of the total morbidity of the aged. In only 5 percent of these diagnoses was the patient referred to a specialist and hospital admission occurred in less than 3 percent. It can be estimated that general practitioners look after something like 90 percent of the disorders of 90 percent of the aged population.

The characteristics of the profile of disease in the elderly can be summarized as follows:

1. The total number of disorders rises rapidly with age.
2. There is a multiplicity of disorders and a predominance of chronic incurable disease.
3. There is a close relationship between

Table 1. *The "Top Twenty" Diagnoses Presented to General Practitioners by Men and Women 65 Years and Older. Prevalence per 1000 per year**

	Men	Women
Obesity	138	250
Arthritis	117	240
Hypertension	89	233
Nervous disorders	74	210
Colds (non-febrile)	131	127
Chronic bronchitis	214	59
Accidents	106	138
Fibrositis, myalgia	109	129
Varicose veins	41	166
Cardiac failure	84	91
Deafness	89	82
Angina pectoris	75	87
Diabetes mellitus	56	89
Acute urinary infections	34	102
Acute bronchitis	93	56
Cerebrovascular accidents	64	66
Febrile colds	46	75
Malignancies	53	59
Earwax	60	41
Myocardial infarction	54	38
Of These Disorders		
Referred to a specialist	*5.1%*	*4.6%*
Admitted to hospital	*2.7%*	*2.5%*

Reprinted by permission from Huygen: J R Coll Gen Pract, May, 1980, Occasional Paper 10.
* Continuous morbidity registration, Nijmegen 1971–1976, number of patient-year observed 7572.

physical illness in the elderly and their social conditions.
4. The hidden part of the "iceberg of disease" is considerably larger than in younger age groups.

The primary care physician caring for elderly patients must be a keen clinician, willing and able to go to his limits within his own talents. He will sometimes have to take calculated risks and he will have to be able to live with uncertainty. It will be more important for him to acquire clinical and human wisdom than special technical skills and a tendency to perfectionism. He must be able to critically appraise the scope and also the dangers and limitations of specialist technology. He must be a generalist, capable of weighing all the pros and cons and assessing the relative importance of various aspects against the lives of his aging patients as a whole.

Wood JK: The role of the family physician in providing psychiatric care in the general hospital. Can Fam Physician 26:263–266, 1980

In 1962, a study was done of family physicians in Saskatchewan concerning practice content, methods of treatment of emotional disorders, patterns of referral, opinions about attitudes toward mental illness, and the use of allied professionals. The study concluded that a large body of emotional disorders never comes to the attention of psychiatrists. It recommended further studies to find out how the skills of family physicians and psychiatrists might be employed in a mutually beneficial way.

In 1979 the same questionnaire was circulated to all 110 Saskatoon family physicians in an attempt to measure any changes in attitudes. A response rate of 38 percent was obtained (42 physicians). Of the respondents, 92 percent indicated that at least 85 percent of their work was family medicine.

Based on the 1979 study, it was found that family physicians continued to express a high level of interest in psychiatry. They perceived an increased, high level of public expectation to have psychiatric illnesses treated by the family physician. The general hospital was usually seen by physicians as the most appropriate facility for inpatient treatment, as opposed to admission to a mental hospital. More physicians in 1979 indicated they wanted to treat their own patients. The lack of consensus about the preferred mode of collaboration with psychiatrists points out the importance of indicating clearly to the consultant how the family physician wants the responsibility for care shared.

It was estimated that the number of hospital patients treated solely by family physicians in a year was 2480 in 1979, with 1280 treated by family physicians with a psychiatric consultation, and 200 treated solely by a psychiatrist.

As a result of this survey of family physician opinion, and a review of events over the past 17 years pertaining to the family physician and the provision of inpatient psychiatric care, the following ideal modus operandi was proposed for family physicians, taking into consideration the patient's needs and expectations, the perceived role and the limitations of the general physician, the expertise of the consultant psychiatrist, and the constraints of the hospital system:

1. Almost all the family physicians' psychiatric patients requiring admission to hospital should be admitted to the general hospital where the family physician normally admits his nonpsychiatric patients.

2. Psychiatric patients should be admitted to hospital under the care of their personal physician.
3. Psychiatric consultation should be readily available, but not mandatory.

4. The level of remuneration for physicians' in-hospital services must be brought up to a realistic level.

Cartwright A, Anderson R: Patients and their doctors 1977. Occasional Paper 8, J R Coll Gen Pract, March, 1979

This is an extensive report comparing changes in British general practice between 1964 and 1977. The study was carried out by the Institute for Social Studies in Medical Care, and a report was prepared for the Royal Commission on the National Health Service. This study is based on a sample of 836 patients with 365 general practitioners in England and Wales. Both patients' and physicians' views are represented with respect to expectations and strategies for health care, the roles of general practitioners and consultants, quality of care, and related subjects.

Several brief excerpts of this study are included here regarding the use of general practitioner services. For example, comparison of patients' estimates of their number of consultations in the previous 12 months (Table 1) shows a decline in the proportion who had not had any consulta-

tions, and therefore suggests an increase in consultation rates. However, the national average consultation rate in the most recent National Morbidity Survey was 3.0 compared with one of 3.8 in the earlier 1955–1956 study. On balance the direction of the change seems doubtful, and the size of the change is probably small.

The evidence on home visits from these two studies in 1964 and 1977 is more clear-cut and points to a definite decline. The proportion reporting a home visit in the previous year fell from 23 percent in 1964 to 19 percent in 1977; the proportion with five or more dropped from 7 to 4 percent.

The proportion of patients who thought a general practitioner was a suitable person to talk to about problems such as children getting into trouble or difficulties between husband and wife had declined from 40 percent in 1964 to 30 percent in

Table 1. *Patients' Estimates of Number of General Practitioner Consultations in Previous Twelve Months*

	1964 (Percent)	1977 (Percent)
None	34	25
One	15	18
Two–four	26	30
Five–nine	11	14
Ten or more	14	13
Number of patients (=100%)	1394	825

1977. But the proportion who said they would discuss a personal problem that was not strictly medical with their own doctor if they were worried about it was 28 percent on both studies. So while people are apparently less likely to regard general practitioners as appropriate for dealing with family or relationship problems, the proportion who feel they would turn to their general practitioner with a personal problem had not changed.

Ninety-four percent of the doctors in the 1977 sample thought that it was appropriate for them to be consulted for depression. (No comparable question was asked about this in 1964.) Among the patients, the proportion who thought they would consult their general practitioner in this circumstance had risen from 54 percent in 1964 to 69 percent in 1977. During this period the number of prescriptions for antidepressant drugs rose from 3.5 million in England and Wales in 1965 to 7.9 million in England alone in 1975. General practitioners' feelings about the appropriateness of consultation for depression may well be a reflection of their feelings that there is something they can do for it. Their less positive reactions to consultation about family problems may result from lack of confidence in their ability to help in such circumstances.

Garg ML, Skipper JK Jr, McNamara MJ, Mulligan JL: Primary care physicians and profiles of their hospitalized patients. Am J Public Health 66(4):390–392, 1976

Few studies focus on the correlation between profiles of hospitalized patients and the specialty of attending physicians. Although a precise definition of the primary care physician remains elusive, by most present day standards it refers to internists, family practitioners, and pediatricians. The purpose of this paper is to describe the type of hospitalized patients cared for by primary care physicians and to analyze differences among the three primary care specialties.

Data were collected from a 5-percent random probability sample drawn from a list of discharges from all nine short-term general hospitals in Lucas County, Ohio, in 1970. Discharges were used instead of admissions since primary diagnosis is more precise at discharge than at admission. After eliminating newborns (377) and deaths (79) from the sample, 4599 patients remained concerning whom there were sufficient data for analysis.

The primary care physicians were responsible for 45 percent of the discharges; the other specialties for 52 percent. Three percent of the patients were under the care of physicians whose specialty was either unspecified or unknown. Among the primary care physicians, internists accounted for a mean of 145 discharges per year per physician; pediatricians, 133; and family physicians, 129.

Patients of internists had the longest mean stay in the hospital, 12.1 days, compared to those physicians in family practice, 8.9 days. Internists on the average had 4.8 patients per day per physician; family practitioners, 3.1; pediatricians, 2.4; and other specialists, 3.6. Analysis by primary diagnosis indicated that the patients of family physicians were fairly evenly divided among a variety of diagnostic categories. However, 42 percent of the pediatricians' patients were hospitalized for diseases of the respiratory system, and 33 percent of internists' patients' for diseases of the circulatory system. The hospital practice of internal medicine was concentrated mostly in the age group of 35 and above, whereas the patients of the family practitioners were more evenly distributed in the age group 25–64. While both internists and family practitioners discharged a high percentage of patients 65 years of age and over, the figure for internists, 38 percent, was higher than that for family practitioners, 26 percent.

Among the primary care physicians it is the internist who on the average discharges the most patients, sees more patients per day, and whose patients stay longest in the hospital. This may be due to the type or seriousness of the cases with which the internist is most likely to come in contact. For example, diseases of the circulatory system, the most frequent category of illness seen by internists, may require multiple hospitalizations and longer stay than diseases of the respiratory system. The difference may also be related to a variation in age of the patients seen by the three types of specialists, the internist seeing more older patients than other primary care physicians.

Although this study is limited to hospitalized patients, it indicates that different primary care physicians may serve distinctly different populations. The practice characteristics of primary care physicians should be examined further on a larger scale in order to help develop a meaningful definition of primary care; more precisely define our needs in the area; and provide guidelines for a national health policy.

Warburton SW, Sadler GR: Family physician hospital privileges in New Jersey. J Fam Pract 7(5):1019–1026, 1978

This paper reports the results of a study of hospital privileges of family physicians in 95 of the 98 acute care, short-stay general (nongovernmental) hospitals in the state of New Jersey.

Of the 95 hospitals, only two did not have any family physicians on their staff.

General medicine was the area in which family physicians were most commonly granted hospital privileges. Eighty of the 93 hospitals granted all family physicians admitting privileges in the area of general medicine, while 12 of the remaining hospitals granted such privileges to at least a

Table 1. *Hospitals with Family Physician Privileges**

Area of Privileges	All FPs	Some FPs	No FPs	Not Applicable	Unknown	Total
General medicine	80	12	1	2	0	95
General pediatrics	52	20	9	12	2	95
ICU	59	14	17	3	2	95
CCU	56	12	21	4	2	95
Newborn nursery	30	27	18	18	2	95
1st Assistant surgery	23	23	39	7	3	95
Routine OB	15	29	31	18	2	95
Operative surgery	14	18	56	4	3	95
ICU newborn	0	7	25	61	2	95
Operative OB	5	3	59	26	2	95

Reprinted by permission from Warburton, Sadler: J Fam Pract, 7(5):1019, 1978.
* Privileges = ability of an MD or DO to admit and treat patients in certain areas of the hospital as of July 1, 1977; N = 95 hospitals.

Table 2. *Expected Family Physician Privileges**

Area of Privilege	Yes	No	Not Applicable	Unknown
ICU	73	14	5	3
CCU	71	17	5	2
General medicine	92	2	—	1
Operative surgery	20	63	8	4
1st Assistant surgery	34	46	11	4
Newborn nursery	61	12	18	4
ICU newborn	8	28	55	4
General pediatrics	74	7	12	2
Routine OB	50	21	18	6
Operative OB	5	58	26	6

Reprinted by permission from Warburton, Sadler: J Fam Pract, 7(5):1019, 1978.
* New board-certified family physician; N = 95 hospitals.

portion of the family physicians on their staff. Intensive Care Unit (ICU), Coronary Care Unit (CCU), and general pediatric privileges were granted in approximately 70 of the hospitals. Operative surgery was granted in 32 hospitals. Thirty percent of the hospitals placed no restriction on the family physicians' privileges. The absence of restrictions had no correlation to size of hospital or location in the state. Table 1 summarizes the extent and type of hospital privileges for family physicians in these 95 hospitals.

The hospitals were asked to indicate the areas in which a new board-certified family physician could expect to receive admitting privileges. As shown in Table 2, the privileges for new board-certified family physicians are quite similar to those which already exist. Small increases are anticipated in the areas of CCU, newborn nursery, general pediatrics, and routine obstetrics, with decreases anticipated in operative surgery and operative obstetrical privileges.

Johnston MA, Tweedie T, Premi JN, Shea PE: The role of the family physician in hospital, Part 2: Use of hospital privileges. Can Fam Physician 26:215–220, 1980

A study on the hospital involvement of family physicians was done with the active staff members of the Department of Family Medicine at St. Joseph's Hospital, Hamilton, Ontario, in 1977. This paper deals with the reasons why family physicians attend hospital, what they do there, how much time they spend there, and their use of hospital privileges, both attending and procedural. A discussion of the study's im-

plications for general understanding of the family physician role, and necessary education for this role, is included.

Table 1 shows the reasons given for practicing in hospital. The replies were spontaneous expressions, not suggested answers. Topping the list are the "patient care" reasons.

The family physicians spent an average of 7.1 hours in the hospital each week. Ac-

Table 1. *The Major Reasons for Family Physicians' Involvement in Hospital*

| | Number of Doctors Giving Reasons in Order of Priority | | | | | |
| | 1st | | 2nd | | 3rd | |
	(frequency)	(percent)	(frequency)	(percent)	(frequency)	(percent)
Patient care Quality of care Necessity for patient care	62	70.4	18	20.4	1	1.1
Continuing education Upkeep of skills	12	13.6	34	38.6	26	29.5
Duty–habit	7	7.9	2	2.3	12	13.6
Patient advocate	4	4.5	9	10.2	3	3.4
Public relations Meet other doctors Contact specialists	1	1.1	11	12.5	15	17.0
Challenge Personal satisfaction Influence future medicine	1	1.1	6	6.8	2	2.3
Remuneration Access to facilities	0	0	4	4.5	8	9.1

Reprinted by permission from Johnston, Tweedie et al: Can Fam Physician, 26:215, 1980.

cording to time spent, the priorities again seem to be, in order of importance: patient care, continuing education, and professional communication.

Four levels of care (total, concurrent, supportive, and referral) were assessed across 12 departments or similar units, spanning the major hospital services. All 88 staff members were asked to estimate the percentage of their patients that they would usually treat in each of the four levels of care in each department. Table 2 shows how many physicians assign half or more of their patients to each level of treatment, displayed as 50 to 90 percent and 90 to 100 percent of patients. For the sake of brevity the figures under 50 percent are not shown. Since all these figures were quick estimates of actual practice, there was some overlap in each level of care, causing increased totals for the number of physicians across the table.

Looking at the attending privileges in a general way, family physicians do rela-

tively little entirely on their own (except obstetrics) and also totally refer relatively little, but because of the proportions of time spent in hospital on patient care (61 percent), they must be considerably involved in concurrent and supportive care. The family physician is often at the center of a communication network of patient, consultant, family, hospital staff, and perhaps community agencies.

A characteristic pattern of current hospital practice for family physicians at St. Joseph's Hospital seems to emerge. When this is compared to the only other similar study (done by the Hamilton Academy and McMaster University in 1966) a distinct change is seen in the volume and type of hospital work. Family physicians still appear to be very active in the hospital but much more in a support role in the major specialties. Some areas are paradoxically deficient in family physician involvement, notably psychiatry and rehabilitation. This is at variance with their responsibility in

Table 2. *Estimated Levels of Care for 50% and 90% of Patients, According to Hospital Department or Units*

	Total Care		Concurrent Care		Supportive Care		Complete Referral	
	50–90%	90–100%	50–90%	90–100%	50–90%	90–100%	50–90%	90–100%
Emergency dept.	20	8	7	0	7	4	19	25
Fracture room	16	6	0	0	0	0	30	46
Obstetrics (normal)	1	54	1	5	1	4	1	21
Neonatal (normal)	2	82	1	0	0	1	0	2
Premature infants	29	3	9	20	10	9	13	12
Pediatrics (general)	30	22	11	4	9	14	5	4
General medicine	35	1	19	6	16	11	10	1
General surgery, Orthopedics, Gynecology	3	0	8	12	18	37	13	9
Surgery: plastic, eye and ENT	3	0	4	7	10	35	12	26
Intensive care unit cardiac monitoring	1	0	13	7	17	39	8	12
Rehabilitation and Stroke	14	1	21	10	15	27	12	8
Psychiatry	1	0	5	3	11	28	7	36

Reprinted by permission from Johnston, Tweedie et al: Can Fam Physician, 26:215, 1980.

those fields outside the hospital. The use of the emergency room and fracture room implies a selective process, most likely being used if the doctor is actually in the hospital but being referred if he is not. Priority for patients booked in the office seems probable.

Tarrant M: What price admitting privileges? A study of hospital admissions by two family physicians. Can Fam Physician 23:837–846, 1977

This is a descriptive retrospective study of the hospital practice of two Calgary family physicians. The intent was to study their hospital practice in relation to their total practice experience and to demonstrate any differences in the two years, especially since the principal acute care general hospital to which they admitted their patients, Foothills Hospital, changed from a brand new provincial hospital with no resident medical staff in 1967 to a fully operational teaching hospital with final year clinical clerks involved in the patient care by 1971.

Table 1 compares the "crude" admission rates for the two physicians in 1967 and 1971. The physicians followed the general trend to admit more of the patients seen.

Most patients were admitted as emergencies (84 percent in 1967 and 86 percent in 1971). Admissions in the elective and urgent categories were low because the physicians had excellent laboratory and x-ray facilities to investigate patients outside hospital where their surgical privileges were restricted, so that they referred all patients except those requiring minor surgery (e.g., D&C's, tubal ligation). Other members of the Department of Family Practice within the hospital with more surgical experience were allowed to perform

Table 1. *Comparison of Number of Admissions in Relation to Total Number of Patients Seen for Each Year*

	1967	1971
Number of admissions	302	352
Number of people admitted	263	317
Total number of people seen in whole year	4,074	4,313
"Crude" admission rate	6.5%	7.4%

Reprinted by permission from Tarrant: Can Fam Physician, 23:837, 1977.

more operations, e.g., herniorrhaphies, so they would have a higher number of elective admissions. Although over 80 percent of the total doctor/patient contacts were conducted at the office, it was found that 50 percent of the patients admitted were seen outside the office, either in the home (16 percent in 1967 and 12 percent in 1971) or in the Emergency Room (34 percent in 1967, 35 percent in 1971).

Since all obstetric patients were delivered in hospital, it is not surprising that the commonest reason for admission in both years was related to pregnancy. In 1967 gastrointestinal problems ranked second, but in 1971 it was miscellaneous problems. Comparison with the corresponding "pro-file" for the two years showed that respiratory diseases were more prevalent but managed principally outside hospital. Trauma, however, was roughly proportional in the profiles both in and out of hospital. Most neuroses were treated outside hospital, while roughly the same proportion of patients with depression required admission. Abdominal pain seemed to be managed more often outside hospital in 1971 than was the case in 1967.

The percentage of admissions requiring consultations rose slightly from 51 percent in 1967 to 54 percent in 1971. There was a more dramatic rise in the number of admissions requiring more than one consultation, the average per case in 1967 being 1.29; in 1971, 1.42 (two cases in 1971 each required six consultations!). This undoubtedly reflects the influx of subspecialists as the medical school developed (and their popularity with the junior hospital staff—the consultation rate was 1.74 per admission when interns and residents were involved in the care). The family physician can act as the patient's advocate by guarding against overzealous or inappropriate treatment by junior or even consultant staff. This study shows that these physicians freely took advantage of this readily available consultation.

Geyman JP, Brown TC, Rivers K: Referrals in family practice: A comparative study by geographic region and practice setting. J Fam Pract 3(2):163–167, 1976

This paper reports the results of a recent study of referrals in eight family practices representing urban, suburban, and rural settings in central and northern California. This study was undertaken to determine the referral/consultation patterns over a 30-day period, permit a lapse of time, and then repeat the study on the same practices during another 30-day period. This allows a comparison of referral/consultation patterns by family physicians as influenced by time, geography, practice setting, and season.

The overall referral rate was 1.6 percent of a total of 6409 hospital and office visits. No significant differences were noted among practice settings. Referring family physicians shared responsibility for patient care in a majority of referrals/consultations, thereby maintaining continuity of care. Over one half of all consultations were in the specialties of general surgery, orthopedics, obstetrics/gynecology, and urology. The results of this study are comparable to a smaller study carried out in New York State in 1971.

A seasonal difference in referral rates was noted. A total of 55 referrals occurred during the month of February, whereas only 48 referrals occurred during May, even though more patients were seen in May than in February. Corresponding referral rates for both periods reflected a higher number of referrals during February, 1.89 percent, while during May, when more patients were seen, the referral rate was 1.36 percent.

In an effort to better understand the type of consultations requested by the family physicians particpating in this study, the researchers asked them to identify each consultation/referral in one of three ways: (1) family physican maintaining full pa-

tient-care responsibility; (2) family physician and consultant sharing patient-care responsibility; or (3) consultant assuming full responsibility for care of the patient's problem requiring referral. A summary of referrals/consultations by type is shown in Table 1. It shows that the family physician maintained full responsibility 3 percent (3 of 103) of the time. In 38 percent of the instances (39 of 103), the consultant assumed full responsibility for the care of the referral problem; most of these referrals involved referral to a consultant in another community. The most frquent type of referral, 59 percent of all referrals (61 of 103), involved a team approach whereby the consultant and the family physician shared responsibility for patient care.

These data indicate that family physicians most frequently refer to general surgeons, obstetricians/gynecologists, and surgical subspecialists. Referrals by family physicians to general internists and pediatricians are relatively infrequent and are exceeded by those to subspecialists.

Table 1. *Type Referral/Consulation by Practice for Two Sample Months*

Physician	Maintained Total Responsibility		Physician and Consultant Shared Responsibility		Consultant Assumed Full Responsibility for Care of Problem Requiring Referral		Total
	February	*May*	*February*	*May*	*February*	*May*	
A	0	0	4	3	3	1	11
B	0	0	3	1	1	7	12
C	0	1	10	11	14	1	37
D	1	0	3	5	3	2	14
E	0	1	10	6	0	3	20
F	0	0	1	4	2	2	9
Totals	1	2	31	30	23	16	103

Morgan S, Folse R, D'Elia G: Referral patterns of family physicians and surgeons in a nonmetropolitan area of Illinois. J Fam Pract 8(3):587–593, 1979

Physicians in southern Illinois were surveyed to determine their referral patterns, rates, and types of problems requiring assistance. The survey involved 31 physicians in a 16-county area.

Twenty family physicians and twelve surgeons were included in the survey of physician office practices. Seven family physicians were board-certified and four were board-eligible. Two of the general surgeons had a subspecialty in thoracic surgery. Of the family physicians, eight were in solo practice, ten in small group practices, and two in large, multispecialty clinics. Six surgeons were in solo practice, two practiced in small groups, and four practiced in large, multispecialty clinics.

The decision to refer is only one method a physician may choose to handle what he/she believes to be a difficult patient problem. Ninety-seven percent of the physicians studied prefer to use other means of solving difficult problems before referring to another physician. The first response of family physicians would be to seek consultation from a physician in a specialty other than general or family practice. The responses for the surgeons were somewhat less clear-cut, although the first choice was to look to a personal library for handling difficult problems. In an effort to determine whether the solo practice arrangement encouraged the physician to rely more on his own resources and, as a corollary, if physicians in groups have more resources available, the responses were separated by practice arrangement. The choices were ranked with a value of 5 being the first choice, 4 the second, and so on, and the mean responses were calculated. The results are presented in Table 1.

Problems most frquently referred by family physicians were cardiac, orthopedic, and general surgical. Opthalmologic and neurologic problems were also among the most commonly referred problems. Neurologic, neurosurgical, and cardiac problems led the list of problems *always* referred by family physicians. Nearly 60 percent of the surgeons *always* referred neurologic, neurosurgical, and cardiac problems. Overall, more referrals and consultations were made for surgical problems than for medical, primary care, or other reasons. Table 2 displays the rank, ordering, and distribution of referrals and consultations in this study.

It appears that nonmetropolitan medical

Table 1. *Choice for Handling Difficult Problems by Specialty and Type of Practice**

| | Type of Practice | | | | | |
| | Solo | | Small Group | | Multispecialty Clinic | |
Choice	FP	GS	FP	GS	FP	GS
Consult personal library	2.63	4.66	2.20	1.00	1.00	3.33
Consult medical/hospital library	1.63	1.50	1.80	3.00	2.00	.33
Consult MD in own specialty	.38	2.00	2.10	2.00	3.00	3.33
Consult MD in other specialty	3.88	2.33	4.10	5.00	5.00	2.66
Refer	3.13	3.50	3.20	2.50	4.00	1.00

Reprinted by permission from Morgan et al: J Fam Pract, 8(3):587, 1979.
* Family physicians (FP) $N = 19$, general surgeons (GS) $N = 11$.

Table 2. *Rank Ordering and Percentage Distribution for Which Referrals or Consultations Were Sought, by Physician Specialty*

Type of Problem	Family Physicians Rank	Family Physicians Percent	General Surgeons Rank	General Surgeons Percent
Cardiac	1	13	3	9
Orthopedic	2	9	1	16
Neurologic		8	6	5
General surgical	3	8	5	6
Ophthalmologic		8		1
Psychiatric	4	6	9	1
Dermatologic		5		1
Neurosurgical	5	5		4
Urologic		5	7	4
Pediatric		4		4
Otolaryngologic	6	4	8	2
Trauma	7	3	4	7
Obstetric-gynecologic	8	3	9	1
Oncologic		2	2	10
Allergic	9	2	8	2
Internal medicine		2	9	1
Thoracic surgical		2	7	4
Hematologic	10	2		—
Colonic and rectal surgical		2		—
Vascular surgical	11	1	4	7
Diagnostic		1		—
Radiologic		0.5	6	5
Respiratory		0.5		—
Pathologic	12	0.5		—
Endocrine		0.5		—
Dental		0.5		—
Podiatric		0.5		—
Chemotherapy		—	7	4
Chemotherapy-pediatric		—	9	1
Plastic surgical		—	8	2
Burns		—	9	1
Nonmedical	10	2		1
Total	**178 responses**		**82 responses**	

Reprinted by permission from Morgan et al: J Fam Pract, 8(3):587, 1979.

practices are somewhat self-contained. This reflects the traditional view of rural medicine as more isolated than urban. The physicians in southern Illinois provide a broad range of services, perhaps a greater range than in other places where family physicians refer more frequently. Family physicians in other areas are referring more for general surgery, while these study physicians referred for more specific reasons, i.e., cardiac, orthopedic, ophthalmologic, and neurologic. Practice arrangement, size of community, and the number of other medical resources available do not appear to be the key to establishing different referral rates. Of greater importance is the fact that referrals are made through the colleague network.

Moscovice I, Shortell SM, Schwartz CW: Referral patterns of family physicians in an underserved rural area. J Fam Pract 9(4):677–682, 1979

This paper examines the rates and patterns of referral of four family physicians in an underserved rural area of Washington State. This research is part of a three-year study examining the impact of several innovations in the organization and delivery of care in the eastern portion of a county in southwestern Washington State. The area covers approximately 300 square miles, has a population of approximately 12,000 with two major towns, one having a population of 3,000 and the other 1,500. The principal industries relate to the growth of timber.

Prior to August 1977, the area had three physicians serving its approximately 12,000 residents. These physicians were 62 (Dr. A.), 57 (Dr. B.), and 57 (Dr. C.) years of age and had been practicing in the community for 33, 22, and 22 years, respectively. All three were solo general practitioners and only one of them (Dr. B.) provided obstetrical care. The area had been designated as a Critical Health Manpower Shortage Area by DHEW Region X in 1975. In August 1977, Dr. C. died, thereby making the need for new primary care providers critical. In October 1977, a NHSC physician (Dr. D.) who had completed a family practice residency began a practice in the area, as did a foreign medical graduate (Dr. E.), who essentially took over the practice of Dr. C. The foreign medical graduate had been trained as a general surgeon, but was delivering primary care in this rural area and did not have hospital privileges to perform complicated surgical procedures. The area has a small rural hospital (26 beds).

The rates and patterns of referral of the four physicians were studied during the three-month period April through June 1978. Based on previous research, each physician filled out a form for every referral to or from other physicians during the study period.

The majority of referrals made by the family physicians were for management of a particular problem outside the scope of practice of the physician. The referral rates ranged from 1.8 to 3.2 percent of all patient visits and were comparable with those previously reported.

The National Health Service Corps physician had the highest rate of referral and the foreign medical graduate had the lowest rate of referral. These results may be explained by practice building incentives as well as the ability to establish ties with the referral network.

Almost 90 percent of all referrals were initiated by the physicians. In examining characteristics of patients who initiated their own referrals, the rate of self-referral was highest (23 percent) among the elderly on Medicare. Failure of the patient to respond to treatment was listed by physicians as the reason for referral 24 percent of the time for self-referred patients as com-

Table 1. *Referrals to Specialties for All Physicians*

Specialty	Referrals	
	Number	*Percent*
Orthopedics	34	21.1
Surgery	31	19.3
Otolaryngology	17	10.6
Neurology	12	7.5
Obstetrics	8	5.0
Urology	8	5.0
Cardiology	7	4.3
Dermatology	7	4.3
Ophthalmology	6	3.6
Other	31	19.3
Totals	161	100.0

Reprinted by permission from Moscovice et al: J Fam Pract, 9(4):677, 1979.

pared to 10 percent of the time for physician referred patients.

Table 1 presents the specialty of the providers who received referrals from the four physicians during the study period. As compared with previous referral studies, these physicians refer considerably more to orthopedic specialists and considerably less to obstetricians. The former may be due to accidents associated with the extensive logging industry in the area and the latter may be due to the sizable obstet-

rical load managed by Dr. B. and Dr. D., as well as the direct use of physicians outside the area by local residents.

The fact that no referrals were received by providers in the rural area from providers outside the area indicates that the referral process goes in one direction. Local physicians refer patients to physicians whose status in the "colleague network" is higher than their own. Over one half of all referrals were to only three specialties— orthopedics, surgery, and otolaryngology.

Elliott C, Backstrom D: Referral patterns in general practice. Aus Fam Physician 1:155–156, 1972

This is probably the first actual study of referral patterns in Australian general practice. A one-month study period involved 16 participating general practitioners.

Of almost 11,000 patient visits during the month, the average referral rate for these physicians was 3.4 percent. Table 1 gives a breakdown in terms of types of referrals.

The pattern of referral varied considerably from one physician to another; e.g., four physicians referred a total of 27 obstetrics/gynecology patients, the remainder contributing only 11; one physician referred 8 to cardiologists, while two other physicians referred one each. On the other hand, referrals to general surgeons, orthopedic surgeons, E.N.T. specialists, and ophthalmologists were fairly constant by all referring physicians. A low level of referral for pediatrics, psychiatry, and allergy was noted.

Needed now are larger studies involving more physicians. It is intended to conduct

a larger survey covering the referral of sixty city and country practices in Queensland for three months.

Table 1. *Breakdown of Referrals by Specialty*

Ophthalmology (excluding for refraction only)	48
Ophthalmology for refraction only	36
Obstetrics and gynecology	41
Orthopedics	40
General surgery	39
General medicine	34
F.N.T.	34
Dermatology	16
Neurology	15
Cardiology	10
Pediatric medicine	8
Pediatric surgery	4
Psychiatry	7
Urology	7
Others	30
Total	**369**

Reprinted by permission from Elliott, Backstrom: Aus Fam Physician, 1:155, 1972.

Fischer PM, Smith SR: The nature and management of telephone utilization in a family practice setting. J Fam Pract 8(2):321–327, 1979

The telephone is an important part of medical practice in the United States. Twenty-five percent of new diseases are reported by telephone, 24 percent of all medical care contacts take place by telephone, and 12.5 percent of a physician's time is spent on the telephone. While these data indicate the importance of the telephone in medicine, there have been few studies on the telephone care system.

Four sites were selected for study representing a variety of family practice settings in Connecticut, including rural, suburban and urban sites. During a three-month study, 2120 telephone calls were logged. These included 1533 (72 percent) which were received by the receptionist staffs and 587 (28 percent) which were logged by the participating physicians.

Table 1 reports the disposition data by chief complaint for the receptionist-logged data. The telephone calls from all four sites were pooled to generate this data. Table 2 reports the chief complaint and disposition data for the physician-logged telephone calls. The 25 most common chief complaints account for 80.0 percent of all of the logged patient complaints. An

Table 1. *Disposition Data for Receptionist-Managed Calls**

	Information	Refer to non-MD	Refer to MD	Urgent Visit	Nonurgent Visit
URI	4	1	9	68	19
Fever	2	1	8	77	13
Ear pain	1	0	7	71	20
Rash	10	3	20	45	23
Flu	30	3	10	40	16
Abdominal pain	1	0	18	64	16
Nausea, vomiting	2	0	32	58	8
Back pain	2	0	19	54	25
Swollen glands	0	0	4	76	20
Skin infection	7	2	17	54	20
Headache	8	0	17	47	28
Diarrhea	11	0	36	42	11
Joint pain	10	0	3	57	30
Eye infection	0	4	11	61	25
Lumps, masses	0	0	4	42	54
Chest pain	0	0	21	58	21
Dysuria	0	0	9	73	18
High blood pressure	0	0	5	25	70
Strain, sprain	10	0	5	65	20
Question of fracture	0	0	0	89	11
Dizziness	0	0	0	78	22
Dyspnea	6	0	28	55	11
Fatigue	0	0	24	18	59
Laceration	0	0	12	88	0
Urinary frequency	0	0	19	56	25

Reprinted by permission from Fischer, Smith: J Fam Pract, 8(2):321, 1979.
* Percentages of total ($N = 1533$).

Table 2. *Chief Complaint Profile and Disposition Data for Physician-Managed Calls**

	Total	Prescription	Information	Urgent Visit	Nonurgent Visit
URI	21.6	35	35	21	9
Flu	7.5	16	60	0	5
Fever	6.0	20	48	20	11
Rash	3.9	43	35	0	22
Nausea, vomiting	3.9	48	43	9	0
Headache	3.4	20	20	40	20
Chest pain	3.2	5	26	63	5
Abdominal pain	3.2	21	32	37	11
Diarrhea	3.1	39	61	0	0
Back pain	2.7	31	44	19	6
Limb pain	2.7	31	38	25	6
Anxiety	2.2	38	31	15	15
Earache	1.7	10	20	60	10
Asthma	1.7	30	60	10	0
Constipation	1.5	44	44	0	11
Skin infection	1.5	44	56	0	0
Hematuria	1.4	0	50	38	13
Strain, sprain	1.4	13	25	50	13
Question of fracture	1.2	0	29	57	14
Eye infection	1.2	0	43	29	29
Drug reaction	1.0	50	50	0	0
Urinary Frequency	1.0	33	50	17	0
Dysuria	1.0	50	17	17	17
Laceration	.9	0	0	100	0

Reprinted by permission from Fischer, Smith: J Fam Pract, 8(2):321, 1979.
* Percentages of total ($N = 587$).

urgent visit was the most frequent disposition for only a few complaints: laceration (100 percent), ear pain (60 percent), chest pain (63 percent), question of fracture (57 percent), and strain or sprain (50 percent).

A comparison of the two disposition tables (Tables 1 and 2) show a marked difference in patient management. For the most frequent symptom, upper respiratory tract infection, disposition by the receptionist staff resulted in 87 percent of patients requiring an office visit (urgent or nonurgent). For the physician-managed telephone presentations of upper respiratory tract infection, 70 percent of all complaints were managed without an office visit. A similar difference can be seen for a wide variety of the reported complaints.

Little difference was observed between the symptoms reported by patients to the physicians as compared to those received by the receptionist staff. Physicians were more likely to use the telephone contact to treat the patient's complaint with home care advice or a prescription. Receptionists were more likely to use the telephone contact for scheduling an office visit.

Freeman TR: A study of telephone prescriptions in family medicine. J Fam Pract 10(5):857–862, 1980

Telephone prescriptions are quite common in North America and have received relatively little attention. This paper examines certain behaviors of the physician and the patient with respect to prescriptions in the office and over the telephone.

This study was carried out at the teaching unit of the Department of Family Medicine of Dalhouise University in Halifax, Nova Scotia. There were five participating practices consisting of five staff physicians, and four first-year and six second-year residents. Each physician was asked to complete a questionnaire every time a prescription was given in an office contact, over the telephone, or in any other type of contact. The questionnaire consisted of identifying data regarding the patient's age, sex, and the nature of the contact. The physician was then asked to rate each patient on a four point scale (1 = does not apply; 4 = definitely applies) for factors previously identified as being characteristic of the "problem patient." The physician also rated his feelings of positivity toward the patient. Also recorded on the questionnaire by the physician were such items as the number of drugs the patient was on, and whether the current prescription was physician or patient initiated or initiated by another physician but continued by the current one. The name of the drug prescribed, days prescribed, and number of refills were also entered.

The results indicate that patients receiving prescriptions over the telephone are demographically distinct, tend to receive large amounts of psychotropic drugs, and are more likely to be seen by their physicians as "problem patients." It was found that the psychotropic drugs were the most common class of drugs in the telephone prescription group (Table 1). Antibiotics were the largest category of office prescriptions. It was found that patients receiving a prescription by telephone were seen by their physicians in a less positive light than patients receiving an office prescription. This difference was statistically significant. Telephone prescription pa-

Table 1. *Drugs Prescribed with Respect to Location**

	Office			Telephone	
	Number	*Percent*		*Number*	*Percent*
1. Antibiotics	41	22.4	1. Psychotropics	29	27.4
2. Antihistamines/ Decongestants	22	12.0	2. Antibiotics	15	14.2
3. Psychotropics	25	13.6	3. Diuretic drugs	11	10.4
4. Miscellaneous drugs	17	9.3	4. Narcotic analgesics	11	10.4
5. Diuretic drugs	14	7.7	5. Cardiovascular drugs	9	8.5
6. Nonsteroidal anti- inflammatory drugs	12	6.6	6. Miscellaneous drugs	7	6.6
7. Gonadal hormones	11	6.0	7. Antihistamines/ Decongestants	6	5.7
8. Cardiovascular drugs	9	4.9	8. Topical steroids	3	2.9
9. Topical steroids	9	4.9	9. Bronchodilator drugs	3	2.9
10. Gastrointestinal drugs	8	4.4	10. Gonadal hormones	3	2.9

Reprinted by permission from Freeman: J Fam Pract, 10(5):857, 1980.
* These represent the ten most frequent drugs in each category. This accounts for almost 92 percent of the prescriptions issued in both locations.

tients were also perceived as (a) behaving in a more helpless and complaining way; and (b) being less cooperative in their own medical care than office prescription patients.

The results of this study suggest that the telephone contact and telephone prescrip-tion may represent a compromise in a strained physician-patient relationship. Further studies in this area could be use-fully directed toward more clearly identi-fying the habitual telephone prescription patient.

Koffman BD, Merritt K: Analysis of after-hours calls and visits in a family practice. J Fam Pract 7(6):1185–1190, 1978

The after-hours encounter is an important aspect of primary care. This study exam-ined the pattern of patient behavior after hours in a rural Ontario setting serving a mixed white and native population. The types of patients and the problem they presented were examined. By studying both calls and visits, it was possible to assess some of the interesting and unexpected factors that influence a physician's decision to see an after-hours caller.

An encounter sheet was completed by the attending physician for every patient contact. The reason for the encounter was documented using a modification of a clas-sification of illness behavior developed by McWhinney. Necessity was rated on a 5-point scale, with 1 as least necessary and 5 most necessary. This item reflected the physician's subjective impression of the need for a call or visit at that time.

During the week, there averaged less than one telephone call a night, with only one of eight occurring after midnight. The weekends saw nine calls on the average. Approximately three out of every five calls and visits were from females. Almost two thirds of the calls and visits came on the weekends. Thirty-one percent of the calls and 37 percent of the visits were for acute infections. Only eight percent of the calls and five percent of the visits were made for primarily psychosocial problems. Acute medical problems made up the bulk of the after-hours work. Almost half the contacts

Table 1. *Characteristics of Problems in Off-Hours Calls and Visits*

		Calls Total* (Percent)	Visits Total† (Percent)
Nature of Problem			
New		70	76
Continuing		30	24
		100	100
Problem Content			
Trauma		19	25
Acute Infection		31	37
Acute Organic		19	17
Chronic Organic		19	7
Psychosocial		8	5
Obstetric		10	7
Other		3	2
		100	100
Reason for Contact			
Limit of Tolerance		59	75
Limit of Anxiety		30	17
Signal Presentation		4	—
No Illness		3	3
Other		4	5
		100	100
Necessity	1–2	16	11
	3	37	29
	4	28	31
	5	19	29
		100	100

Reprinted by permission from Koffman, Merritt: J Fam Pract, 7(6):1185, 1978.
* N = 83.
† N = 59.

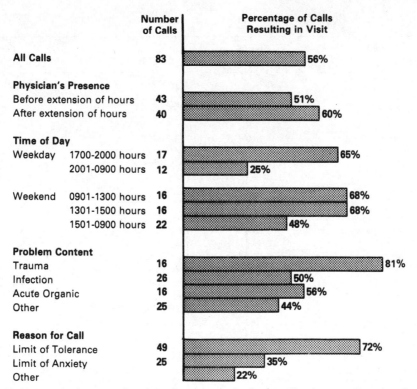

	Number of Calls	Percentage of Calls Resulting in Visit
All Calls	83	56%
Physician's Presence		
Before extension of hours	43	51%
After extension of hours	40	60%
Time of Day		
Weekday 1700-2000 hours	17	65%
2001-0900 hours	12	25%
Weekend 0901-1300 hours	16	68%
1301-1500 hours	16	68%
1501-0900 hours	22	48%
Problem Content		
Trauma	16	81%
Infection	26	50%
Acute Organic	16	56%
Other	25	44%
Reason for Call		
Limit of Tolerance	49	72%
Limit of Anxiety	25	35%
Other		22%

Fig. 1. The impact of various factors on whether a caller is seen. (Reprinted by permission from Koffman, Merritt: J Fam Pract, 7(6):1185, 1978.)

were rated 4 or 5 on the necessity scale. Table 1 summarizes the characteristics of after-hours calls and visits.

Figure 1 illustrates the relationships between several factors and the physician's decision to follow a telephone call with a visit. Most likely to result in a visit were high necessity calls. A patient at the limit of his tolerance of symptoms or presenting with trauma was very likely to be seen.

Calls placed after 12 PM on a weeknight had less chance of being seen. The sex of the patient did not prove to be an important factor.

The decision to see a patient after a telephone call is received is influenced by many factors. Whether or not the physician is at the office is not a factor. Time of the call, problem type, reason for the call, and perceived necessity all play a role.

Curtis P, Talbot A: The after-hours call in family practice. J Fam Pract 9(5):901–909, 1979

Patient care after hours continues to be an important part of the work of family physicians, in spite of the trend toward increasing Emergency Room utilization. In this paper the literature concerning after-hours care in family practice is reviewed in terms of definition, demography, utilization, morbidity, and patient stereotypes.

Table 1. *Morbidity Profile of After-Hours Contacts (rank order of frequency)*

Symptom	Percent of Total	Problem	Percent of Total
Fever	12.0	Acute URI	10.2
Skin wounds	6.1	No diagnosis made	5.8
Pain, swelling, injury of leg	6.0	Viral infection	4.3
Sore throat	5.8	Laceration/wound	3.3
Nausea and vomiting	5.7	Intestinal infection	3.3
Abdominal pain	5.5	Anxiety neurosis	3.2
Cough	4.4	Acute otitis media	3.0
Earache	4.1	Bruise/contusion	2.6
Cold	4.0	Asthma	2.2
Headache	4.0	Cystitis/UTI	2.2
Pain, swelling, injury of arm	3.8	Influenza	1.9
Allergic skin reaction	3.6	Abdominal pain	1.9
Entry of "None"	3.4	Advice and health instruction	1.6
Diarrhea	3.0	Adverse effects of drugs	1.3
Back pain	2.9	Strep throat	1.2
Medication	2.9	Insect bites and stings	1.2
Other respiratory problem	2.7	Fever, cause unknown	1.1
Chest pain	2.7	Prescription problem	1.1
Pain, swelling, injury of face	2.3	Low back pain	1.1
Nasal congestion	2.1	Depression	1.0
Total number of symptoms recorded: 5,608; 1.3 symptom per contact.		Total number of problems recorded: 4,700; 1 problem per contact.	

Reprinted by permission from Curtis, Talbot: J Fam Pract, 9(5):901, 1979.

In the Family Practice Residency Program of the University of North Carolina, 4760 after-hours calls were recorded over two years by residents and faculty physicians. Seventy-two percent of the calls were handled purely on the telephone with little variation for patient age groups. The overall call rate was 474 calls per 1000 patients per year. Fever and skin wounds were the most frequent symptoms recorded, and respiratory tract infections, minor trauma, and anxiety were the commonest diagnoses. Acute respiratory tract infections and minor trauma accounted for 32 percent of all the diagnoses. Asthma appeared to be the most important medical condition presenting relatively frequently after hours. Behavioral and psychiatric problems were identified in 6 percent of all the contacts. The rank order of frequency of symptoms and diagnostic problems is shown in Table 1.

The physicians handled 72 percent of the 4760 contacts using telephone consultation alone. The remaining 28 percent were seen either in the Family Practice Center (16 percent), in the Emergency Room (8 percent), or sometimes in other settings (4 percent). The percentage of calls handled strictly on the telephone varied only moderately between patient age groups; from 67 percent of calls in the 15 to 24 years age category to 75 percent in the 0 to 4 years age category. There was, however, considerable variation between physicians in the extent to which calls were handled exclusively by telephone. The percentage of calls handled by "telephone care" ranged from 60 percent to 93 percent for individual physicians.

Thirteen percent of the contacts engendered anger or frustration in the physician. A survey of patients calling after hours demonstrated a lack of congruence between physician and patient concerning the main reason for the call in over 30 percent of contacts.

Matthews WC, Crum HP, Andrus LH: Doctor's Other Office, an alternative to the emergency room. J Fam Pract 4(5):943–945, 1977

Doctor's Other Office is a group of ten family physicians which offers after-hours and weekend health care to noncritical patients who might otherwise go to a hospital Emergency Room, even though their medical problems do not require its expensive, elaborate facilities. The primary purpose of Doctor's Other Office is to provide continuous care to the member physicians' regular patients for noncritical medical emergencies after hours, that is, situations that need immediate attention but do not require Emergency Room care.

In practice, patients who are treated include some who cannot and do not wish to contact their regular doctor after hours; many, such as transients and newcomers, who have no regular doctor; those who find doctors' regular office hours inconvenient or impossible; and some who simply do not wish to wait for an appointment during regular hours. Cost to the patient is about one half what the same treatment would cost in an Emergency Room because there is no charge for the Emergency *Room*.

One of the family physicians rents his office to the corporation for these off-hours. A physician is present every weekday evening from 7 to 11 PM and weekends and holidays from 10 AM to 11 PM. A receptionist assists the physician on duty during these hours by taking phone calls, registering patients, taking temperatures, "chaperoning" gynecological examinations, and preparing examination rooms. She also maintains financial records, completes insurance forms, and types medical reports. On weekends and holidays, when patient loads tend to be heavier, a nurse is present from 10 AM to 6 PM. The history, physical examination, and treatment program are recorded by the physician on duty and a copy is sent to the patient's own physician.

After 11 PM calls are infrequent, so an answering service refers them to the home phone of the physician on call that evening. Most of these late calls can be handled over the telephone. Those that cannot be so easily resolved are usually of a truly emergent nature and require ER facilities or hospitalization.

Experience has shown that the Doctor's Other Office is a viable alternative to the expensive, inappropriate, and overutilized ER for the care of most nonemergent patient needs after-hours and on weekends. Because the office is located in the area served by the physician members, and because of the effective patient record reporting system, care has continuity and prevents the fragmentation caused by the ER "one-shot" care of episodic illnesses. The Doctor's Other Office presents an efficient method of handling patients at odd hours. The record system provides rapid information to the patient's family physician, and an efficient, predetermined system of referral and hospitalization has been worked out by each physician for his own patients.

Warburton SW Jr, Sadler GR, Eikenberry EF: House call patterns of New Jersey family physicians. J Fam Pract 4(5):933–938, 1977

This paper reports the results of a study of house call attitudes and practice patterns of New Jersey family physicians. The 290 participating physicians (41 percent of the total membership) were considered to be a representative sample of the New Jersey Academy of Family Physicians.

House calls were offered by 82 percent of the 290 physicians in the sample; no difference was noted between rural and urban or between younger and older physicians. The average number of house calls per week was 6.05: 4.71 scheduled, and 1.34 emergency. Patients who were elderly, homebound, had suffered a stroke, had cancer or congestive heart failure made up the majority of those receiving house calls. This survey also showed that many of the physicians who stated that they do not "offer" house calls to their patients, did in fact perform them.

The physicians were asked to review a list of medical problems and indicate those which they perceived to be appropriate reasons for making a house call. Their responses are presented in Table 1, along with the frequency with which they listed them as reasons for their last three house calls. There appeared to be a direct relationship between these two variables.

In order to gain a further insight into the physicians' attitude toward nonmedical problems which might necessitate a house call, they were also asked whether "social (nonmedical) factors" ever necessitated a house call. Twenty-four percent (69) of the sample responded either "moderately often" or "frequently." Additional questions aimed at better defining the physicians' general attitude concerning house calls and the physicians' responses to these questions are shown in Table 2.

Table 1. *Medical Problems Considered To Be Appropriate for House Calls*

Problem	Reporting Appropriate*		Reported Among Reasons† for Last 3 House Calls	
	Number	*Percent*	*Number*	*Percent*
1. Death pronouncement	245	84	30	4
2. Stroke	187	64	63	8.5
3. Cancer	162	56	35	5
4. Congestive heart failure	156	54	53	7
5. Emotional problems/family crisis	119	41	18	2
6. Chronic lung disease	116	40	16	2
7. Pneumonia	113	39	25	3
8. Chest pain	113	39	16	2
9. High temperature (104F or more)	104	36	10	1
10. Shortness of breath	97	34	0	0
11. Vomiting	71	24	6	0.8
12. Complications of pregnancy/delivery	57	20	0	0
13. Trauma	43	15	17	2

Reprinted by permission from Warburton et al: J Fam Pract, 4(5):933, 1977.
* N = 290.
† N = 739.

Table 2. *Physicians' Attitudes Concerning House Calls*

Attitude	Strongly Disagree or Disagree		Neutral		Strongly Agree or Agree	
	Number	*Percent*	*Number*	*Percent*	*Number*	*Percent*
1. Important part of comprehensive continuing care	49	(17)	28	(10)	211	(73)
2. Family relationship knowledge just as well obtained in office	133	(46)	35	(12)	107	(37)
3. Only for acute crisis care	169	(58)	26	(9)	89	(31)
4. Keep infectious disease out of office	186	(64)	50	(18)	52	(18)
5. Nuisance and waste of time	113	(39)	33	(11)	140	(48)
6. Moneymaking part of practice	242	(83)	26	(9)	30	(7)
7. Number will increase over 5 years	214	(74)	37	(13)	31	(11)
8. Physician's prerogative to make unsolicited house calls	172	(59)	35	(12)	77	(27)

Reprinted by permission from Warburton et al: J Fam Pract, 4(5):933, 1977.
N = 290. Unanswered questions will cause some totals to be less than 100 percent.

Taylor RB, Burdette JA, Camp L, Edwards J: Purpose of the medical encounter: Identification and influence on process and outcome in 200 encounters in a model family practice center. J Fam Pract 10(3):495–500, 1980

This paper describes a study of various aspects of the covert agendas that may or may not be addressed during the physician-patient encounter. The study concerned two questions: Why does the patient come to the physician? And, how does patient-physician agreement as to the primary purpose affect the process and outcome of the medical encounter?

Questionnaires were completed by patients and resident or faculty physicians immediately following medical encounters at the Bowman Gray School of Medicine Family Practice Center. Patient-physician dyads to be questioned were selected on a random basis and were first informed of their selection when presented with questionnaires following the visit.

Separate interviews of patients and physicians following 200 medical encounters revealed a preponderance of visits for continuing care, a paucity of visits for social and emotional problems, and a number of visits in which "concern" as the patient's primary purpose was misperceived by the physician. Table 1 lists the distribution of encounter purpose as stated by patient and physician. According to patients, most visits (46.5 percent) were for continuing health care, including health maintenance, follow-up visit, prenatal care, and prescription refills.

Physician and patient were considered in concordance when both indicated the same category as their single choice reflecting the primary purpose of the visit. The

Table 1. *Distribution: Purpose of the Medical Encounter as Perceived by Patient and Physician*

Purpose	Patient Perception	Physician Perception
Continuing care	91	96
Administrative purpose	5	6
Physical problem	53	68
Emotional problem	7	6
Social problem	1	4
Concern or worry	41	17

Reprinted by permission from Taylor, Burdette et al: J Fam Pract, 10(3):495, 1980.

Table 2. *Patient-Physician Concordance of Primary Purpose of Encounter*

	Cases	Percent
Concordance	137	69.5
Nonconcordance	60	30.5

Reprinted by permission from Taylor, Burdette et al: J Fam Pract, 10(3):495, 1980.

visit purpose was compared with education level of the patient or with physician perception of the patient's intended compliance. In both concordance and nonconcordance groups, physicians underestimated both patient satisfaction with the encounters and intended compliance.

The physician and patient may have different perceptions of the purpose of the visit—differing agendas, priorities, and objectives. Early open discussion of the primary purpose of the visit can prevent the misperceptions of purpose revealed in this study, amounting to more than 30 percent of encounters. In many instances, such an early transaction will allow the physician to focus appropriately on a concern or psychosocial problem rather than searching for an elusive, and perhaps nonexistent, physical disease.

total numbers of patient-physician dyads in concordance and non-concordance are listed in Table 2.

There was no statistically significant relationship when agreement (or lack of agreement) between patient and physician as to the purpose of the encounter was compared with patient age and sex, number of previous visits of the patient to the physician, and subsequent patient-physician agreement as to the diagnosis, prognosis, therapy, and satisfaction. There was also no statistically significant relationship when patient-physician concordance as to

Hyatt JD: Perceptions of the family physician by patients and family physicians. J Fam Pract 10(2):295–300, 1980

The professional definition of the family physician has not been based on research that considers both patient and family physician perceptions. This study explores whether patients and family physicians agree or disagree in their perceptions and expectations of the family physician. Results that identify areas of conflict can be used to improve the family physician-patient relationship and family practice.

Questionnaire responses from 86 family physicians and 287 patients from ten family practices in Los Angeles were analyzed

to compare their attitudes, perceptions, and expectations of the family physician. Both groups agreed the family physician could handle most medical problems (including hospital care), should provide continuity, should emphasize preventive medicine, and should be caring. The physician's manner and skill were felt equally important. Family physician and patient expectations conflicted in four major areas: referral, the handling of emotional problems, concern with and care of family, and the issue of autonomy.

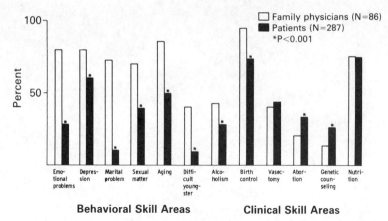

Fig. 1. Problem areas a family physician should handle *without referral,* assessed by family physicians and patients. (Reprinted by permission from Hyatt: J Fam Pract, 10(2):295, 1980.)

Almost 50 percent of the patients see their family physician for all medical care, and only 16.5 percent also have an obstetrician-gynecologist. Seventy-one percent of the other adults at home also see the same family physician, ranging from almost 90 percent in a prepaid multispecialty group to 6 percent in the newest solo practice.

Over 90 percent of patients and physicians agree that a family physician (1) could handle most medical problems; (2) should care for the patient who is hospitalized; and, importantly, (3) should encourage a patient to take steps to preserve his health, such as to stop smoking, exercise, and lose weight. Significant differences exist, however, when assessing specific skills a family physician might handle without referral, especially regarding most emotional and behavioral matters which patients accept much less often than physicians (Figure 1). More agreement exists over certain clinical skills such as vasectomy, nutrition, genetic counseling, drug abuse, and abortion.

Disagreement exists within the power relationship between patients and physicians. Compared to only 14 percent of the family physicians, 38 percent of the patients feel the doctor should not try to pressure the patient who chooses not to accept the physician's advice (P < 0.005). More patients, 36 percent, insist that a patient should be seen by his family physician even though he/she may be short of time; only 14 percent of the physicians strongly agree (P < 0.005). More than 70 percent of the physicians feel a patient prefers to be told what to do, while only half of the patients would agree (P < 0.001). Ninetenths of the physicians believe in using their own discretion in deciding how much is good to tell a patient about his illness, but over half of the patients disapprove. Only when a patient is seriously ill do almost all patients agree with the family physician's role to help the family adjust.

By including both physicians and patients in the present study, concordant and conflicting views of the family physician can be identified. Intervention designed to change perceptions and improve patient satisfaction could be directed to two areas: patient education about family physicians and physician education to improve physician attitudes and conduct. In this way, family practice will develop by taking into account the perceptions and expectations of its patients.

SECTION TWO
Graduate Education in Family Practice

COMMENTARY

THE papers and abstracts in this section deal with the development of graduate education programs in family practice over the last ten years. Particular attention is focused upon graduate education in the United States, but a number of papers provide comparative views of similar training programs in Canada, England, Scotland, Australia, and New Zealand. Together these papers provide a collective view of energetic progress over the last ten years to formally train family physicians in structured educational programs beyond medical school.

There are more similarities than differences in the objectives and content of graduate training for family practice among the various countries represented here. It is of interest, however, that widely divergent approaches are taken to the organizational structures for graduate training. For example, continuity of care by residents over a full three years of training is a fundamental requirement of family practice residency programs in the United States, whereas continuity of care is relatively de-emphasized in the training of family physicians in the other countries. There is, as yet, no evidence whereby the outcomes of these various training systems can be compared in terms of the knowledge, skills, attitudes, and performance of the graduates of these different kinds of programs.

Many of the issues involved in providing effective teaching and learning in specific curricular areas are common to graduate programs regardless of their organizational structure. Of special interest in this respect are papers which deal with teaching strategies in pediatrics, obstetrics-gynecology, human sexuality, geriatrics, medical ethics, sports medicine, office surgery, behavioral science, and community medicine.

The content and quality of graduate teaching clearly has much to do with the extent and ways in which family practice will contribute to each country's health care system. There is already solid evidence that the developments in graduate education for family practice during the 1970s are meeting public expectations and societal needs for the primary health care of families. The closing paper of this section describes important benchmarks of progress of family practice residencies in the United States over the last ten years, and the final abstract summarizes some of the findings of recent regional and national graduate followup studies involving more than 3,000 graduates of these programs.

Graduate Education in Family Practice*

Thomas L. Leaman, John P. Geyman, Thomas C. Brown

As noted previously, there are organized family practice programs in over three quarters of the medical schools in the United States and in all of the medical schools in Canada at the present time. Each of these programs has developed, or is in the process of developing, residency training programs in family practice.

The development of a family practice residency program in a university setting involves a particular set of problems and opportunities not encountered in community hospital settings. A number of basic issues must be addressed, such as the clinical role of the department in the medical school, its relationship to other clinical departments and to residency programs in other specialities, the mechanisms for inpatient care and for teaching by family practice faculty and residents, and the relationship to affiliated community hospitals.

Three well-established and respected departments, which reflect different approaches to the above-mentioned kinds of issues, have been selected for the present study. They are: (1) the University of Minnesota, (2) the Medical University of South Carolina, and (3) the Medical College of Virginia. During the authors' site visits to each institution, discussions were held with departmental faculty and residents, chairmen of other departments, the Dean of the medical school, and others involved with the family practice residency program. All involved facilities were visited, methods of teaching, patient care, and administration were discussed, and related written materials were reviewed.

This report will present sequentially the three programs, beginning with an overview of the resources and programs of each department, followed by a description of the highlights of each department's residency training programs, and educa-

tional and administrative approaches. Subsequent discussion will focus on the commonalities and differences among the three programs.

University of Minnesota

Introduction and Overview

A precipitous decline in the number of family physicians serving the state, particularly in rural areas, became apparent in the early 1960s. In response to this, the University of Minnesota began feasibility studies for a program in family practice in 1966. A program was instituted as a division of the Department of Internal Medicine in 1969. A mandate from the state legislature that year, accompanied by substantial funding, resulted in the establishment of the Department of Family Practice and Community Health in 1972. The Department has grown rapidly since then to become the largest family medicine department (in numbers of faculty and residents) in the United States today.

The faculty of the Department has been recruited from a variety of disciplines. Of the 30 full-time faculty, 21 are physicians (17 family physicians, 1 internist, 2 pediatricians, 1 psychiatrist); 2 are educational psychologists; 1 is a clinical psychologist; 1 a specialist in business administration; 1 a family counselor; 2 are communication specialists; 1 is a psychologist; and 1 a research fellow. Also, there are 103 part-time faculty members from all the major disciplines of medicine. The volunteer

* Reprinted by permission from *The Journal of Family Practice*, 5(1):47–61, 1977.

clinical faculty consists of 442 physicians in the state who participate in the program as preceptors. These faculty serve 215 residents and a medical school with a class of approximately 250 which, during 1976–1977, had 140 of the third and fourth year students tracking in family practice.

UNDERGRADUATE LEVEL. The Department conducts teaching programs for medical students at three levels. At the first-year level, it is responsible for a large part of the instruction in the "Introduction to Clinical Medicine" course. This course is directed toward history-taking, interview techniques, physical examination, and diagnosis. Second year students take a required preceptorship in a family physician's office in the Twin Cities area for a series of 16 half-day sessions. The Department also contributes to the "Patient Assessment and Advanced Interviewing" course conducted during the students' "Introduction to General Psychiatry." Third and fourth year students may participate in the "Rural Physician Associate Program" which provides a one-year elective experience in rural family practice. Students tracking in family medicine take a six-week preceptorship with a family physician, as well as elective courses or rotations on such subjects as Management Concepts, Family Dynamics, Clinical Laboratory, Surgery for Family Practice, Alcohol and Drug Abuse, Medical Ethics, and Independent Study. Further, the Department provides advisors for all of the students who are tracking in family practice.

GRADUATE LEVEL. A three-year family practice residency teaching program is conducted in a variety of settings. Six model family practice clinics have been established in conjunction with the University Hospital and six community hospitals in the Twin Cities area, to form the University of Minnesota Affiliated Hospitals Residency Training Program in Family Practice and Community Health (the Affiliated Program). In addition to the Affil-

iated Program, the two county hospitals in the Twin Cities area (Hennepin County General Hospital and St. Paul Ramsey Hospital) also offer three-year graduate training programs in family medicine. The county hospital programs are academically related to the Department of Family Practice and Community Health, and their faculty members are part of the Departmental faculty, although the programs are administered separately. A new training program in family medicine at the University of Minnesota-Duluth Medical School holds a similar relationship. As of July 1, 1976, there were 215 family practice residents in the entire residency system, which consisted of 131 in the Affiliated Program, 61 in the two county programs, and 23 in Duluth.

POSTGRADUATE LEVEL. An annual one-week "Family Practice Refresher" course is offered, which attracts over 200 physicians each year. A variety of shorter courses is also offered. The Department conducts a unique Master of Science Program in Family Practice and Community Health. This academic degree program is available for residents wishing future training in areas of teaching, research, administration, or political science. As of July 1, 1976, there were 22 students enrolled in the Program, all of whom were family practice residents.

Description of the Affiliated Program

The Department of Family Practice and Community Health decided early to develop a cohesive, centrally located program involving the University Hospital and six community hospitals within a 25-mile radius in the Twin Cities area. This decision was based on an interest in maximizing university support and responsibility. Table 1 presents an overview of the component units of the Affiliated Program.

The close professional relationship between the Departmental faculty and the af-

Table 1. *The University of Minnesota Affiliated Hospitals Residency Training Program in Family Practice and Community Health**

Family Practice Center	Hospital	Number of Residents	Year Started
Bethesda Family Physicians	Bethesda Hospital	24	1971
Hazel Park Family Practice Center	St. John's Hospital	18	1972
Smiley's Point Clinic	Fairview/St. Mary's Hospital	30	1971
St. Louis Park Medical Center	Methodist Hospital	18	1971
North Memorial Family Practice Clinic	North Memorial Hospital	23	1972
University Family Practice Clinic	University Hospital and Affiliated Hospitals	18	1971

* All of the units in the Affiliated Program are located in Minneapolis or St. Paul within a 30-minute radius of the University.

filiated community units permits the graduate training program to emphasize community experience and service as well as academic learning. The six family practice clinics provide the future family physician with a representative model of group practice in an urban setting and an insight into a team-oriented approach to primary care. Residents are associated with one of the six units for the full three years of their specialty training. Each clinic provides a unique experience of ambulatory care, depending on the ethnicity, age, and income levels of its surrounding community. In addition to ambulatory care experience, each unit is designed to present a complete, well-balanced, core curriculum for the development of the basic primary care requisites: obstetrics/gynecology, internal medicine, surgery, pediatrics, emergency and behavioral medicine.

Some of the community hospitals in the Affiliated Program previously conducted rotating internships prior to developing family practice residency training. None of these hospitals presently offers other specialty residency training, although obstetrics/gynecology and surgical residents from the University rotate through some of the hospitals. The following further describes each of the six residency units.

BETHESDA LUTHERAN HOSPITAL. This private, 300-bed, general hospital is located near the state capitol in St. Paul. The Bethesda Family Physicians Clinic is located in a large suite of offices in a modern professional building nearby, with internal access to the hospital. The clinic includes 12 examination rooms, a minor surgery and orthopedics room, a conference room, video-tape facilities, and an x-ray unit, and its support areas. The hospital has both coronary and intensive care units, a fully staffed Emergency Room, and a new, 15-bed crisis intervention center.

ST. JOHN'S HOSPITAL. This 400-bed, community-based hospital is located on the east side of St. Paul. The hospital has a full range of facilities available, including a large, chemical-dependent treatment center. Over half the members of the active medical staff are family physicians, who provide 85 percent of the hospital admissions. The associated Hazel Park Family Practice Center is located 2½ miles away and draws its patient population from the surrounding middle-class neighborhood. The clinic building was once a neighborhood grocery store but has been totally remodeled to provide modern, efficient facilities. This unit is the only one in the Program in which the Unit Director's practice was converted to a teaching practice. It is interesting to note that 75 percent of this physician's practice remains with the teaching program.

FAIRVIEW AND ST. MARY'S HOSPITALS. Located across the Mississippi River from the University of Minnesota, these are two private hospitals, with a combined capacity of 908 beds. They are well equipped and well staffed, with 523 physicians, including both family physicians and a full range of other specialists. Fairview Hospital is particularly active in social service, adolescent crisis, geriatric inpatient, and orthopedic follow-up. St. Mary's Hospital is particularly active in cardiac rehabilitation, chemical dependency, and a mental health and drug treatment community outreach program. The Family Practice Center is located across the street from its affiliated hospitals in a Victorian building—a community landmark—and is known as Smiley's Point Clinic. The Center offers a program in gerontology, which provides health care to senior citizens in the neighborhood, and also services a school health service for students of a nearby liberal arts college.

METHODIST HOSPITAL. This private, 470-bed hospital is located in a western suburb of Minneapolis. This hospital contains complete facilities and, since 1975, has been designated as a regional cancer center. Its Family Practice Center has been located at the St. Louis Park Medical Center, one mile away. This is a large, multiple-specialty clinic with 90 physicians. Patient population is drawn from the surrounding suburban area and is largely young and middle class. Increasing administrative and conceptual difficulties between the family practice group and the large multidisciplinary group have resulted in a reassessment of this location. Thus, as of July 1977, this unit will relocate to the neighboring community but will continue its relationship with Methodist Hospital.

NORTH MEMORIAL HOSPITAL. This private, nonprofit hospital, with 550 beds, is located in northern Minneapolis. The hospital has several unique features which add to its strength as a family practice training center. These include an unusually busy Emergency Room, an obstetric service that averages nearly 200 deliveries a month, a special care nursery for premature or severely ill newborns, and a 35-bed acute psychiatric and crisis intervention center. North Memorial's Family Practice Center is located about two miles from the hospital. Recently it has been remodeled to provide up-to-date facilities, including x-ray and laboratory capabilities.

THE UNIVERSITY OF MINNESOTA HOSPITAL. This hospital provides complete secondary and tertiary health-care facilities. Some of the usual family practice resident rotations, such as general internal medicine, are not available in this setting, and residents have access to a number of other hospitals in the Twin Cities area. The University Family Practice Center is located on the campus. The current space available is quite compact, but a greatly enlarged family practice area is under construction. The majority of patients seen at the Center are neighborhood residents who live within a one-mile radius of the University. Additional patients include faculty and students from the University.

Common Educational Approaches

While each unit of the Affiliated Program is uniquely designed to best fit its particular cadre of residents, Unit Director, and affiliated hospital and community setting, the administrative structure and many educational aspects are common to all units. The common educational goals of the Affiliated Program are: (1) to produce family physicians able and willing to provide comprehensive and continuous medical care within the context of the patient's family and community, and (2) to produce family physicians who will locate to the geographical areas of need within the area of responsibility of this Program.

Curricular objectives and program standards are being derived from these goals and, presently, a detailed set of core curricular objectives, which define the minimum competencies expected of all residents, is being completed and piloted in two of the affiliated units. Also, the Affiliated Program is presently involved in the development and implementation of a common set of standards and policies applicable to all units of the Program.

The "typical" curriculum in the Affiliated Program includes eight months of internal medicine, four months of pediatrics, four months of obstetrics/gynecology, three and a half months of surgery, one month of emergency medicine, two months of orthopedics, one month of otolaryngology, two months of neurology, two months of psychiatry, one month of community health, and six months of electives. Each unit, however, has instituted a number of variations to meet particular needs and opportunities. These differences allow the program to fit into a wide range of community settings and meet a variety of resident and faculty needs.

All the units of the Affiliated Program use the University's resources extensively. All residents are required to take the same courses in behavioral science, business management, and research which are offered predominantly by university-based faculty and are taught at the University campus. Required courses cover such topics as Communications, Psychosomatic Medicine, Dynamics of Marriage and Family, Quantitative Methods, Practice Management, and Community Health.

As part of the required behavioral science teaching program, all residents throughout the Affiliated Program are recorded on video tape with a patient on two occasions during the first year. The taped interaction is then reviewed and critiqued by a group which includes the respective resident, faculty members, practicing family physicians, and a behavioral scientist. Immediate feedback and written evaluations are subsequently provided to the residents.

Family Practice Grand Rounds are held at the University on a weekly basis for all residents, and facilitate a multidisciplinary approach to common clinical problems encountered in family practice.

The Affiliated Program uses a series of evaluational systems. Each part of this series is designed for data collection to assist in making decisions based on all available information. The decision-maker may be a resident concerned about his or her own strengths and weaknesses, or a Unit Director asking about a Unit's program, or a course instructor concerned about teaching effectiveness, or the Program Director concerned about where best to place funds to meet overall needs of the Affiliated Program. To collect information to help answer such questions and make subsequent decisions, the Affiliated Program uses a series of evaluational systems including: (1) a periodic internal review, (2) a criterion-referenced system, (3) a norm-referenced system, and (4) special forms of evaluation (not regularly scheduled), including an interviewing checklist, resident profile, chart audit, and special project evaluation.

The periodic internal review seeks information from a wide variety of sources about the conduct of the entire program, including administration, residents, faculty, and patients. The results of these reviews are examined and used as a basis for making appropriate changes in the Program. The criterion-referenced system, currently in the developmental stage, compares residents' and teachers' abilities to well-defined, expected competencies. The norm-referenced system compares residents, teachers, and services to other residents at the same level, to other teachers, and to other services. Chart audit is used as an evaluational strategy as well as an educational tool, providing residents with immediate feedback on their record-keeping skills and decision-making abilities. Much emphasis is placed on chart audit throughout the Affiliated Program, and regular audit conferences are held. One unit requires precepting family physicians to audit every chart in the Family Practice Center on a daily basis.

Emphasis has been placed on data retrieval in all of the Family Practice Centers. In four centers, the data retrieval is automated and tied to the billing system, which is able to provide regular reports, the age/sex profile, the clinical problem register, the longitudinal patient care report, and a category analysis of problems encountered. Data are provided both for the practice as a whole and for each individual provider. The system has practical applications in management, program evaluation, resident education, and clinical research.

Administrative Aspects

The Chairman of the Department of Family Practice and Community Health is the Program Director of the Affiliated Program. He is responsible for the conduct of the Program, accountable to the accrediting agency and to sources of programmatic funding, and holds the final authority for making decisions relative to the conduct of the Program. With a program of this size and complexity, no single individual can personally plan, implement, and evaluate all the many aspects of this multifaceted program. Thus, while the entire faculty is responsible for the educational aspects, the Department's Graduate Education Committee, which consists of the Program Director, Unit Directors, and other faculty, proposes policies and programmatic guidelines for the Affiliated Program. Also, the Department has identified faculty members with specific administrative roles; these individuals relate with the Program Director in implementing approved policies and guidelines.

Application and selection procedures for new residents are centrally coordinated. A single NIRMP matching number is used throughout the system, and applicants are then internally matched to their desired unit through negotiations of the Program Director and Unit Directors. To date, interview visits are scheduled for all resident applicants so that each may be interviewed in any of the six units of the Program in which they have an interest. Preference is accorded to residents from Minnesota or with Minnesota ties.

Financial support for the Affiliated Program comes from state appropriations, the affiliated hospitals, federal funds, and clinic-generated monies from patient care. The Program Director determines the allocations of these funds with input from the Budget Committee composed of Unit Directors, hospital representatives, medical school representatives, and others. A nonprofit professional corporation has been established at each unit to provide a mechanism for handling patient-generated income.

The annual budget for all programs related to the Department of Family Practice is about $7 million. In the first few years the state funding was provided for both the Department and the Graduate Program on a special appropriation's basis, but as of 1976–1977, the Department funds have been incorporated into the annual budget for the School of Medicine. The annual budget for the Affiliated Program is in excess of $4 million per year.

The following analysis represents the approximate contributions to total costs of the Affiliated Program during the years 1973–1976: one third from state funds, one third from patient care income, one sixth from hospital contributions, and one sixth from federal grants.

It is estimated that the total cost per resident is approximately $33,000 per year. With this in mind, state funding was provided on the basis of $15,000 per resident per year during 1975–1976, when there were 100 residents enrolled in the Program. However, this level of funding was held constant during the 1976–1977 year, when there were 131 residents enrolled, so that capitation per resident was substantially reduced. Further, since the termination of a 2¼-year Department of Health, Education, and Welfare grant as of July 1976, no federal funds have been available to support the Program. Efforts to provide adequate funding in light of these decreases include an increase in each affiliated hospital's contribution to a level of $6,000 per year for each resident in its unit. Also, it is anticipated that greater efficiencies in patient care and closer scrutiny of indirect costs now being allocated to each Family Practice Clinic can increase the proportion of funding from patient care revenue to approximately 40 percent of total Program cost. While these efforts have maintained the Program for the past year, federal funding is necessary and has been applied for.

Comment

The Department of Family Practice and Community Health is now recognized and respected as a major clinical department in the School of Medicine. Effective liaison with other departments has been established, and the contribution to the teaching of medical students is substantial. The Department's residency programs are attracting a large number of qualified applicants. The affiliated hospitals are convinced that their residency programs are contributing to improvements in the quality of patient care and the continuing medical education of their staff.

Further, there is every evidence that the state's needs are being effectively addressed by this Department's coordinated efforts. The proportion of graduating medical students from the University of Minnesota who choose family practice residencies is impressive. In 1977, 28 percent of the graduating medical students matched with family practice residency training programs. During the past three years, the two major fields selected by medical school graduates from the University of Minnesota were family practice and internal medicine. A preliminary estimate in 1972 suggested that the State of Minnesota would require 125 new family physician graduates each year for the next ten years to meet its needs. It is predicted that there will be a total of 72 physicians in each year of the residency training programs in Minnesota. This growth in programs clearly represents an effective response to the state's needs for graduate training in family practice.

An excellent record has been demonstrated by program graduates. Of 239 former residents in family practice residency programs affiliated with the University of Minnesota, 168 (70 percent) are now in private practice; of these, 110 (65 percent) practice in Minnesota and an additional 25 (15 percent) are in practice in the surrounding region (Dakotas, Iowa, and Wisconsin); 19 have changed specialties; two have entered academic medicine; and the remaining are primarily in the military or public service.

The most pressing problems affecting the continued development of the Department are in three areas. First, faculty recruitment continues to be a challenging problem, as in many other family medicine departments. The difficulty is in the identification, recruitment, and development of experienced family physicians with interest and skill in teaching. Secondly, the Department is heavily dependent upon the continued flow of a high level of state funding. Any reduction of this level could have a major impact on the Department's efforts and effectiveness. Thirdly, while much progress has been made in the development of mutually productive interrelationships between the University and its affiliated community hospitals, further sharing and cooperative efforts in teaching, quality control, and research remain to be developed. In particular, the affiliated relationships with Hennepin County General Hospital, St. Paul Ramsey Hospital, and the Duluth Program can benefit from an increased level of cooperative interaction to meet mutual needs.

On a national basis, the Department has recognized from its beginning the opportunity and responsibility to contribute to the total knowledge of education in family medicine. It has shared information freely through publications and national meetings. The contributions of the Department have been many and are continuing, but three areas should be particularly noted.

1. Working relationships have been developed with community hospitals to provide mutual benefits for the institutions and to strengthen teaching capabilities. These relationships include the establishment of the Family Practice Centers as nonprofit corporations.
2. The development of evaluational instruments and systems has been a major thrust of the Department and continues at all levels.
3. Within the behavioral science teaching program there has been a concerted effort toward teaching communication skills. New methods are constantly being investigated and evaluated and the results shared.

Medical University of South Carolina

Introduction and Overview

In 1969 South Carolina was 48th of the 50 states in physician/population ratio. The greatest need was for family physicians. The Medical University of South Carolina, then the only medical school in the state, accepted the responsibility of meeting the shortage of family physicians by establishing a full-status, major Department of Family Practice in May 1970. There has been a remarkable degree of encouragement and financial support as well as excellent cooperation from all other departments in the establishment of this new Department.

Currently there are 25 full-time faculty members including 15 physicians. The full-time members of the Charleston faculty represent a wide range of expertise in such areas as: (1) nutrition, (2) geriatrics, (3) behavioral science, (4) medical ethics, (5) anthropology, (6) social work, and (7) computer technology.

The Department of Family Practice has as its objectives the teaching of the concepts of family practice at graduate and undergraduate levels, the demonstration of the modern specialty of family practice,

the pursuit of relevant research, and the support of the Affiliated Family Practice Residency Programs throughout the State. The divisions within the Department function primarily in Charleston, but each Division Chief meets regularly with his or her counterpart in the affiliated residencies throughout the State.

The Department of Family Practice is now organized into six divisions, each headed by a senior faculty member. There is a division to address each of the following areas: (1) undergraduate education, (2) graduate education, (3) behavioral science, (4) research, (5) evaluation, and (6) geriatrics.

DIVISION OF UNDERGRADUATE EDUCATION. This Division has 60 hours of required curriculum time in the first year. During this period the clinical rationale for the specialty of family practice, the common disorders seen in family practice, emergencies, and diagnostic anatomy are covered through family and patient presentation with a multidisciplinary approach. The curriculum will use the family life cycle as a lattice for the entire course next year, beginning with pediatrics and ending with geriatrics. The Department also offers a variety of electives, including both preceptorships and clerkships for third and fourth year students.

DIVISION OF GRADUATE EDUCATION. This Division is responsible for the curriculum of the Charleston Residency Program and for defining and achieving its educational objectives. The operation of the Family Practice Model Unit and all of the hospital rotations and other learning opportunities within the Medical University program are managed by this Division.

DIVISION OF BEHAVIORAL SCIENCE. This Division includes eight full-time faculty members who give formal presentations, supervise residents in their care of patients, serve as co-counselors with residents, and manage selected problems at the residents' request. Television monitoring is used extensively and is available in every examining room. Both a family physician and a behavioral scientist are scheduled to be on duty at all times in the monitoring room of the Charleston Family Practice Center. Immediate feedback can be provided to residents who are observed; in addition, desired segments of their interviews are recorded, reviewed, and discussed.

DIVISION OF RESEARCH. The mission of this Division is to encourage and develop scientific curiosity and investigative skill among the residents and faculty. Members of the Division are available to residents throughout their training. Also, a one-month elective opportunity is available. Many types of research are possible, including an epidemiological study of the community in which a resident might choose to locate. Elaborate computer facilities are also available and are used extensively in the computerization of the medical records in Charleston.

This Division is responsible for all research conducted within the Department and must approve any studies undertaken by faculty members, residents, or other members of the Medical University who may wish access to any family practice patient data. All patient data for the past seven years are stored in the computer and are immediately available for research purposes. There is high interest among the residents, and several faculty members are actively engaged in research.

DIVISION OF EVALUATION. This Division is responsible for the development of procedures for resident and faculty evaluation, and evaluation of the residency as a whole. Procedures for chart audit have been developed. The annual In-Training Examination is a big event during which each resident has an extensive written and clinical examination. This Division provides evaluative services for all residency programs of the Statewide Family Practice Residency System (SFPRS). All residents in the Charleston Program are required to take this examination annually; the affiliated programs are encouraged to participate. The results of the examination are available to the resident and his/her faculty advisor and/or Program Director.

DIVISION OF GERIATRICS. This is the newest Division. It is developing a teaching program in a nearby nursing home as well as didactic presentations for undergraduates and residents.

Statewide Family Practice Residency System

The Department is deeply committed to the success of the Statewide Family Practice Residency System (SFPRS). In 1973 the Governor urged the training of more family physicians. This prompted a proposal by which a SFPRS would be developed that would include the three existing programs and add four new programs. To provide one family physician for each 2,400 persons in the state by 1985 would require a system which could produce 67 family physicians each year or have the total capacity of 201 training positions. The program was to be implemented over a period of four years at a total cost of approximately $22 million. Total capital funding and 60 percent of the teaching operational costs were to be provided. This was approved and funded.

The capacity and development of each Program is shown in Table 2.

Development of the system has been slower than planned because of lengthy start-up times and difficulty in recruiting directors and faculty. In the fourth year of the project 128 positions are filled, which represents about 64 percent. The system will be completely developed by 1979. The following describes each of the five currently operational programs.

CHARLESTON. The University-based Family Practice Residency Program at Charleston is now well established with a total of 45 residents—15 in each year. The Family Practice Center is an attractive, one-story facility of 30,000 square feet located within easy walking distance of the 500-bed Medical University Hospital, three affiliated community hospitals, and a large Veterans' Administration Hospital.

First year residents are assigned to the Family Practice Center their first two months. The curriculum in the Medical University-based program includes approximately eleven months of internal medicine and medical subspecialties, five months of pediatrics and its subspecialties, two months of obstetrics/gynecology, four months of surgery and surgical electives, two months of emergency medicine, and eight months of electives. Two separate one-month behavioral science rotations are required in the second and third years of the Program.

The 45 residents are divided into five practice groups, each with a family physician, behavioral scientist, dentist, pharmacist, physician assistant, nurse, and LPN as faculty members. A computerized problem-oriented medical record is used. All information is available from cathode-ray terminals—located in every room—and also from computer typewritten paper records. A computerized life-events program has been developed for use in patient care,

teaching, and research. The computer is also used for management of appointments and the billing of patients for services. Residents spend one half-day per week in the Family Practice Unit during the first year, three half-days during the second year, and four half-days during the third year.

SPARTANBURG. The Spartanburg General Hospital Family Practice Residency Program is located in a modern office setting in the ambulatory care building, which is attached to the 500-bed hospital. It is designed to accommodate 12 residents per year or a total of 36. There has been a problem of attrition which has reduced the number of senior residents appreciably. The three-year curriculum includes 12 months of internal medicine and 6 months of pediatrics. A wide variety of electives is offered and a two-month rotation is required in community medicine. Also required is two months in "psychiatry and ambulatory psychological medicine," an offering made possible by a half-time psychiatrist on the faculty. Residents spend three half-day sessions per week in the Family Practice Center during the first year, four during the second year, and five during the third.

GREENVILLE. The Greenville General Hospital Family Practice Residency Program began in 1971. The Family Practice Center

Table 2. *Statewide Family Practice Residency System, Medical University of South Carolina*

	Established	New Residents per Year	Capacity	Residents Now in Training
Spartanburg General Hospital	1970	12	36	29
Greenville General Hospital	1971	12	36	29
Richland Memorial Hospital, Columbia	1975	10	30	11
Anderson Memorial Hospital	1975	8	24	14
Medical University Program, Charleston	1970	15	45	45
Self Memorial Hospital	1978	4	12	—
McLeod Hospital, Florence	1978–1979	6	18	—
Totals		67	201	128

is presently located one mile from a 600-bed community hospital, but a new building is under construction which will place it very near a newly constructed hospital complex where there is ample parking.

Two training plans are offered to residents depending upon their wish to include obstetrics in their practice. Those electing obstetrics include nine months of internal medicine, eight months of pediatrics and six months of obstetrics, with a variety of subspecialty rotations. Those not electing obstetrics have ten months of internal medicine, nine months of pediatrics, and the minimum of two months of obstetrics/gynecology. The residents spend one half-day each week in the Family Practice Center during the first year and one half of each day at the Center during the second and third years.

COLUMBIA. The Richland Memorial Hospital Family Practice Residency Program is located in the State capitol. The Family Practice Center comprises the largest part of a new and modern ambulatory care building adjacent to the newly constructed modern 500-bed hospital. This Program, whose curriculum is patterned after that of the University Program, has a capacity of ten residents in each year.

A new medical school is being developed at the University of South Carolina in Columbia, and the Family Practice Residency Program is expected to form the nucleus of the Department of Family Practice for the new school. This Residency Program will continue to be a member of the Statewide Family Practice Residency System and will maintain its close relationship with the Medical University Program at Charleston.

ANDERSON. The Anderson Memorial Hospital Family Practice Residency Program was established in 1975. A new Family Practice Center has just been completed which provides clusters of rooms around nursing stations, facilitating an interdisciplinary team approach.

This Program has a capacity for 12 residents in each year. The curriculum is similar to that at the University, including the required preceptorship. A one-month, community medicine rotation during the first year is required. Residents are required to spend two half-days per week in the Family Practice Center during the first year, three during the second year, and five during the third year.

Common Educational Approaches

A common characteristic of each of the Programs is the emphasis on quality education. The development of good practice habits is stressed, as well as the utilization of teachers, who are always available in the units. In each, the ratio of teachers to residents is relatively low—averaging five to one or less. While ample time is provided in the practice units for residents to practice, the pace is relatively slow, and direct supervision is always available and encouraged. Some faculty members continue to maintain patient care activities, but in a very small proportion of their time. Resident supervision is conducted through chart review, personal observation, and television monitoring. The use of television for both monitoring and video taping is extensive in all of the Programs. The procedure, thought to be essential as a basic educational tool, has come to be regarded as commonplace by both patients and residents.

A second commonality is the availability of computer resources for medical record storage and data analysis. At Charleston, extensive experimentation has been conducted with computer storage of all medical record data. The entire dictated note and all data are entered into the computer. All computer services are available to all programs within the Statewide System, but they are used less extensively in the other Programs.

Behavioral science is taught in all of the Programs. A major goal of the Department, from the beginning, has been to achieve a balance between teaching in the behavioral and biological sciences. The Division of Behavioral Science provides teaching at the University Program and also serves as a resource for statewide members. Within the system, each Program is free to choose its faculty to meet its own identified needs, and each Program has chosen to appoint a behavioral scientist as one of the full-time faculty members. These persons are of varying backgrounds, but most are clinical psychologists. The activities in most Programs include didactic teaching and working with patients, usually with the resident involved. Faculty members usually do not serve as consultants for referral, but provide patient care only through the residents. Each is responsible to the Program Director at his/her own location and not to the Division of Behavioral Science. When faced with a clinical-behavioral problem, residents in all of the Programs report that the usual procedure is first to consult with a seasoned family physician from the staff. A second source is the behavioral scientist in the resident's own Program. The ultimate source for the most complex problems is consultation with a psychiatrist.

Evaluative procedures are available to all the SFPRS Programs and are used by all to varying degrees. As described earlier, the Division of Evaluation in Charleston has developed a series of instruments designed to provide a broad measurement of achievement, including patient management skills. Continuity of care is a major concern and has resulted in a fixed policy affecting all residents in the system. It is required that every resident spend at least 33 of his or her 36 months maintaining some activities in the Family Practice Centers. Thus, a resident is not able to take elective courses away from the Family Practice Center for more than a total of three months during the training program.

All of the Programs have developed regular, daily conferences at noon, which vary widely in type and purpose, and which are frequently conducted by residents. The many patient-centered conferences are used to demonstrate the different approach of the family physician. Attendance is expected.

Administrative Aspects

Each of the Programs of the SFPRS is almost autonomous, having been separately accredited by the Residency Review Committee and having its own matching number in the National Intern and Resident Matching Program. The Departmental Chairman shares the overall responsibility for all of the educational programs but each may determine its own curriculum within broad limits, taking full advantage of community resources and characteristics of the hospital and staff. This flexibility and the varied curricula offered permit applicants to choose a program which will suit their individual needs. All full and part-time teachers must be reviewed and approved by the Medical University Appointments and Promotions Committee for appointment in the Department of Family Practice. Faculty members at the Medical University are available for consultation and for teaching in the affiliated programs. Likewise, teachers in the community hospital-based programs are welcomed teachers at the University.

SFPRS monies are distributed to the various programs according to a formula, based largely on the number of residents in training, which covers all capital costs and 60 percent of the costs of the educational program. Costs such as nurses' salaries are not covered. Each program contributes substantially to the operating costs from its sponsoring hospital, federal grants, fees from patient care, and the Area Health Education Center (AHEC). Also, some faculty support is available through the Medical University consortium, which provides for undergraduate educational experiences in several of the sponsoring hospitals. Statewide funding provides for a teacher-resident ratio of one to six in addition to the Director and Assistant Director. An even lower ratio is projected for the future. Some Programs presently use funds from other sources for additional full and part-time teaching. In South Carolina, AHEC functions statewide and has contributed $318,000 to family practice education during the current academic year.

The cost per resident at the present time is estimated to be $31,000 per year. When the system is completely developed there should be greater cost effectiveness, so it is projected that in the future the figure will be decreased to $28,000.

Comment

One obvious and great strength of the South Carolina system is its abundant and apparently dependable funding, which has provided an opportunity for imaginative advanced planning. Total funding is available for capital development and a matching arrangement with community hospitals for operating expenses. The question must be raised as to the future of the Program if legislative funding should suddenly cease even though any abrupt termination would seem extremely unlikely because of the success of the Program in approaching its goals. The system is designed to provide considerable financial strength, since operating budgets include funding from multiple sources. So it could be anticipated that if state funding should cease, these Programs could continue, although at a markedly curtailed size.

The SFPRS has proven to be a sound working relationship between community hospitals and the university, with advantages to both. Resources (talent, consultation, direction, initiatives, funding) are available to community hospitals, without stringent controls. This arrangement has encouraged variability among programs while at the same time maintaining quality control. The University benefits by the exchange of ideas and through the advantages of increased size and statewide impact. Funds are used by the University Program to develop new ideas—possible only within an academic center—which are then shared with community programs.

The attrition problems of two of the community hospital programs are puzzling and not yet fully explained. Within the University Program the attrition rate is one of the lowest in the nation. Numerous explanations are possible and will warrant further investigation.

Although the projected number of residents in the SFPRS at the present time is less than originally planned, the development seems to be proceeding at an acceptable pace. The high retention rate of physicians in the state may well offset the lower than anticipated number of graduates. To date there have been 79 graduates of the Statewide Family Practice Residency System, including 41 from the Charleston Program, 19 from the Greenville Program, 8 from the Spartanburg Program, and 1 from the Anderson Program. Of these graduates, a total of 45 (57 percent) have established practice in South Carolina. Almost one half (46 percent) of Charleston graduates have remained in South Carolina, whereas over two thirds of graduates from the other programs in the SFPRS have stayed in the state.

The University Program at Charleston has accepted responsibility for exercising leadership in developing educational methods in family medicine. While the contributions of this Program have been many, two of the most notable are in the development of an emphasis on behavioral science teaching in family medicine and in the use of the computer in medical records. The fact that each of the community hospitals has chosen to include at least one full-time behavioral scientist in its faculty is evidence of the success of the parent program in demonstrating the value of the contribution of these faculty members to the teaching of family medicine. The use of the computer has been less well accepted by community hospitals, partially because many aspects are still developmental and partially because both the future funding and direct benefits are less clear.

One of the most outstanding strengths of this Program is the evident enthusiasm and strong support from other disciplines within the University and within the community hospitals. This kind of support is also much in evidence from the administrative arms of these institutions.

It is interesting to note that the directors of the Programs are individuals who have had extensive personal experience in private family practice prior to entering into their present roles. This is also true of most of the senior faculty who serve as the chiefs of the various divisions.

Another great strength of this entire system is the overwhelming emphasis on teaching. Ample evidence for this is shown in the teacher/resident ratios, in programs for instructing teachers, in the close supervision of residents at all levels, in the extensive use of chart audit, in the daily conferences at noon, and in the all-pervading use of the video camera. Other evidence includes the carefully paced patient schedule—typically one patient per half hour. The stated reason for this is to provide adequate time for discussion, reading, recording, and reflection.

Another growing aspect of this Program is an emphasis on evaluation, demonstrated by the full Division designed for evaluative purposes. That Division has developed extensive instruments, currently being validated, which should provide both a measure of success and a useful teaching tool.

One of the greatest contributions of this Program that may, perhaps, be of national interest, is the demonstration to legislators that meeting the need for family physicians can be accomplished through the development of the highest quality programs at predictable times and costs.

Medical College of Virginia

Introduction and Overview

In Virginia the need for primary care physicians was first recognized as reaching crisis proportions in rural areas. The Virginia Academy of Family Physicians joined with the Farm Bureau and the Virginia Council for Health and Medical Care (a private foundation) to seek legislative help in finding a solution to the problem. This triad began efforts to educate the legislature in 1966. Every legislator was contacted by his or her family physician. The coalition began to gather data and to educate both the legislature and the public concerning the need to replenish Virginia's family physician population.

In 1968 the Virginia State Legislature appointed a subcommittee to study the shortage of family physicians and subsequently documented both the shortage in numbers and the discrepancies in distribution. In 1969, following a period of data gathering, documentation, and public education, specific funds were made available to the two medical schools in Virginia —the University of Virginia and the Medical College of Virginia—for the purpose of family practice training. The legislature did not specify administrative structures but permitted the schools to develop their own programs.

The Medical College of Virginia chose to establish an autonomous Department of Family Practice which became a reality in July 1970. A family physician was identified who was in active practice in Virginia and who had written articles concerning the need for family physicians, criticizing the University for not attending to the training of family physicians. A search committee nominated this physician as a person with the necessary leadership skills and motivation to head the new Department. He was confronted by the Dean with his own criticisms and challenged to "put up or shut up."

He accepted the responsibility, and the

first priority identified in the development of the Department was the establishment of informational systems which would provide data in two areas: (1) the population of existing physicians in all forms of primary care in relation to the patient population in each political subdivision of the state, and (2) the content of primary care in terms of numbers and kinds of problems presented to primary care physicians.

The first collection of data was completed in 1972 and provided a basis for projection of Virginia's primary care physician needs over the next 20 years. It has been generally accepted as accurate, reasonable, and achievable. It calls for an annual production over the next 20 years of 111 primary care physicians per year for Virginia, of which 75 should be family physicians. The Medical College of Virginia's proportionate responsibility of this expressed need is considered to be between 36 and 42 family physicians per year. A resurvey was conducted and the projections updated in 1975.

About the same time, a massive study was begun to identify the numbers and kinds of problems Virginians present to primary care physicians. A coding and data retrieval system was developed. Data were collected on the primary care experiences of 88,000 patients in 26 practices representing a variety of both private practice and academic settings. A careful analysis was made of over 500,000 patient encounters.* One of the interesting conclusions drawn from this study was that in the urban, suburban, and rural areas studied, the same patterns of medical problems existed, and that these were identifiable and relatively constant within and between practices.

Having identified the needs in terms of numbers, kinds, and distribution of physicians, a program was developed to meet

these needs. It was decided to begin at the residency-training level because of the possibility for earliest results. Family practice was established as a full and autonomous Department of the College of Medicine of the Medical College of Virginia. The Chairman, Associate Director, and staff represent the Department, which is physically located at the College of Medicine at Richmond. It was decided to establish four Residency Programs at first, based geographically in the shortage areas identified in the data collection study: Fairfax, Blackstone, Newport News, and Virginia Beach. A Program was not established initially at Richmond—the location of the Medical College—because the study indicated Richmond as an area having the least need for family physicians.

While the Department's major focus is in the resident program, it is also directly involved in teaching at other levels. At the *undergraduate level* the Department has responsibility for conducting a third-year, required community hospital rotation. While students may elect various specialties with which to associate in these rotations, a large number choose family medicine and the course is coordinated by that Department. The Department also plays a major part in the human behavior course offered by the Department of Psychiatry for first and second year medical students. A variety of electives are offered for first, second, and fourth year students. These electives combine carefully designed experiences in teaching practices with conferences at the medical center involving students, faculty, and clinical faculty.

A variety of *continuing education* opportunities for practicing physicians is also provided through the Department of Family Practice. In all of the Residency Programs, noon conferences have been approved for category I credit and are often attended by practicing physicians. At the rural location of Blackstone, Virginia, the resident journal club has become a major continuing education attraction for physicians from throughout the area. The De-

* Marsland DW, Wood M, Mayo F: A data bank for patient care, curriculum, and research in family practice: 526,196 patient problems. J Fam Pract 3:25, 37, 1976.

partment also participates in the primary care continuing education activities of other clinical departments.

The Affiliated Residency Programs

Each of the five Residency Programs has unique features forming an individual personality, but all have some common features also. The patient populations are demographically typical of the various localities in which they are situated. The total number of patients served by the five Family Practice Centers is 75,000. Data from the 23 practicing physicians in Virginia whose practices were studied, indicate that the spectrum of problems encountered in the Centers is almost exactly the same as the spectrum presented in private practice. Each Residency Program is related to a full-service hospital, and each has modern office facilities with appropriate laboratory and x-ray services. All maintain problem-oriented records and have an informational system which allows immediate identification of patients and particular problems for use in preparing for the daily conferences. This information is also collected in Richmond and computerized for use in statistical and epidemiological studies for educational planning and research purposes. Table 3 presents an overview of the five Affiliated Family Practice Residency Programs.

BLACKSTONE. The Blackstone Family Practice Center is located predominately in a rural section of southern Virginia, approximately one hour from the Medical College of Virginia (MCV) in Richmond. It is the only medical facility in the town of Blackstone and delivers all primary care services to the community. The three physicians who were located in the community developed the Family Practice Center and constitute the full-time teaching faculty. The Center provides ongoing family care for approximately 11,000 people from the area.

During the first year, residents rotate through MCV hospitals in Richmond in all the clinical areas, and each resident spends a full day every two weeks in the Family Practice Center with patients to whom he or she has been assigned.

After finishing the first year, residents physically move to Blackstone but spend four months in elective hospital rotations either in MCV or in community hospitals in the Richmond area. Residents spend approximately half their time in patient care and the other half in teaching conferences and other academic pursuits. Patients from Blackstone are hospitalized primarily in Richmond. Referring residents make rounds to in-hospital patients approximately twice weekly, but referred Blackstone patients are usually seen daily by family practice residents who are on rotation in Richmond. First year residents see approximately five patients per day, and second and third year residents, about eight to twelve.

The Center teaches a total of 18 residents: six each in the second and third years, who spend most of their time in the Center, and six first year residents, who are there briefly.

FAIRFAX. The Fairfax Family Practice Center is located in Vienna, Virginia, and

Table 3. *The Affiliated Residency Program* Medical College of Virginia*

Program Sites	Number of Residents	Year Started
Blackstone	18	1971
Fairfax (Vienna)	18	1971
Newport News	36	1970
Virginia Beach	18	1973
Chesterfield (Richmond)	18	1976
Total	108	

* There is not a full University-based Program (including a Family Practice Center) on the Medical College of Virginia campus. Most of the inpatient clinical rotations for the Blackstone Program are conducted at the University Hospital. The Family Practice Centers and their related community hospitals provide the major teaching settings for family practice residents during the entire three-year Program.

occupies an entire second floor of a modern office building in a suburban business area. The Center includes a large conference room and offices for each resident, as well as laboratory and x-ray facilities. The Center, with an enrollment of 11,000 people, serves approximately 2,000 patients from the area per month. There are 12 residents: six in each of the second and third years, plus an additional six first year residents who are in attendence at the Center one half-day per week. Each resident provides care for approximately 100 families.

All hospital work is performed at the Fairfax Hospital, a 600-bed, general hospital located nearby.

NEWPORT NEWS. The Riverside Family Practice Center is located at Newport News and was the first model training center affiliated with the Medical College of Virginia. Riverside Hospital is a community facility with more than 600 beds.

The Program provides educational opportunities for 36 residents in family medicine, plus an additional six first year family practice residents who receive their first-year in-hospital training in this program, with the family practice training at Virginia Beach. Riverside residents spend one half-day per week in the Family Practice Center during the first year and approximately half time during their second and third years. Third year residents have a one-month required rural experience with a practicing family physician.

The Family Practice Center is in a recently constructed modern building and provides 14 examining rooms, although there are plans to almost double this space in the near future. Both x-ray and laboratory facilities are available within the unit. Care is provided for 14,000 patients through approximately 2,300 encounters per month. Unlike the other three MCV programs, the patient population here is largely indigent, with only about 25 percent paying privately. The practice profile of problems presented, however, is compa-

rable with that of other MCV programs and with private family practices in the area.

VIRGINIA BEACH. The First Colonial Family Practice Center is located in the city of Virginia Beach. Six residents per year are accepted in this Program. The first year is spent at Riverside Hospital at Newport News, during which time residents return to the First Colonial Family Practice Center in Virginia Beach one half-day each week. Second and third year residents receive their family practice training in the Virginia Beach Center and the General Hospital of Virginia Beach, a 400-bed, full-service hospital.

During the first year, residents see an average of six patients per day. During the second and third years, residents are assigned responsibility for 100 to 200 families. Approximately half the residents' time at the Center is spent in patient care and the other half in academic pursuit. While the residents spend a large part of their time during the second and third years in the Family Practice Center, four months are available each year for elective rotations.

Family practice patients are usually hospitalized at the General Hospital in Virginia Beach and cared for by the family practice residents from the Center. The patient population includes approximately 20,000 people and is representative of all social groups.

CHESTERFIELD FAMILY PRACTICE CENTER. The newest member of the MCV residency family group is the Chesterfield Family Practice Center, located in the southside of Richmond, six miles from the Medical College of Virginia. Its associated hospital is the Chippenham Community Hospital, a full-service hospital with bed capacity approaching 400 at the present time.

This Program also accepts six residents at each level and provides teaching in the same general format as the other MCV programs. Residents spend one half-day per week in the Family Practice Center during the first year and two thirds of their time there during the second and third years. Elective opportunities are available for four months in both the second and third years in both the Chippenham Hospital and in the MCV hospitals in Richmond.

Common Educational Approaches

The basic philosophy of the Department continues to advocate a systems approach: identify the data needed, devise the systems to collect the data, collect and analyze the data, and develop programs based on the analysis. This has been the approach used for (1) developing a system of Residency Programs in geographical locations of physician need and (2) for developing an educational program based on an ongoing analysis of what family physicians need to know.

The initial curriculum had been developed on the basis of the opinion of the faculty as to the needs of family physicians. The faculty is convinced, however, that this method of determination is faulty and that curriculum ought to be based on the problems encountered in practice. A major effort has been expended to develop the necessary data base for curriculum closely related to known content of practice. The curriculum was organized in accordance with the "special requirements for residency training in family practice" of the Essentials of Approved Residencies.* It is currently being modified by the actual experience as recorded in the data system; and ongoing efforts are being made to complete a set of objectives and an evaluative mechanism based directly on the data accumulated.

A general review of the curriculum of

* American Medical Association: Special requirements for residency training in family practice. In Essentials of Approved Residencies. Chicago, American Medical Association, 1975.

the five component members of the Medical College of Virginia system reveals a typical rotating program with the greatest emphasis on internal medicine, plus blocktime in pediatrics, obstetrics/gynecology, surgery, and emergency medicine, a short elective, and minimal time in the Family Practice Center. The most striking departure from the usual curriculum occurs in the second and third years, during which the major emphasis in teaching all disciplines occurs in the Family Practice Centers. Active teaching is conducted by regularly scheduled daily consultants and by the family physician faculty. In these two years there are only eight months of required in-hospital rotations and eight months of elective time, which may be both inpatient and outpatient experiences.

As in many programs, there is an absence of any required rotation in psychiatry. In-hospital psychiatry is available as an elective at most member Programs, but basic teaching occurs in patient-oriented conferences on a longitudinal basis with generous use of both psychiatric and behavioral science consultants.

In the management of psychological or emotional problems, residents turn first to faculty family physicians and secondly, to consultants in behavioral science or psychiatry, depending on the availability of particular consultants.

Opportunities are made available for participation in special research projects, community activities, and practice management. Practice management techniques are taught through the offices of a fulltime faculty member in practice organization and management. This person is charged with the responsibility of providing each resident with the opportunity to participate in the actual unit management and to provide access to information regarding practice locations, building plans, methods of financing, legal arrangements, insurance, accounting methods, office procedures, personnel policies, and the related basics of practice management.

This general curricular plan, with diminished inpatient teaching, expanded specialty teaching in the Family Practice Center, and only outpatient psychiatric teaching, corresponds precisely with the Department's commitment to a curriculum based on practice content. Teaching methods in the past have often been on an apprenticeship basis. The leadership of this Department believes that this is not the best method—in fact, the apprentice is not likely to learn more than his or her instructor knows. Consequently, new methods are being sought and are relying heavily on the consultant-conference in the family practice setting and on clinical investigation projects.

The Audit and Evaluation Procedures of the Medical College of Virginia Programs are similar in each Program: original, extensive, and continuing. Philosophically, the attitude is that "episodic audit leads to episodic care." Evaluation of residents in the teaching/learning process is based on the standard of patient care delivered by each resident over the three year continuum. The attempt is made to develop in the physician's mind the continuing appropriateness of self-examination and assessment of patient outcomes as the most valid measures of personal success. It is actually a process of continuing education.

An additional precept is the belief that to be effective in the field of health maintenance, family physicians need detailed knowledge of their practice community in terms of number of patients by age, sex, distribution, and kinds of problems which affect them. This information permits the physician to identify various high-risk groups for specific health educational purposes. It permits the physician to see his or her patients as members of family groups making up the larger community, where the largest proportion of health care usually remains unsupervised and unmonitored until the patient chooses to return to the office. Effective health maintenance requires complete practice information for adequate practice monitoring.

The methodology that has been estab-

lished to permit this ongoing evaluation consists of: (1) a problem-oriented medical record adapted to family practice, (2) a census tract filing system, (3) an age and sex index with a record of demographic characteristics for a diagnostic index classification (soon to be converted to the International Classification of Health Problems in Primary Care System), (4) a physician's daily work sheet, permitting the recording of biological, behavioral, and social problems of identified patients for classification with the diagnostic index, and (5) an E-book, maintained for the resident by a staff coder.

These instruments form an ongoing evaluative system which is functioning in all MCV programs and is funded by the educational component. Data from the daily work sheets are keypunched (through a unique arrangement with the State Penal System) and entered into the computer at the Medical College. In order to check the similarity of residency practices with those of private physicians, additional data are being collected from 23 separate nonteaching practices in the state. This provides a total patient population base of greater than 100,000.

This system has permitted evaluations of a resident's performance in three ways: (1) structural adequacy and completeness of the resident's problem-oriented medical record; (2) measurement of the resident's capacity to achieve the minimum critique, established by faculty and residents, for *diagnosis* of a condition; and (3) measurement of the resident's capacity to achieve the minimum critique, established by faculty and residents, for *management* of a condition.

The resident's strengths and weaknesses are identified, allowing for adjustment of patient and elective experiences to repair any deficiencies. An additional capacity of this system, which is currently being pursued by a number of residents on an elective basis, is the "longitudinal audit." In this form of audit all patients with a particular problem at one practice location are identified. The patient charts are analyzed in detail for both process and outcome, and for associated additional problems. The information generated provides new insights into the value of various procedures and identifies previously unsuspected but related problems. It is then available for curricular modifications.

Administrative Aspects

Each of the five Residency Programs is under the direct leadership of a full-time, family physician Program Director. The key to the relationships throughout the system is a very personal one in which each of the component programs is considered a partner to the others. Functionally, this system operates through three standing committees: the Records and Research Committee, the Curriculum and Evaluation Committee, and the Practice Organization and Management Committee. Faculty from each Family Practice Center and residents from each level of training constitute the membership of these committees. The faculty at the Medical College of Virginia coordinates the activities of these committees. The Chairmen of each of these committees plus the Program Directors and Chairman and Associate Director of the Department form the Executive Council. These committees are advisory to the Council and, functionally, they serve as full partners in all decision-making areas within their purview.

The full-time faculty of the affiliated programs have been largely recruited from the communities in which they serve. Frequently, faculty members have brought their practice into the educational system. The faculty is chosen on the basis of clinical excellence and educational interest, and members serve as partners in the management of the educational system as well as directors of patient care within the Residency Program.

A carefully selected consultant faculty in all appropriate specialty areas is available in each Residency Program. These faculty members are compensated financially and, after a trial period, offered faculty rank. Consultants provide patient care advice and daily clinical conferences. The conference is of several hours duration and is part of a planned curriculum covering the entire spectrum of problems which have been identified as important in family practice.

Payment for all full-time faculty salaries, consultants, and second and third-year stipends and clerical personnel is funded through the educational system itself rather than the participating hospitals in all but one Residency Program. Because of this mechanism, it is possible to make decisions regarding reallocation of funds by educational rather than institutional needs.

Each of the affiliated programs has received individual accreditation and therefore each has separate matching number in the National Intern and Residency Matching Program. While resident applicants have increasingly come from Virginia medical schools, there are also highly qualified applicants from out of state.

The funding mechanism for this Program began with an initial allocation by the state legislature of $228,000 in 1969 for the biennium 1970–1972. The state continues to be the major source of support for the entire system, currently appropriating approximately $1.8 million per year, provided by direct line-item budget to the Department of Family Practice. Initially there were some difficulties within the institution apparently related to a lack of appreciation of the University's need to train a new type of physician to meet Virginia's rural needs. However, as it became apparent that the Department of Family Practice was not subtracting from the University's total resources but adding to its capability by developing affiliated programs, these difficulties greatly diminished.

Approximately 88 percent of the state funds are distributed to the member Residency Programs. The formula for this distribution provides full support for resident stipends at each location only in the second and third years. The first-year stipends are paid by the affiliated community hospitals. State funds are distributed by the Department of Family Practice and pay for a portion of faculty salaries plus full support of an educational and secretarial staff; an additional $60,000 is distributed to each Program for consultants in a variety of clinical fields. The general formula for support in each Program is for approximately three full-time faculty members and two secretaries per each 12 residents in the second and third years. (Since first year residents spend little time in the family practice unit, they are not included in the formula.) The allocation for consultants amounts to approximately $240 per day per program throughout the year.

The three Departmental faculty persons and staff located in the medical school are funded by the College of Medicine with Departmental and grant funds. Each of the component Programs receives additional support in varying degrees and methods from the hospital in which they are situated and through federal grants. The approximate cost per resident per year at the Medical College of Virginia is $30,000.

Comment

The Department's statistical determination of Virginia's family physician needs over the next 20 years comprises the only data available. It has been generally accepted by all authorities as accurate, reasonable, and achievable. It calls for an annual production over the next 20 years of 111 primary care physicians per year for Virginia, of which 75 each year should be family physicians. The Medical College of Virginia's proportionate responsibility of this expressed need is considered to be between 36 and 42 family physicians per year. The Department's five present Programs ac-

cept 36 physicians each year for residency training.

An analysis of the family practice graduates from the MCV Programs through 1976 indicates that 62 percent of the total of 76 graduates have chosen to stay in the state of Virginia. An additional 22 percent have located in nearby areas. Sixty percent of these graduates have chosen to practice in nonmetropolitan areas.

The major goal of the Department of Family Practice is to increase the availability and quality of primary health-care services for the people of Virginia. While this has been the primary goal, the leadership of the Department has recognized the need for academic pursuits as well. While these activities have enriched the Program and assisted in achieving its primary goal, they have had an even greater impact on the development of the new discipline of family medicine through better definition, understanding of process, and development of innovative educational methods. The Medical College of Virginia's family practice program has made enormous strides in a very short period of time, based on a carefully planned systems approach.

Several interesting or potential problems have arisen and are currently being addressed:

1. The teaching of behavioral sciences in these Programs through intermittent use of consultants rather than through their constant availability has been identified by program directors as a problem.
2. Since a major portion of the funding is derived from the state legislature, any funding decrease would present a hazard to further progress. But because the funding base is built on multiple components it would be anticipated that the Program could continue, although at a seriously reduced size.
3. The educational process described here may be seen to vary considerably from those described elsewhere. This raises the question of determining the value

of this educational approach and is one of the most basic of all questions facing the entire discipline of family medicine —how can the results of educational efforts be measured?

The contributions of this Program to the discipline of family medicine and, indeed, to the whole field of medical education, have been considerable and are most notable in two areas—innovative educational methods and ambulatory care research.

The most creative aspect of the curriculum under development at MCV is its foundation upon carefully measured data of the content of family practice. Rarely have curricula been developed on such a rational base.

The extensive research program in ambulatory care has, of course, been instrumental in the development of the curriculum. However, there are other aspects of the Program which are also of great value. The methodology developed is of use to other programs and practitioners in primary care. The size of the sample and the care with which the information has been collected make the "Virginia Study" a standard to which other data may be compared.*

The use of these methods has already proven an excellent educational tool for residents within the MCV system, and faculty and residents are experimenting with new applications of the system—eg, the "longitudinal audit." The publication of this process and its results have served as a positive motivational factor for residents in other programs as well.

Discussion

The history of the three programs is similar. In each, there was a study measuring

* Marsland DW, Wood M, Mayo F: A data bank for patient care, curriculum, and research in family practice: 526,196 patient problems. J Fam Pract 3:25, 37, 1976.

the need for primary care physicians within the state and projections of this need during the foreseeable future. In each instance, a university accepted a measure of responsibility for meeting the need and established a full Department of Family Medicine, under various titles, and under the leadership of a strong personality.

In each of these programs there has been direct, abundant, and predictable funding. The funding has been carefully earmarked to provide direct support for the family practice program. While this assistance has provided the necessary lifeblood for these programs, the danger of future loss of funding is recognized. In each instance, multiple financial sources have been identified, involving some federal and private funds, but involving community hospital funds to an even greater extent. It would seem likely that if state legislative funding diminished, these programs could continue, although at a considerably reduced level.

Each of the three Departments, while focusing a major effort on the residency program, is also actively involved in family medicine teaching at other levels. All offer some teaching at the predoctoral level and some continuing education activities. All of these various activities are seen as a continuum of the effort to meet health-care needs through the teaching of family medicine.

Each of the programs involves a network with a number of other hospitals, and each has a considerable degree of autonomy. This autonomy has encouraged the development of a variety of educational programs—deliberately attempting to meet resident needs and to provide for experimentation in the development of new teaching methods. These networks have been able to identify some areas of activity which are best conducted jointly: research efforts, educational objectives, general curricular outlines, funding sources, teaching patterns, and methods of evaluation. In each instance there is some organization which promotes communication both with the parent university and among the various members. Through this organizational arrangement there is active input from all community hospital partners, and, in most cases, active input from residents at all levels of each hospital.

Each of these university programs has accepted a role of innovator of new ideas both in research and in teaching methods. In each program this thrust has been different: for example, South Carolina has incorporated behavioral scientists in the faculties; MCV has emphasized careful compilation of problem and demographic data on each encounter; Minnesota has developed a new series of evaluative techniques.

The teaching of behavioral science has been approached quite differently by the three programs. At MCV the teaching is conducted by behavioral scientists or psychiatrists, who are engaged as consultants by the individual program and combine patient care consultation with conferences on a scheduled basis. At Minnesota there is a didactic series of behavioral science presentations, usually conducted at the university, in which residents are expected to participate. This is supplemented by various conferences at the member hospitals. At South Carolina a behavioral scientist is a member of each Program's faculty and teaches through guiding residents in their patient care, as well as through conferences and didactic presentations.

There are two common denominators among the three programs with regard to behavioral science. These are (1) a commitment by each program to include behavioral science as a major component of the educational program, and (2) a consistency of the residents' approach to seeking help when handling human behavioral problems. When asked, residents consistently report that their first source of help is a seasoned faculty family physician. The second resource is a behavioral scientist, either in the program or as a consultant. Their third source of help, for the most

complex problems or deeply disturbed patients, is consultation with a psychiatrist. This pattern has been reported by residents with great consistency at all three programs.

There is interest in all three programs in evaluation through a variety of approaches. Two of the programs, South Carolina and Minnesota, have groups of faculty members whose prime responsibility is the development of evaluative techniques. In all programs the various evaluative instruments are supplemented by the personal evaluation of those with whom the residents work—and this measurement is given great weight.

In each program, although in varying degrees, there is active participation by residents in all phases of the organization and of the decision-making process. This includes various teaching conferences, of course, but in nearly all instances includes programmatic decision making, curricular change, evaluation, and residency selection.

Even though the three statewide systems represent a much larger number (16) of residency programs, the consistently high quality of the programs is quite evident. This quality is manifested both in the University-based programs and in the affiliated community hospital programs, lending strong support to the concept that both are better because of their interrelationships. Along with this high quality there is an attention to the detail of the known ingredients of successful programs—attention to selection, curriculum, evaluation, etc. There is also a strong sense of stability and "belonging" among the faculties of the various programs.

Through a wide array of mechanisms—including work with the legislature, development of nonprofit corporations, and the use of consultants and rotations from other clinical departments—each of the programs has developed a variety of relationships with other institutions and groups. For just one example, at South Carolina the behavioral science division in the Department of Family Practice has now been asked to teach behavioral science to other departments as well. This type of willingness to explore relationships with new groups and with new means of relating is common to all three programs.

In addition to the attainment of legislative funding for the programs, each organization has successfully sought and found support through a variety of other mechanisms and systems. In South Carolina there is an Area Health Education Consortium which has provided strong financial support. At the Medical College of Virginia an arrangement has been worked out with the state penal system enlisting its assistance in the coding process. At Minnesota the Family Practice Center at each of the community hospitals is being handled through the development of nonprofit corporations. This variety of support systems adds additional stability.

In each program, there is a tendency to consider some aspects a sine qua non for a successful program, as exemplified by the inclusion of a behavioral scientist in each program at South Carolina, the extensive use of consultants on a daily basis, and the total coding system at MCV, and the various mechanisms for personnel and group evaluation at Minnesota. But since none of these programs uses all of the emphasized features of the other programs, either the educational products are less than optimal or the features are not, after all, totally essential.

It is of interest to look for the various common denominators of these three excellent programs, of which there appear to be at least six: (1) an enthusiastic and committed faculty, possibly the most important factor, (2) dedication, skill, and interest in the educational process, (3) adequate funding, (4) careful screening of applicants in the selection process, choosing those who would fit best in the particular program, (5) family practice physicians who are able to serve as genuine role models, and (6) an "accepting" environment, both in the university and in the community hospital.

Comparative Content of Three Family Practice Residency Programs*

John Whewell, Geoffrey N. Marsh, Robert B. Wallace,
J. Christopher Shank

A method of collecting physician-patient encounter data is described and applied to the comparison of the clinical content of residents' experiences in the family practice office. Comparisons were made of over 1,000 consecutive unselected encounters in each of the three family practice residency programs. Considerable differences between the patients encountered by the three programs were observed and between program patients and patients attending family physicians in Iowa. It is important to monitor the demography and diagnostic status of patients attending family practice residency programs to ensure the authenticity of the residents' experience.

Curricula for family practice residency programs have been well reported on in the literature. The model office in such programs has similarly been studied, and Rakel[1] has suggested that it should "imitate as realistically as possible the private practice of medicine." Although several papers on the content of family practice have been published,[2-4] there have been few assessments of the range of diseases and problems encountered in model offices.

Johnson and Wimberly[5] compared problems encountered in one residency program with problems characterizing practice in Minnesota and concluded they were similar, but the differences in age of the patients would appear to throw some doubt on this. Shank[6] noted considerable differences between his experiences as a resident and that of practitioners and residents taking part in the Virginia Study,[2] although stressing that differences in method may have accounted for some of the apparent discrepancies.

In Great Britain information on the range of problems seen in general practice training schemes is similarly sparse. Richardson and Howie[7] felt that the experience of general practice trainees was similar to

that of practicing physicians, but O'Flanagan[8] found considerable deficiencies in his experience in a training program.

To investigate this further in a standardized, comparative fashion, it was decided to study patients presenting to family practice residents in the model offices of three residency programs in the United States and to compare them with existing information on patients attending family physicians. The programs under study were those sponsored by the Universities of Arizona and Iowa and the independent community hospital program in Cedar Rapids, Iowa. The University of Arizona program in Tucson has one model office in close proximity to the University Hospital. The University of Iowa has two offices, the smaller one being on the outskirts of Iowa City and the larger one being in Williamsburg, a rural community 20 miles away where the practice was relatively unopposed. The Cedar Rapids program has three model offices, the primary one close to Mercy Hospital with a smaller one in the rural town of Mechanicsville several miles away. There is also a clinic in St. Luke's Hospital, Cedar Rapids, dealing only with visits for pregnancy, gynecology, and family planning.

The aims of the study were to compare the epidemiology of problems and the de-

* Reprinted by permission from *The Journal of Family Practice,* 9(4):613–619, 1979.

mography of patients presenting at the model offices with the range of problems and patients seen by 25 established family physicians in Iowa.[9] An analysis of the latter showed considerable correspondence to the National Ambulatory Medical Care Survey and was considered to be suitably representative of family practice in the community. An additional objective was to compare the process of the physician-patient encounter in the model offices of the three programs with the process of encounter experienced by Iowa family physicians.

Methods

A physician-patient encounter form was utilized which had been previously used in a study comparing Iowa family physicians and British general practitioners.[9] The patient's age, sex, and main reason for presentation (either specific illness or preventive or routine examination) were recorded. Space for up to four diagnoses was available on the form, and the diagnoses were arranged in order of time spent on each. History, extent of examination (none, local, system, or complete), time taken, and the nature of any diagnostic tests were also recorded. Follow-up intentions, referrals, and admissions to the hospital were noted, and residents were asked to record if anti-

biotics or psychotropic drugs were prescribed. All diagnoses were coded by the same person using the classification of the Royal College of General Practitioners to ensure comparability with the previous study.

The study was carried out in Arizona in January and February 1977 and in the two Iowa programs in August and September 1977. As the seasonal and climatic conditions in Arizona were so very different from those in Iowa, it was not considered essential that the studies in Arizona and Iowa should be concurrent. Encounters recorded were consecutive and so were completely unselected.

Results

There were 1.696 recorded encounters in Arizona, 1,739 in the University of Iowa program, and 1,819 in Cedar Rapids, Iowa. One or more items of information were missing in a few encounter forms in each program.

Table 1 shows the age-sex distribution of patients. The University of Arizona and the Cedar Rapids programs both showed a preponderance of females, distributed mainly in the 19 to 44-year age group. Both of these programs, particularly Cedar Rapids, encountered a lesser proportion of patients over 65 years of age.

Table 1. *Age-Sex Distribution of Encounters*

	University of Arizona		University of Iowa		Cedar Rapids		Iowa Family Physicians	
	Number	*Percent*	*Number*	*Percent*	*Number*	*Percent*	*Number*	*Percent*
Male	554	33.0	773	44.8	488	26.9	994	40.3
Female	1,125	67.0	953	55.2	1,327	73.1	1,472	59.7
Age (years)								
0–1	74	4.4	81	4.7	97	5.3	107	4.3
2–4	83	4.9	109	6.3	126	6.9	154	6.2
5–18	199	11.7	348	20.2	418	25.8	432	17.5
19–44	875	51.6	663	38.4	841	46.3	864	35.0
45–64	285	16.8	269	15.8	167	9.2	523	21.2
65+	180	10.6	256	14.8	116	6.4	386	15.7

Table 2. *"Well" and "Ill" Encounters*

	University of Arizona		University of Iowa		Cedar Rapids		Iowa Family Physicians	
	Number	*Percent*	*Number*	*Percent*	*Number*	*Percent*	*Number*	*Percent*
"Well"	253	15.1	276	16.0	610	33.6	369	15.0
"Ill"	1,422	84.9	1,451	84.0	1,206	66.4	2,097	85.0

The Cedar Rapids residents saw considerably more "well" patients than the other programs or the Iowa family physicians (Table 2). They also saw relatively fewer "chronic" patients but a higher percentage of repeat acute visits (Table 3).

Table 4 shows the average time taken with each patient. Residents in Cedar Rapids corresponded more closely to the Iowa family physicians in the amount of time spent with patients, the Arizona residents in particular taking more time per visit than the practicing family physicians. This correlated well with the volume of patients seen in the office. Although the number of residents in each program was similar, in the Cedar Rapids model offices 3,290 patients were seen per month compared with 1,300 and 1,200 in the Iowa and Arizona programs, respectively.

Table 5 shows that the established Iowa family physicians saw more cardiac and respiratory disease than the residents. Many more cases of pregnancy were seen in Cedar Rapids than in other programs. In this respect the Iowa program was particularly deficient. Arizona residents saw less trauma than the others. The top ten specific diagnoses are listed in Table 6. The Cedar Rapids list is dominated by pregnancy but correlates most closely with the experience of the Iowa family physicians.

The extent of examination of "ill" patients is shown in Table 7. In all programs there is a greater tendency for residents than for the Iowa family physicians to carry out a full examination. Residents in the University of Iowa program were less likely to carry out specific diagnostic procedures than were residents in the other two programs; this was particularly true in the case of pelvic and rectal examinations, urinalysis, bacterial culture, and blood pressure determinations. Table 8 represents an example of how residents handled a particular problem, in this case, first visits of tonsillitis. The use of antibiotics and psychotropic drugs is shown in Table 9. All the residency programs were more conservative in the use of drugs than were the Iowa family physicians.

Discussion

Differences clearly exist between the various programs. Many of the differences were due to the local conditions in which the programs operate. Residents can see

Table 3. *Type of Illness*

	University of Arizona		University of Iowa		Cedar Rapids		Iowa Family Physicians	
	Number	*Percent*	*Number*	*Percent*	*Number*	*Percent*	*Number*	*Percent*
Acute first visit	594	41.8	662	42.9	478	39.3	961	45.8
Acute repeat visit	431	30.3	456	31.4	534	43.9	675	32.2
Chronic visit	397	27.9	373	25.7	204	16.8	461	22.0

Table 4. *Duration of Visits—All Patients*

	University of Arizona		University of Iowa		Cedar Rapids		Iowa Family Physicians	
	Number	*Percent*	*Number*	*Percent*	*Number*	*Percent*	*Number*	*Percent*
Minutes								
0–5	164	9.9	279	16.5	640	35.5	766	31.1
5–10	553	33.4	827	49.0	860	47.7	1,206	48.9
10+	941	56.7	583	34.5	304	16.9	492	20.0

only those patients who present themselves. In Arizona the family practice office is adjacent to the University Hospital and is in competition with the surrounding physicians and university departments, not the least of which is the Emergency Room. In addition, Medicaid is not applicable in the state of Arizona, and such patients are referred to the County Hospital. The Cedar Rapids program is somewhat different because its office is in St. Luke's Hospital where only maternity, gynecological, and contraceptive problems are seen; in addition, this program also cares for many Welfare patients (Title 19), who are not seen by the Arizona residents. Two thirds of the patients seen in the University of Iowa program were seen in the Williamsburg office which, because of its relatively unopposed position, conformed most closely to an Iowa family practice office.

The age-sex structure and local conditions are reflected in the range of diseases seen. The younger female element seen in the Arizona and Cedar Rapids programs presented more pregnancy and genitouri-

Table 5. *Distribution of All Diagnoses Made in "Ill" Patients**

Diagnostic Category (RCGP)	University of Arizona N = 1,844	University of Iowa N = 1,827	Cedar Rapids N = 1,515	Iowa Family Physicians N = 2,757
Infective	5.5	5.3	5.4	4.1
Neoplasms	2.0	2.8	2.2	2.4
Allergic, metabolic	6.3	7.6	6.6	5.9
Blood disorders	0.3	0.5	0.4	1.0
Mental and emotional	4.8	5.9	5.6	5.6
Diseases, nervous and special senses	7.7	10.2	7.5	8.2
Circulatory disorders	9.8	12.4	9.2	15.3
Respiratory disorders	13.2	9.9	7.9	15.4
Gastrointestinal tract	7.5	7.1	6.1	4.2
Genitourinary	11.4	8.2	10.5	7.0
Deliveries and pregnancy	6.2	2.5	17.6	5.8
Skin diseases	5.3	7.8	5.6	5.5
Digestive disorders	7.5	7.1	6.1	4.2
Musculoskeletal	8.3	6.6	3.6	6.0
Congenital deformities	0.6	0.1	0.4	0.4
Perinatal morbidity	0.2	0.0	0.1	0.0
Ill-defined symptoms	4.4	2.4	1.8	1.5
Accidents, poisonings	4.1	10.7	8.1	10.3
Prophylactic procedures	1.2	1.3	1.5	0.3

* Figures represent percentages of *N*.

Table 6. *Top Ten Diagnoses*

Diagnosis	Number
University of Arizona	
1. Common cold	116
2. Pregnancy	102
3. Hypertension	93
4. Acute otitis media	69
5. Abdominal pain	48
6. Urinary tract infection	45
7. Tonsillitis	45
8. Vaginal discharge	44
9. Depression	38
10. Headache	35
University of Iowa	
1. Hypertension	140
2. Minor trauma	118
3. Tonsillitis	58
4. Acute otitis media	57
5. Urinary tract infection	53
6. Anxiety	46
7. Depression	44
8. Allergic rhinitis	38
9. Warts	37
10. Common cold	37
Cedar Rapids	
1. Pregnancy	236
2. Hypertension	75
3. Minor trauma	72
4. Diabetes	41
5. Tonsillitis	40
6. Vaginal discharge	39
7. Acute otitis media	34
8. Urinary tract infection	25
9. Common cold	24
10. Depression	23
Iowa Family Physicians	
1. Hypertension	241
2. Pregnancy	138
3. Minor trauma	132
4. Common cold	128
5. Tonsillitis	97
6. Acute bronchitis	81
7. Sprains and strains	77
8. Acute otitis media	73
9. Diabetes	66
10. Anxiety	57

nary problems, while the relative lack of older patients, particularly in Cedar Rapids, resulted in a comparative shortage of patients with cardiovascular and musculoskeletal disorders. With an increasingly aging population, the supervision of chronic degenerative diseases will occupy an increasing proportion of the family physician's time. It is therefore important that future family physicians be exposed to sufficient cases of illness of this kind. Residents in the University of Arizona program saw less trauma than the other residents because the Emergency Room of the University Hospital was directly across the street and the family practice office was frequently bypassed.

This raises the whole question of how closely should the conditions seen in a model office approximate to those seen in a typical family practice office, if such an establishment indeed exists. How many common colds does a resident have to see before he is comfortable in treating them? Would the resident receive a better educational experience if he were exposed to more cases of the type which are going to constitute a more serious problem to him in his subsequent professional career? Seen in this light the higher proportion of pregnant patients seen in Cedar Rapids is educationally sound but not if it is at the expense of older patients with chronic diseases. It must, however, be remembered that with the greater work load in the Cedar Rapids program a smaller percentage does not necessarily reflect a smaller overall figure.

How closely should the behavior and work patterns of residents approximate to those of established practitioners? Parkinson's Law[10] states that "work expands so as to fill the time available for its completion," and to some extent this appears to apply to residency programs. Residents in Cedar Rapids saw considerably more patients per month than did residents in the other two programs, and consequently took less time with each patient. In this they closely followed the Iowa family physicians. Obviously, in his initial training a resident must be expected to work more slowly because of his relative lack of experience, need for increased supervision, and lack of detailed knowledge of the patients. But

Table 7. *Procedures Performed on "Ill" Patients*

	University of Arizona N = 1,417		University of Iowa N = 1,449		Cedar Rapids N = 1,190		Iowa Family Physicians N = 2,099	
	Number	*Percent*	*Number*	*Percent*	*Number*	*Percent*	*Number*	*Percent*
No examination	118	8.3	98	6.8	50	4.2	40	7.9
Local examination	573	40.4	653	45.1	621	52.2	894	42.6
One system examination	450	31.7	392	27.0	290	24.4	946	45.1
Full examination	261	18.4	290	20.0	214	18.0	204	9.7
Other	15	1.1	16	1.1	15	1.3	15	0.7
History taken	1,308*	91.9*	1,281†	88.3†	1,082‡	89.7‡	1,519§	72.4§

* *N* = 1,422.
† *N* = 1,451.
‡ *N* = 1,206.
§ *N* = 2,099.

what of the resident who is approaching the end of his training? Should he be able to work at the rate which might be expected of him in his future practice? If this is desirable, he will have to be provided with sufficient patients to stimulate him to do so. But patients cannot be supplied which do not present themselves. A need for additional medical services in the community would appear to be a necessary requirement for the establishment of family practice residency programs. If newly emergent family practice residency offices are to attract an adequate practice population, they must be located where there is a need and the nature of that need will differ in different areas.

In the handling of specific problems there was little difference between the three training programs. The example of

Table 8. *Selected Procedures in First Visits for Tonsillitis**

	University of Arizona N = 32	University of Iowa N = 45	Cedar Rapids N = 32	Iowa Family Physicians N = 93
Duration of visit in minutes				
0–5	9.4	29.3	59.4	43.8
5–10	59.4	58.5	40.6	5.1
10+	31.3	12.2	0.0	1.1
Follow-up				
Appointment made	18.8	26.3	0.0	20.0
Appointment as needed	78.1	73.7	93.5	70.0
Appointment nil	3.1	0.0	6.5	10.0
Specific procedures				
Thermometer	78.8	86.6	93.8	79.5
Stethoscope	81.8	66.6	78.1	66.6
Otoscope	63.6	86.6	96.9	84.9
Throat culture	69.6	55.0	71.9	15.0
Hematology	6.1	6.6	†	15.0
Antibiotics started	27.2	46.7	43.7	67.7

* Figures represent percentages of *N*.
† Not known.

Table 9. *Prescriptions for Antibiotics and Psychotropic Drugs for "Ill" Patients*

	University of Arizona		University of Iowa		Cedar Rapids		Iowa Family Physicians	
	Number	*Percent*	*Number*	*Percent*	*Number*	*Percent*	*Number*	*Percent*
Started on antibiotics	112	7.9	129	8.9	158	13.1	324	13.5
Maintained on antibiotics	43	3.0	33	2.3	38	3.1	80	3.8
Total on antibiotics	155	10.9	162	11.2	196	14.2	404	17.3
Started on psychotropics	8	0.6	10	0.7	9	0.7	61	2.9
Maintained on psycho-tropics	18	1.3	40	2.7	12	1.0	97	4.6
Total on psychotropics	26	1.9	50	3.4	21	1.7	158	7.5

acute tonsillitis given in Table 8 was typical. Residents appear to follow the conventional academic approach more closely than do the established family physicians. More importance was placed upon bacterial confirmation of diagnosis and less reliance upon antibiotics. Although their exposure to mental and emotional disease was very similar to that of their established colleagues, considerably fewer psychotropic drugs were used by residents. This no doubt reflects the teaching they receive and a willingness to conform to it, at least during their training period.

This study demonstrates that considerable difference existed between the three family practice residency programs in the spectrum of clinical problems seen in the model offices. It also indicates a need to monitor more closely the work done in this setting, not only for the whole program but for each individual resident as well. In this study wide variations occurred between individual residents; for example, female residents saw an even greater proportion of female patients than did the male residents. This may not necessarily be inappropriate, as this may be the pattern of practice they will subsequently be involved in. This sort of information is readily available in every family practice program and the authors agree with Boisseau and Froom[11] that programs should record and use it.

The physician-patient encounter form used in this study is a practical tool for collecting data. It can serve in a standardized way to allow data collection in different residency or practice settings. Comparisons of different settings stimulate healthy questions and improvement for all concerned.

Obviously, the model office experience is not the sum total of the experience of a family practice resident. Rotation and electives in other specialty and subspecialty departments augment and complement it. Identified deficiencies can and should be rectified by participation in appropriate family practice preceptorships where those gaps in experience can be corrected. This, of course, assumes that the family practices associated with a training program maintain the necessary information systems to enable them to do this. Nevertheless, the cornerstone of the family practice residency program must be the model office experience. It is here that the embryo family physician learns what family practice is all about.

Acknowledgments

The authors wish to thank the residents in the three programs for their courtesy in completing the encounter forms; and the heads of the departments in the Universities of Arizona and Iowa, Dr. H. Abrams and Dr. R.E. Rakel; and the head of the residency program in Cedar Rapids, Dr. C.R. Aschoff, for their help and financial support.

REFERENCES

1. Rakel RE: Training of family physicians. J Med Educ 50(12) (pt 2):145, 1975
2. Marsland DW, Wood M, Mayo F: Content of family practice: Part 1: Rank order of diagnoses by frequency; Part 2: Diagnoses by disease category and age/sex distribution. J Fam Pract 3:37, 1976
3. Morbidity statistics from general practice: Second National Morbidity Survey 1970–1971. In Office of Population Censuses and Surveys: Studies on Medical and Population Subjects, No. 26. London, Her Majesty's Stationery Office, 1974
4. Hodgkin K: Towards Earlier Diagnosis. New York, Longman, 1973
5. Johnson AH, Wimberly CW Jr: Comparative profiles of residency training and family practice. J Fam Pract 1(3/4):28, 1974
6. Shank JC: The content of family practice: A family medicine resident's 2½-year experience with the E-book. J Fam Pract 5:385, 1977
7. Richardson IM, Howie JGR: A study of trainee general practitioners. Br J Med Educ 6:29, 1972
8. O'Flanagan PH: One trainee's clinical experience. JR Coll Gen Pract 27:227, 1977
9. Marsh GN, Wallace RB, Whewell J: Anglo-American contrasts in general practice. Br. Med J 1:1321, 1976
10. Parkinson CN: Parkinson's Law. London, Murray, 1958, p 9
11. Boisseau V, Froom J: Practice profiles in evaluating the clinical experience of family medicine trainees. J Fam Pract 6:801, 1978

Family Practice Residency Training in the Community*

A Report on Four Years' Experience

John P. Sherin, Joseph R. Morrissy,
Martin J. Bass, I. R. McWhinney

The Department of Family Medicine at the University of Western Ontario has been training family practice residents in community based group practices for four years. The methods used to select and evaluate the residents and their practice experience are outlined in this article.
Despite difficulties which arose as a result of geographical distance, the experience was felt to be worthwhile by those who participated. The program has been approved by the Department of Family Medicine for expansion and continuation.

Since its inception in 1967, the Department of Family Medicine at the University of Western Ontario has been developing and modifying its residency training program. The first training site was in a hospital setting located in the community. The latest development, the subject of this report, has been to associate residents with group practices.

Residents spend 12 months of their two year program in one of four family medical centres, which are geographically separate from, but affiliated with, the teaching hospitals in London. The teaching hospitals provide core experience in medicine, surgery, pediatrics, obstetrics and gynecology, and selective experiences in the subspecialties.

A number of community practices in London and the surrounding area have been extensively involved in undergraduate teaching.

As early as 1971, discussions were held with some of these practices with the object of incorporating them into the residency training program. It seemed likely that the community practices could offer more patient contact for the resident when compared with the fulltime teaching practices. Undoubtedly, the in-hospital experience would be greater in the community practices because of their association with nonteaching hospitals. It was felt that the resident would be encouraged to follow surgical cases and assist in the surgery.

It was important that the teaching goals of these satellite practices be the same as the parent department and that they devote adequate time to resident teaching. The teaching skills necessary to enable the resident to learn could be acquired on the job with the assistance of experienced teachers from the department. It was critical that the resident's experience be different from that of a locum tenens, especially in terms of staff teaching time. Similarly, it was essential that the resident's individual aims and objectives be discussed and agreed upon by the group, since the situation was very different from that of a young doctor who has joined the group with a view to eventual partnership.

A fulltime member of the department was appointed to organize the formal aspects of the program and to maintain communication between the residents, supervisors, and the department.

Selection of Residents

In 1971, several of the larger group practices, already approved for under graduate

* Reprinted by Permission from *Canadian Family Physician*, 26:595–602, 1980.

experience, suggested to the department that they participate in the postgraduate training program. The details of hospital and departmental funding, curriculum supervision, and the selection of residents were the subject of deliberation and negotiation over the next four years. The Ontario Ministry of Health provided funding specifically to train residents in community facilities. These funds supplemented those already available for training residents in the family medical centres.

The program began in 1975 with the selection and assignment of residents to three practices. The first practice, a group of six family physicians, is located in a small village surrounded by prosperous farmlands and is approximately 50 miles from London. The second, a group of four family physicians, is located in a high density population area in urban London. The third, a larger group of 13 practitioners, is situated on the growing margins of a medium sized city about 70 miles from London. A large multi-specialty practice over 1,000 miles away in northern Ontario, was the fourth practice to join the program.

Residents were admitted to the program in the first three practices after completing a rotating internship. They were given credit for their in-hospital experience and like the other residents, were required to complete 12 months in a family practice setting. The residents in the practices outside London were required to obtain a full license in order to practice in the non-teaching hospitals.

The recruitment of suitable candidates for the community or satellite practices was placed in the hands of the Postgraduate Education Committee and its Subcommittee on Resident Selection. Advertisements were place in the appropriate journals and notices were posted in teaching hospitals. Because of the licensing requirement, it was decided that only those applicants who had completed an approved rotating internship or its equivalent would be considered for appointment to a community practice. The applicants were interviewed both by a member of the department and a representative from the involved practice. The final selection and ranking were made by the full Selection Committee of the department with input from the community practices. In the first year, from a total of nine interested and qualified applicants, three were chosen for the program.

Additional Training

In the first four years of the program, seven of the 11 residents have undertaken further training beyond the family practice year. This further training was based on the resident's needs and future plans. Some of the additional training was arranged because of observed weaknesses in given areas. Other training was undertaken because particular residents had chosen to practice in certain geographical areas where special skills were needed. For example, one of the residents who was going to practice in the Northwest Territories took six months of obstetrics and anesthesia. Other experiences have been in pediatrics, internal medicine, general surgery, and orthopedics.

The Remote Practice

The practice in Northern Ontario was integrated into the program in a different manner from the other three practices. In 1970, it was selected as a teaching practice in the Ontario government's student preceptorship program and, at the same time, appointed as a University of Western Ontario undergraduate teaching practice. Since it was too remote from the main teaching centre to be effectively integrated for the teaching of residents undertaking a "core experience", it was decided to use this resource for third year training. This practice has offered third year residents training and experience in family medicine, surgery, internal medicine, and aspects of community health. Residents have also been able to experience the problems of providing care to more isolated areas such as Indian reserves which are only accessible by air.

Curriculum and Teaching

Each community practice selected from among its membership a physician to be the principal supervisor of the resident's work. The selected physician was responsible for teaching and evaluating the resident with assistance from other members of his group. The curriculum was organized along lines similar to that offered to residents in the established teaching centres. The five major components are:

1. In-practice clinical experience, with evaluation by the resident's supervisor and other members of the practice. Viewing through one-way mirrors and chart reviews are used to assess each resident's performance. Each practice had a one-way mirror installed in one of their examining rooms specifically for this purpose. Each resident is viewed at least one-half day per week by a member of the practice.
2. Half-day teaching and evaluation sessions are conducted by fulltime teachers from the department. These sessions occur once every two weeks; assessment forms are completed by the teacher for each resident/patient contact. Similar cross-viewing sessions are scheduled for all residents in the family medicine program.
3. Attendance for a half-day per week at seminars arranged for all residents by the Department of Family Medicine.
4. Attendance at weekly Balint seminars organized in London for family medicine residents by the Department of Psychiatry.
5. "Enrichments" in a specialty or sub-specialty of the resident's choice are taken on one half-day per week during the

resident's time in the practice. Orthopedics, ENT, and dermatology are common choices.

Clinical Experience

It was important that the residents get exposure to all the common problems experienced in family practice. To monitor the content of the resident's activity, an encounter sheet was completed by every resident after each office, house or emergency visit.[1] These were analyzed in the 25 categories in Table 1. They included most of the important problems seen in practice yet are detailed enough to assess a resident's experience. Table 1 compares the six month experience of the three community practice residents of 1977 with their 12 second year peers practicing in the teaching Family Medical Centres (FMC).

The experience of the two resident groups in Table 1 was similar in number of problems and in problem distribution. Both resident groups saw patients in every category. Striking differences are the higher percentages of respiratory, ear, back and joint problems seen by community residents—all relatively acute problems. Teaching centre residents saw higher percentages of chronic problems: hypertension, cardiovascular, obesity, diabetes. The higher percentage of anxiety problems in the FMCs may reflect a difference in patients or in labelling. While female genital and pregnancy visits were slightly lower in the community, this has improved with time. Initially, the office staffs were reluctant to have the residents see these sensitive problems. As the staffs became increasingly comfortable with the residents' skills, this became less of a problem.

Resident Evaluation

Five parameters are used to assess the resident's experience during his year in the program:

Table 1. *Distribution of Problems Seen by Residents in Community Practices and in Teaching Family Medical Centres, July–December 1977*

Problem Category	Three Community Practice Residents (N = 3,030 Problems) Percent of Problems Seen	Twelve Second Year Residents in Family Medical Centres (N = 11,344 Problems) Percent of Problems Seen
1. Ear	8.0	4.6
2. Respiratory system	23.7	12.4
3. Urinary tract	2.2	3.2
4. Female genital	2.6	3.9
5. Skin	8.6	9.6
6. Digestive system	7.2	6.6
7. Infectious diseases of childhood, hepatitis	1.3	0.7
8. Eye	2.3	1.7
9. Injuries	7.7	9.5
10. Back, joint, arthritis	7.3	3.0
11. Anemia	0.4	0.4
12. Hypertension	1.8	5.4
13. Cardiovascular	2.5	4.9
14. Obesity	1.0	2.6
15. Diabetes	0.5	1.8
16. Neoplasms	0.1	0.4
17. Headache, fatigue	1.6	2.3
18. Anxiety states, depression	2.8	5.1
19. Psychosocial, family problems	1.7	1.9
20. Other mental problems	0.3	1.0
21. Alcoholism, addiction	0.3	0.8
22. Preventive examinations	5.7	4.6
23. Pregnancy	2.4	4.0
24. Office procedures	1.4	0.4
25. Other	6.6	9.2

1. *Assessment of Visiting Faculty:*
   Office visit assessment forms were regularly completed by fulltime departmental teachers after viewing and discussing a resident/patient office contact. Patients are usually booked at half hour intervals, allowing adequate time for discussion. The various skills demonstrated by the residents are scored on a scale of 1–15 in each of eight categories (Table 2).
   At the end of the residency year, these assessments are tabulated to obtain each resident's profile. Using this method, the resident's strengths and weaknesses become apparent and the results can be compared with their peers in the established teaching centres (see Table 2).

2. *Internal Viewing* and weekly assessment is conducted by the resident's supervisor or one of his colleagues. Audiovisual aids, together with records and clinical conferences, are used as a basis for this assessment. The resident's supervisor submits a year end assessment of the resident which includes the resident's effect on and acceptance by the group members and the patient population.[2]

3. *Informal Debriefing Sessions* between the resident and the departmental liaison

Table 2. *Summary of Office Visit Assessments—1975–1976 Second Year Residents*

Performance Skills	Community Practice Residents (2)		Peer Group Residents (23)	
	Number of Patient Contacts Assessed	*Average Score (1–15 Scale)*	*Number of Patient Contacts Assessed*	*Average Score (1–15 Scale)*
Doctor-patient relationship	54	11.2	150	11.7
Problem searching—subjective	54	11.0	151	11.5
Problem searching—objective	54	11.6	145	12.1
Clinical judgment	54	11.4	146	11.6
Management plan	54	11.0	149	11.4
Overall competence	53	11.0	142	11.5
Efficiency	54	12.1	151	12.1

teacher occur at regular intervals throughout the residency year. The resident's personal and professional concerns are often revealed and appropriately handled.

4. *Postgraduate Training Assessment* questionnaires must be filled out by all residents in the program at the end of the residency year. The questionnaire is a seven page detailed evaluation of the program's instruction, content and organization. Assessed and computerized replies reveal a spectrum of opinion from community practice residents. There are several areas in which there is strong agreement, e.g.,
— the resident was made to feel a part of his group.
— the program gave them a great deal more experience than they would have obtained from a second year of internship.
— their supervisors were available for consultation when needed.

5. *Year End Written Assessment* of the program by the resident allowed him to reinforce or communicate other opinions or concerns about the program in areas not dealt with in the formal questionnaire. There were residents who expressed disappointment with the obstetrical experience. It was suggested that residents would benefit from more frequent opportunities to view their supervisor and other members of the practice.

Financial Implications

An arbitrary dollar value can be assigned to the time spent by members of a group in viewing and supervising a resident, together with the time spent as back-up to the resident when he is on call evenings and weekends. The supervisor's loss of time attending departmental meetings has to be taken into account. These expenses were offset to a large extent by fees generated by the resident, together with small grants to the teaching practices from the Department of Family Medicine. In the final analysis, it was felt that the practices neither lost nor gained a great deal financially as the result of taking on a resident for training.

Problems Encountered by Clinical Supervisors

The presence of a resident in the practice was found to be more demanding on the clinical supervisor than the presence of an undergraduate student. In the early stages of the project, the supervisors needed much support in handling the problems which occurred almost daily in this kind of teaching. Fulltime teachers have the support of colleagues with similar problems and comparable experiences, a resource not available to the community practice teachers. The difficulties encountered by these part-time teachers were not initially appreciated by the fulltime teachers. This resulted in a feeling of isolation which did not allow the part-time teachers to develop their teaching skills to their full potential.

Three steps were taken to counter these difficulties. First, the community teachers involved with residents were invited to take part in the monthly faculty development workshops organized for fulltime faculty members. Secondly, a liaison teacher from the fulltime faculty was appointed for each community practice. Following each monthly workshop, the departmental liaison persons and community practice supervisors, together with the program director, met to discuss current problems. Thirdly, the liaison teacher visited his community practice monthly for the dual purpose of teaching and evaluating the resident and to meet with the resident and his supervisor. The community practice teachers were also invited to evaluate and teach the residents in the fulltime teaching centres, i.e. cross-viewing.

As a result of these decisions, the community teachers developed a greater sense of belonging to the department. Their skills and confidence as postgraduate teachers improved visibly month by month. They were able to keep in close touch with the department's objectives and they became less reluctant to consult by telephone whenever necessary.

When group practices become involved in teaching, it is not uncommon for the commitment to teaching to vary widely between members of the group. This has certainly been the case with the four groups involved in the program. While all members of a group must support the decision to have a resident in the practice, some members may not wish to be personally involved with his/her training. At first, we questioned if partial involvement would jeopardize the program. With the passage of time, however, we have discovered that the program can work in the absence of complete participation of all the group members concerned.

The most successful teachers are those who are enthusiastic about teaching. Contact with a physician who teaches grudgingly can only be a negative experience for the resident. To be a good family physician teacher, one must be both a good family physician and a good teacher. However, not all good family physicians are necessarily good teachers. This principle is restated here because failure to appreciate the second part of it was a major block to the establishment of harmonious relationships both within some of the groups, and between those groups and the Department of Family Medicine. Only after the department was able to convince those who did not wish to teach that they were in our eyes still competent family physicians was that problem resolved.

In three of the communities, residents have been using the facilities of the local hospital. These hospitals have not been accredited by the Canadian Council for the Accreditation of Preregistration Interne Training Programs; however, the fully licensed resident is able to apply for hospital privileges as a member of the Department of General Practice.

There are obvious anomalies in this situation. The departments of family medicine in the Ontario medical schools take the position that a full license to practice unsupervised primary care should not be granted before a minimum of two years of primary care are completed. They are supported in this by several of the faculties of medicine. If, at some future date, the licensing authority accepts this position, then community hospitals will presumably have to attain accreditation as teaching hospitals in order to participate in such programs.

In 1976, Curry[3] enunciated principles for the successful incorporation of community facilities into a university based teaching program. Important among these principles were the maintenance of close and frequent face to face communication between the faculty members in the various practices with the fulltime members of the department. With the practices in southern Ontario, we have been able to meet these principles.

Concerning the northwestern Ontario practice, it is clearly more difficult to maintain the frequent personal contact. The clinical supervisor in that practice has, however, been able to visit the university department twice yearly for two days at a time. On these occasions, progress and problems have been adequately reviewed and the supervisor has taken part in faculty development seminars and resident teaching. The resident from that practice has also been able to visit with the program director at least once per year. Once a year one of the fulltime faculty, usually the program director, has visited the remote practice for a few days. The purpose of these visits has been to evaluate and teach the resident, but some time has also been devoted to faculty development activities.

For all the practices, some important benefits have resulted from these activities. These include the development of weekly clinical rounds in which all group members and the resident have participated and presented. More frequent evaluation of the resident's work and redefinition of his objectives has been instituted. Improvements in standards of record keeping have been noted.

While the relative isolation of the practice in northwestern Ontario poses some problems, these have not been insurmountable. Regular written evaluations have been forwarded to the program director by the principal preceptor and the resident, who in this practice has always been a third year resident. In our opinion, it would be unwise to attach a first or second year resident to this practice for a period of longer than three months.

The question of accommodation for the resident attached to these practices needs to be addressed. It has proved very difficult to lease accommodation for a period of less than one year. We believe that this is probably true for most centres in Canada. That being so, it seems likely that for economic reasons, a resident will almost al-

ways have to be located in one centre for a year. We have, in general, not been able to obtain a subsidy for housing. This does not mean that the resident is obligated to spend a whole year attached to the community family practice teaching unit. In future, as the program becomes more flexible, we feel sure that a certain period of time will be spent in family medicine and the rest of it in the different specialty areas associated with the local hospital facility.

In the north, the practice partnership bought a two-bedroom house, situated close to the hospital and the practice. This house is rented at a competitive rate to the resident. The house was furnished with the assistance of the Northwestern Ontario Medical Program (NOMP), a provincial government sponsored program aimed at encouraging physicians to settle in the north. NOMP has also been generous in helping to defray the moving expenses of the residents who have undertaken this rotation. Each resident has personally visited the practice, at the partnership's expense, prior to accepting a position there. The partnership and NOMP have also been generous in providing a travel subsidy enabling the resident to attend appropriate conferences and clinical meetings.

These facilities could be used for shorter rotations by residents. It would be necessary to guarantee the owners of the various living accommodations that the rent would be paid even if a resident is not always present. From the point of view of the resident and the program, this more flexible use of the facilities has a lot to recommend it. A source of finances to cover the guaranteed rental would be difficult to find. This seems to be the most important of the three problems which remain to be solved. The second of these is the necessity of providing each attached resident with his own office, and a suitable area for study. Finally, consideration should be given to finding a way to provide audiovisual equipment such as videotape recorders. This last is clearly a relatively expensive item, because one complete unit i each practice would be available for use by only one resident. In the fulltime teaching centres, such equipment can be used more economically by sharing it amongst three or four residents.

The group members in all the practices and their patients have accepted well the problems encountered by the residents leaving at the end of the year.

Since the program's inception in July 1975, 11 residents have completed the second or third years of the program, for a total of 15 residency training years in community practices. Nine of these 11 physicians have successfully passed certification examinations of the Canadian College of Family Physicians and two of the 11 physicians are completing a third year of the program. The locations of those graduates who have gone into practice range from British Columbia to Prince Edward Island. The majority are in smaller communities with one physician electing to go to northern Ontario (Cochrane), and another to the Northwest Territories.

In conclusion, the Department of Family Medicine of the University of Western Ontario has had four years of successful experience training family physician residents in community group practices. It is undoubtedly a more economical way of pro-

ducing well trained family physicians for Canada and it is to be hoped that individuals in positions of authority or who may be called upon to fund such programs will look closely at this experience.

Acknowledgments

Special thanks are due to Drs. Jim Gall, Keith Gay, Gary Gibson, Ron Gingrich, Ken Hook, Ray Mailloux, Richard Moulton, and Wayne Weston, together with all their partners, for their persistence in and their encouragement of this program. We are also deeply indebted to the residents who have so enthusiastically made the program a success.

REFERENCES

1. Dickie GL, Newell JP, Bass MJ: An information system for family practice. Parts 3 and 4. J Fam Pract 3:633–645, 1976
2. Mollineux J, Hennan B, McWhinney I: Intraining performance assessment in family practice. J Fam Pract 3:405–408, 1976
3. Curry H: The Role of Community Practices in Residency Training. Address given to The Society of Teachers of Family Medicine Annual Meeting, New Orleans, 1976

Postgraduate Training for General Practice in the United Kingdom*

John M. Eisenberg

Although the role of general practice is well established in the United Kingdom's National Health Service, formal postgraduate training for primary care practice is a recent development. Trainees may enter three-year programs of coordinated inpatient and outpatient training or may select a series of independent posts. Programs have been developed to train general practitioners as teachers, and innovative courses have been established. Nevertheless, there is a curious emphasis on inpatient experiences, especially since British general practitioners seldom treat patients in the hospital. In their outpatient experiences trainees are provided with little variety in their instructors, practice settings, and medical problems. The demands on this already strained system will soon be increased due to recent legislation requiring postgraduate training for all new general practitioners. With a better understanding of training for primary care in the National Health Service, those planning American primary care training may avoid the problems and incorporate the attributes of British training for general practice.

In recent years hundreds of training programs have been established in the United States to provide postgraduate training in primary care for residents in family medicine, general internal medicine, general pediatrics, and obstetrics-gynecology. At the same time in the United Kingdom, where general practice is well established as an essential element of the National Health Service, major reforms have occurred in the training of general practitioners. In this article the author reviews postgraduate training in the United Kingdom—its history, status, problems, and prospects—in order to provide insights for American medical educators into the training of primary care physicians in another medical care system.

History

Medical education in Great Britain generally begins at age 18 or 19 with a medical school course of study which lasts five years. After medical school the new graduate completes an obligatory preregistration year (internship), which generally includes six months of hospital work in general medicine and six months in general surgery. The physician then may choose to concentrate in a hospital specialty and enter a lengthy training program of hospital work. Alternatively, the new physician may decide to enter general practice. In the past there were no requirements for postgraduate training in general practice. Some physicians entered practice immediately after the preregistration year, whereas others individually arranged training posts in various hopsital specialties. The Trainee General Practitioner Scheme was established in 1948 and provided an optional year of training in general practice under an established general practitioner. Several innovative programs were initiated soon after. The first program to link hospital training with general practice appointments was developed in the Inverness, Scotland, area in 1952.[1] In Wessex, England, in 1960 Dr. George Swift developed a coordinated postgraduate training program with the support of the Nuffield Provincial Hopsitals Trust.[2]

The growth of these coordinated training programs was slow, however, and by 1968 only 10 centers were operating.[1]

* Reprinted by permission from the *Journal of Medical Education*, 54:314–322, April, 1979.

Even the one-year trainee assistantship began to lose popularity. In 1957, 450 trainees were working with general practitioners, but by 1965 the number had fallen to 124.[3,4] By 1969 a majority of entrants to general practice still had not undergone any planned training to prepare them for general practice, and most who had received postgraduate training had done so in a haphazard manner.[5]

Further development of postgraduate training for general practice was spurred by the Doctors' Contract of 1966, an agreement between physicians and the National Health Service which modified reimbursement schedules to improve the financial attractiveness of general practice, and by the maturation of academic general practice departments. Supported by the increasing strength of the Royal College of General Practitioners, general practice training had clearly begun its resurgence by 1973, and the number of positions had increased to 336, offered by 102 programs.

Current Training

There are now two ways that a trainee can complete three years of general practice training. First, he can independently select a variety of hospital and outpatient posts. Second, he can join one of the planned three-year vocational training programs organized by a regional adviser for postgraduate training in general practice. The adviser is a general practitioner who is usually an officer of the Regional Advisory Subcommittee of the National Health Service for General Practice Training. This subcommittee is similar to advisory committees in other specialties, all of which advise the National Health Service's Regional Committee for Postgraduate Training.[6,7] At the national level policy is recommended by the Joint Committee for Postgraduate Training in General Practice, which is similar to national advisory committees in other specialties.

Approximately half of the doctors currently entering general practice do so after a three-year postgraduate program. In 1976 of 1,766 registered trainees in general practice, 1,261 were entered in three-year planned programs.[7] Because the regional general practice adviser coordinates the various hospital experiences with the trainee's apprenticeship in a general practice, these programs are said to be "linked" or "packaged." The advantages for the trainee of the package program include the convenience of having the regional adviser arrange the various experiences, the assurance of being located in one area for three years, coordinated educational activities (including special courses), and the ability to work with a general practitioner early in the traineeship. On the other hand, the self-constructed programs potentially offer more flexibility and self-determination for the trainee. For the package programs hospital posts are evaluated and approved by either the regional adviser in general practice or the Joint Committee on Postgraduate Training in General Practice.[4] The programs usually include six-month rotations in four hospital specialities, most commonly general medicine, pediatrics, geriatrics, psychiatry, emergency medicine, gynecology, or occasionally obstetrics.[8,9]

The rationale for hospital training of general practitioners, who will rarely manage inpatients after the completion of their training, includes the following: the concentration of patients with serious aspects of diseases; the ability to develop problem-solving skills under close supervision; the opportunity to learn the services available in the hospital; graded degrees of clinical responsibility; and more didactic teaching than is possible in general practice because of time constraints. Practically, another major reason for including inpatient training for up to two-thirds of the program is that hospital posts are generally available, since funds have been allocated to support trainees in National Health Service hospitals. In contrast, funds are available for only one year of training with general practitioners in their practices. From the hospital specialists' point of view, general practice programs offer a ready and regular supply of house staff, especially in those peripheral hospitals where it has been difficult to attract trainees.

In most programs the trainee completes two years of hospital training and then joins a training general practice for a year. In one study the average trainee was seeing 93 patients weekly with no obvious socioeconomic difference between the trainee's and the preceptor's patients and with a representative array of diagnostic categories.[10]

Most trainees spend one or two sessions weekly away from the practice when they meet with other trainees for special educational programs. Some of these "day-release courses" run throughout the three years of training, but the great majority are confined to the general practice year. They deal with clinical topics, subjects in health care organization, and psychosocial topics.[11] In addition to providing the most substantial academic contribution to general practice training, the day-release courses bring trainees together regularly, thus reducing the effects of professional isolation.[7]

Preceptors

By 1976, 1,766 physicians were training in three-year general practice programs in the United Kingdom. At that time there were 1,475 preceptors available to accept trainees.[7] Because the estimated need for preceptors will increase further, there has been some concern about the ability to recruit more teachers of high quality. Certainly, the incentive exists for general practitioners to accept trainees: the trainee's salary is paid by the National Health Service, the preceptor is paid 1,300 pounds yearly, the trainee sees large numbers of patients, and an allowance for an extra automobile and for telephone expenditures is available. The task, therefore, has been

to choose the preceptors wisely and to enable them to improve their ability to teach. During the past several years general practitioners applying for approval as preceptors have been subjected to careful scrutiny, as have their practices.[12] The new preceptors must pass the membership examination of the Royal College of General Practitioners.

In addition to carefully choosing the preceptors, leaders in general practice training in the United Kingdom have developed a number of programs to teach the preceptors how to teach. The first three of these programs were established in 1966 in Manchester, in Liverpool, and at the Royal College of General Practitioners in London. Another early course was developed by the British Postgraduate Medical Federation.[13] These courses have emphasized interpersonal communication, role-playing, self-awareness, and teaching methods.[13-15] The focus has been on discussing psychological elements of teaching rather than clinical aspects of general practice or mechanical factors such as lecture style.

With the current need for more well-trained teachers in general practice, many regional advisers require that new preceptors complete a brief course in teaching methods. These short courses usually meet for a half-day weekly and are often led by general practitioners who were themselves trained in the more intensive London and Manchester workshops. Because more course leaders are required, the Nuffield Provincial Hopsitals Trust has supported a series of six-week courses to train them and course organizers, who, in turn, are responsible for training the general practitioners.

Evaluation

Competence in general practice is evaluated by the membership examination of the Royal College of General Practitioners. The examination consists of three written parts, which are prerequisites to an oral examination. The written papers consist of multiple-choice questions, essay questions based on the trainee's own patients, and a traditional essay paper.[7] The oral examination consists of two parts: one is based upon the trainee's diary of 50 consecutive cases and often includes questions on practice administration; the second concentrates on clinical problems presented by the examiners. While about 75 percent of those taking the college examination pass it, nearly all of those who have completed three-year training programs are successful. Membership in the college is not required for all registered general practitioners.[8]

In an uncontrolled study of the effectiveness of general practice training, Freeman and Byrne[16] studied 80 trainees and their trainers in seven training programs. Before the training program they found that (a) there was no significant difference between the scores of trainees and their trainers in a test of medical knowledge; (b) trainers scored better than trainees in essay questions relating to problem-solving; and (c) trainees who were ranked highest in their problem-solving skills and knowledge scored better in measures of personality such as self-confidence and security. After the three-year training program the investigators found that (a) there was a general increase in scores of knowledge for the trainees; (b) there was an even greater improvement in scores relating to problem-solving; (c) there was a tendency for the trainee's score to approximate that of the preceptor; and (d) differences in scores among the trainees decreased during the training period.

Problems

Despite the impressive progress made during the past 10 years—developing planned programs, training teachers, and working on evaluation tools—there are a number of difficulties facing general practice training today.

Inpatient Training

A number of questions have been raised regarding the appropriateness of hospital training for general practitioners, and several difficulties exist in the organization and curriculum of the hospital posts:

1. Appropriateness of inpatient training. Trainees themselves have complained that too much time is spent in the hospital training experience.[16] Since British general practitioners rarely have hospital privileges, hospital training may not be the best way to train physicians who eventually will be responsible only for outpatients.[17]

2. Content. There is also doubt that the administrators of general practice training programs have sufficient control over the content of inpatient experiences to assure that they are appropriate.[9] Since the general practice trainee must enroll separately in each clinical rotation, the training is directed by the hospital specialist who accepts the trainee, even though a joint Royal College of General Practitioners and Royal College of Physicians committee approves many of the posts. At present national standards are being developed and all posts will be visited. However, since each post is effectively the property of the consultant, he will continue to control the content of the program even though he may not appreciate the needs of general practice trainees.

3. Schedules. Even when the educational content of the posts is appropriate, it is often difficult to schedule the posts so that all trainees obtain the experience they desire. In some areas the general practice program organizer is allowed to identify which trainee will rotate through which service at which time, but even then the available positions are often limited by the specialists.[16,18] In addition, it has often been difficult to ensure free time for trainees to attend conferences relating to general practice while they are on their hospital rotations.[18]

4. Status of general practice trainees. Although one might anticipate that general practice trainees would be treated as

second-class citizens when they work in collaboration with specialty trainees there is little evidence to support this contention. It has been suggested, however, that the faculty enjoy teaching specialty trainees more than general practice trainees.[18]

5. Hospital-based outpatient training. In addition to their inpatient services, hospital consultants are responsible for specialty outpatient clinics; but, ironically, little of the trainees' time is spent in the hospital outpatient setting.[17] By spending more time in the clinics, not only would trainees see a concentration of problems they are more likely to encounter in practice but also the specialists could educate the trainees in the proper use of and communication with the consultant.

6. Work load. One reason that trainees do not spend more time in the hospital outpatient setting is that their services are needed on the inpatient services. In fact, many trainees complain that their inpatient-service responsibilities are disproportionate to the teaching they receive and that little formal training occurs in the hospital specialities.[6,16–18]

7. Reinforcement of career goals. Another problem with the emphasis on inpatient training during the first few years is the possibility that trainees lose sight of their orientation toward general practice.[18]

8. Limited number of posts. Even if hospital training were ideally suited for the education of British general practitioners, there would remain another problem— there does not seem to be a sufficient number of positions available. Positions have been especially hard to find in general medicine, pediatrics, and psychiatry.[6]

Training Practices

By the mid 1950s the Trainee General Practitioner Scheme initiated in 1948 had developed a reputation for exploiting the physician in training.[4] Whitfield pointed out that training for general practice was inadequate and that the trainee year was often little different from being a hired assistant.[4] Some have argued that training has changed little since Whitfield's study;[19] and, indeed, there are a number of criticisms which can be leveled at the training practices.

1. Insufficient time. The corollary of the criticism that too much time is spent in inpatient training is that too little is spent in outpatient training. The Royal College of General Practitioners has proposed the development of programs which give more time in general practice, but funds to extend the trainee year are not available.[7]

2. Insufficient teaching. At its best, the traineeship can be considered a tutorial in the traditional style of British higher education, but a common complaint is that the preceptors spend too little time with their trainees. In the Oxford area, only 33 of the 45 trainees received any regular training throughout the traineeship year.[20]

3. Exploitation of trainees. The median number of visits per week by trainees in one survey was 107, high enough to raise doubts about whether the trainees were being exploited to provide service.[14] Some observers, however, point out that trainees see half the number of patients as their preceptors; and it is often said that preceptors with trainees see fewer patients themselves than when they are without trainees. These observers conclude that the trainees "are not being used as ordinary assistants".[10] On the other hand, preceptors estimate that they spend a median of 9.8 hours weekly with their trainees, whereas the trainees estimate less than half that figure, 4.5 hours.[21]

4. Limited responsibility. The opposite extreme of exploitation occurs when the preceptor is unwilling to allow the trainee to accept personal responsibility for patient care. In one survey 36 percent of preceptors had the trainees simply observe them during the entire training period.[9]

5. Insufficient variety. One explanation for the absence of more rigorous teaching lies in the complaint that the teaching practices often do not encounter enough

medical problems to support teaching discussions.[16] This perceived problem might be overcome by more sharing of patient problems with the trainee by other members of the practice or by trainees working in other practices. In fact, many trainees have expressed the desire to work in more than one practice.[22] In addition to offering the chance to learn the diagnosis and management of more problems from physicians with different approaches, such variety would allow the trainee to observe various ways of organizing a practice.[19]

6. Publicity of available posts. Another problem has been the difficulty of communicating the availability of various posts to potential trainees.[9]

7. Poorly equipped practices. A major disability of many training programs is the lack of adequate practice premises. Despite efforts to place trainees only in well equipped practices, one investigator described one-third of all training practices in Scotland as having inadequate premises; there were no reference books in 60 percent of the practices, and 70 percent had no journals relevant to general practice.[19]

8. Overemphasis on psychosocial aspects. Another defect in the training of British general practitioners is at the same time one of its strengths. The leaders of general practice training have encouraged the teaching of psychosocial aspects of primary care. However, in writing their guide to training, *The Future General Practitioner*,[23] they have emphasized psychosocial aspects almost to the exclusion of biomedical aspects of primary care. They have placed relatively less emphasis on the different types of medical problems seen in outpatient practice, the difficulties of early diagnosis, and the principles of prevention.

Prospects

The Royal Commission on Medical Education of 1968 proposed five years of postgraduate training which would be divided between three years of general professional inpatient training common to all specialties (one of which would be the preregistration year) and two years specifically designed for general practice.[1] This recommendation was in keeping with the Royal College of General Practitioners' preference for five years of postgraduate training. The British Medical Association disagreed, suggesting that three years was sufficient; but there was agreement that postgraduate training for general practice needed an overhaul.[7] Despite this agreement, no legislation was forthcoming and another study committee was convened. The Merrison Committee, reporting in 1975, suggested that general practice should be regarded as a specialty for which an appropriate term of specific training was necessary. British medical educators agreed with the proposal that all prospective general practitioners should undertake a minimum of three years of suitable training—two years in recognized hospital appointments and one year as a trainee in an approved general practice.

In response to this perceived need for required training of general practitioners, Parliament passed the important National Health Service Vocational Training Act of 1976, which allows the secretary of state to prescribe the medical experience required of a doctor entering general practice. If a physician does not complete the mandatory training, he may not become an unrestricted principal general practitioner, but he may serve as an assistant to a principal. The regulations will probably require three years of postregistration training which, in addition to the preregistration year, will comprise four years of postgraduate experience. A minimum of 12 months will probably be spent as a trainee in general practice, with the remainder of the three years in hospital posts. The preliminary regulations stipulate that not less than six months be spent in three of the following hospital specialties: general medicine, chest medicine, geriatric medicine, rheumatology, traumatic surgery or accident and emergency medicine, obstetrics-gynecology, pediatrics, psychiatry, otorhinolaryngology, dermatology, ophthalmology, anesthesiology, and rehabilitation.[24] The required training law is expected to become effective in 1980; thus, trainees have three years from the late 1976 passage of the law to complete their training.

Implications

On the one hand, general practice is well established as a major component of British medicine and is frequently described as an international model of primary care delivery. However, postgraduate training of general practitioners in the United Kingdom is still in its adolescence. Its successes and its failures offer lessons for primary care educators in the United States.

One of its successes, increased reimbursement for British general practice, has heightened the attractiveness of primary care, in contrast to American payment mechanisms which compensate well for diagnostic procedures and surgery but poorly for primary care. The day-release courses are an admirable model of a planned curriculum in nonclinical aspects of primary care. Few American residencies have developed such programs, and even fewer have developed cooperative courses offered to all residents within a region. The day-release course idea also could reinforce the resident's interest in primary care during the inpatient training experience. The extensive use of a network of community physicians with whom residents can serve apprenticeships is also more well developed in the United Kingdom. Furthermore, the careful screening of physicians and their practice sites and the formal training which the teachers receive in educational techniques are reforms which American educators might well adopt.

On the other hand, the emphasis in these teachers' workshops on psychosocial aspects of medicine might be complemented by educational strategies for teaching clinical skills, such as physical examination or the use of diagnostic tests. Other disadvantages of British training for general practice which American primary care educators might avoid include the limited experience which trainees have because they are assigned to only one general practice. Residents can be exposed to several physicians as preceptors, various practice settings, and different groups of patients. In addition, the deployment of residents as observers is unacceptable; they should be actively involved in patient care.

The exploitation of British trainees by hospitals which otherwise would have difficulty attracting house officers may occur in this country and should be detected as a result of careful scrutiny of training programs by the certifying bodies in medicine, pediatrics, and family practice. The dependence of general practice training upon hospital-based training in the United Kingdom limits it ability to develop its own curriculum and schedules. However, in any interdisciplinary training program there will be some dependence upon other specialities. In order to integrate the training experience, there should be joint development of goals, objectives, curricula, and evaluation programs by educators from each discipline.

The disproportionate amount of inpatient training for British general practitioners is less of a problem in the United States, where primary care physicians generally maintain hospital privileges and where there are significant differences in the goals of primary care training in medicine, pediatrics, and family practice.

Acknowledgments

The author was supported in part by the Clinical Scholars Program, Robert Wood Johnson Foundation, and in part by the National Health Care Management Center at the Leonard Davis Institute of Health

Economics, University of Pennsylvania (Public Health Service grant HS 02577, National Center for Health Services Research).

REFERENCES

1. Hasler J: The development of vocational training for general practice. J R Coll Gen Pract 24:613–616, 1974
2. Swift G: Postgraduate preparation for general practice. Br Med J 2:590–595, 1963
3. Watson J: A review of the trainee practitioner scheme. Health Bull. (Edinburgh) 33:191–197, 1975
4. Whitfield MJ: Training for general practice: Result of a survey into the general practitioner trainee scheme. Br Med J 1:663–667, 1966
5. Eaton G, Parish P: Medical training and experience of doctors new to general practice in 1969–1970 (England and Wales). J R Coll Gen Pract 27:11–15, Supplement, 1977
6. Reports from General Practice XIV. The Future General Practitioner, Part I. Problems of Organizing His Practice. London: Journal of the Royal College of General Practitioners (publisher) 1971
7. Irvine D: Education for General Practice. In Fry J (Ed.): Trends in General Practice. London: Royal College of General Practitioners, 1977, pp. 158–182
8. Horder JP: The education of the general practitioner in the United Kingdom. Intern J Health Serv 2:183–191, 1972
9. Irvine D, Russell I, Taylor G: The accreditation of vocational training programmes—results of a pilot survey. J R Coll Gen Pract 24:617–629, 1974
10. Richardson IM, Howie JGR, Berkeley JS: A further study of trainee general practitioners. J R Coll Gen Pract 24:661–665, 1974
11. Swift G: A course in vocational training for general practice in Wessex. Br J Med Ed 2:63–70, 1968
12. Council of the Royal College of General Practitioners. The selection and remuneration of teachers in general practice. J R Coll Gen Pract 22:79–86, 1972
13. Byrne P: The history of a course. Update 1:547–553, 1969
14. Harris CM, Long BEL, Byrne P: A teaching methods course in Manchester for general practitioner teachers. Med Educ 10:193–197, 1976
15. Marinker M: A teachers' workshop. J R Coll Gen Pract 22:551–559, 1972
16. Freeman J, Byrne P: Reports from General Practice No. 17: The Assessment of Vocational Training for General Practice. London: Journal of the Royal College of General Practitioners (publisher) 1976
17. Smith A, Walker J: Vocational training—some problems. Update 11:468–471, 1975
18. Byrne PS, Freeman J: Vocational training for general practice: Some problems of implementation. Br J Med Educ 4:268–270, 1970
19. Donald JB: The trainee year—a critical appraisal. Br Med J 1:672–675, 1975
20. Training in Practice. (Editorial) Br Med J 4:959–960, 1976
21. Irvin D, Russell I, Taylor G: The accreditation of vocational training programs—results of a pilot study. J R Coll Gen Pract 24:617–629, 1974
22. Drinkwater CK: Vocational training for general practice: A comparison of the views of trainees and teachers. Br. Med J 4:96–98, 1972
23. Working Party, Royal College of General Practitioners: The Future General Practitioners. London: British Medical Journal (publisher) 1972, pp. 1–265
24. Department of Health and Social Security: Consultation Paper. Vocational training for new general practitioners. Br Med J 2:1549, 1977

Training Family Doctors in Australia*

Wesley E. Fabb

As the crow flies, it is 1,800 miles from Cairns in the far north of Australia to Hobart in the southern island state of Tasmania, and traveling across Australia, almost 2,000 miles from Sydney on the east coast to Perth on the west coast. Trainees in The Royal Australian College of General Practitioners' (RACGP) vocational training programme for family practice— the Family Medicine Programme (FMP)— are scattered over this vast area, obtaining their training in family practice training posts and hospitals. Some are located in the major capital cities, whilst others are situated in the remotest parts of the continent.

At the beginning of 1974, the first trainees were enrolled. By June 1978, there were 1,450 active trainees in the Programme (Figure 1). Of these, over 600 were in family practice posts working and training with general practitioners in the community. The rapid growth of this national Programme has been facilitated by the injection of Australian government funds. In 1973, the then Australian government established the Hospitals and Health Services Commission which invited community groups to make submissions for funds to improve community health. The RACGP, which prior to this was able to carry out vocational training in only a limited way because of lack of funds, applied for a grant to set up a national programme of vocational training for family/general practice. In October 1973, the first grant was made, and by January 1974, offices in the six state capitals and in Canberra, the federal capital, were established, state directors and staff appointed, and the first trainees enrolled.

* Reprinted by permission from *The Journal of Family Practice*, 9(4):741–743, 1979.

208

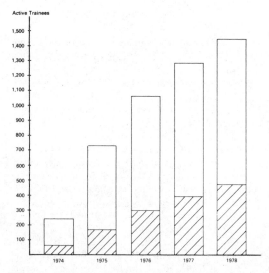

Fig. 1. Active trainees in the Family Medicine Programme at June 30 of each year (proportion who are females shaded).

Organization of the Programme

Because of the size of Australia, it was recognized from the outset that the Programme would have to be a decentralized one which could provide training opportunities even in remote parts of the country. Accordingly, the country was divided up into training areas, there being now 87 such areas. In each area, an area coordinator, who is usually a practicing general practitioner, has been appointed to work half to one day a week for the Programme. His functions are to identify hospital and family practice training posts, to ensure that these posts provide adequate training opportunities for the trainees in them, and to provide advice, support, and educational courses and resources for the trainees in his area. These coordinators, called ARCs on the local scene, have been specially trained to carry out their important role, as the ARC network is considered to be the rock on which the Family Medicine Programme is built.

At a state level, the area activities are coordinated by a state office where there is a medically trained state director, one or two medical educators, and administrative support staff. The state office is responsible for trainee recruitment, career counseling, placement of trainees in family practice training posts, teacher education, the provision of educational resources, seminars, workshops and courses, and liaison with hospitals and state health departments to secure the best possible training opportunities for family medicine trainees.

At a national level, the state activities are coordinated at the headquarters of the Programme in Melbourne. A medically trained Director and three national educators, supported by library, administrative, and technical staff provide educational, evaluational, and research expertise and resources, and administrative support. Grant monies are administered through the national office, the grant for the 1978–1979 financial year being just under A$5 million. The national office houses a Resource Centre which contains the most comprehensive collection of educational resources on family and community medicine in Australia. This collection is augmented continually with audiovisual material developed in the Programme's colour television studio, and with printed material created by the Programme and produced in the printing department. All of the national activities are situated in the same building. The Director of the Programme is responsible to the Council of the RACGP for its successful management. A National Advisory Board advises the Director and the Council on the operation of the Programme.

The Programme may be likened to a wheel with the national office the hub, the state offices the spokes, and the periphery the training areas, where trainee family doctors are trained in hundreds of family practice and hospital posts. There are now over 700 family practice posts and 137 hospital posts involved with the Programme (Figure 2). In each family practice post one of the general practitioners is appointed a supervisor to oversee the training process. He acts as an advisor, tutor, model, and counselor to the trainee and his or her spouse. Training for this role is provided by the Programme's area coordinators and educators. At present there are no special training practices which provide a high level of monitoring of the trainee through one-way glass or by videotape, but it is anticipated that some existing training practices will undertake this role on a pilot basis during 1979.

Whilst in a family practice, the salary of the trainee is paid by the practice, but the Family Medicine Programme provides a salary subsidy which amounts to a little over 50 percent for the first three-month terms, reducing for second and third

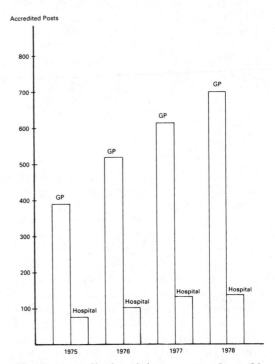

Fig. 2. Accredited training posts at June 30 of each year.

terms. A teaching allowance is also paid to the supervisor, and trainees who train in rural or metropolitan areas of health care need are paid an additional incentive allowance.

Reorientation Programme

One part of the Programme which has been very successful has been the reorientation programme, which provides an opportunity for those who have been absent from clinical practice for some time to rejoin the work force after a period of special training and updating. It has been mostly middle-aged women who have joined this programme and women coordinators were appointed in five states to supervise its conduct. The programme is now winding down as most of those requiring reorientation have been through the programme. However, an increasing number of trainees, both male and female, are seeking part-time training, and the coordinators are now focusing their attention on the special problems of part-time training. At present, one third of the trainees in the Family Medicine Programme are female.

Educational Philosophy

The Programme extends over four years, the first two being spent mostly in hospitals rotating through posts relevant to family practice and the second two being spent mainly in family practice posts. The educational philosophy of the Programme is to encourage self-directed learning and evaluation and to provide patient centered, problem oriented learning opportunities. The principles of adult learning[1] are applied and are accepted by trainees and trainers alike. A participatory management style is used which involves staff at all levels of the Programme, as well as

trainees. Most trainees take the Fellowship examination of the RACGP at the completion of their training.

Impact of the Programme

The effect of the Programme in the five years of its existence has been substantial. Interest in training for family practice has heightened, the numbers entering family practice have increased sharply, and the severe shortage of general practitioners existing in the early 1970s has been relieved, although the Family Medicine Programme would not take all the credit for this as many other factors have influenced the situation. Perhaps the greatest challenge now facing the Programme is to ensure that with the threatened surplus of medical graduates, *all* those who wish to enter family practice receive adequate training so that they can make an effective and efficient contribution towards satisfying the health care needs of the Australian community.

Acknowledgment

The Family Medicine Programme is funded by the Australian government through its Community Health Programme, Project No. 73CAV 1.

Author's Update

By June, 1980, there were 1476 full-time trainees in the Family Medicine Programme, 30 percent of whom were female, with a further 238 trainees involved in part-time or re-orientation training (84 percent female), a total of 1714 trainees. Since the Programme first began taking trainees in early 1974, 3874 full-time trainees have been enrolled.

At present, there are almost 150 hospitals associated with the Family Medicine Programme, and of the 700 accredited family practice posts scattered round Australia, 246 are currently occupied by a trainee.

Provided funds are available, the Programme will continue to expand to an anticipated 2,000 trainees, and an annual intake exceeding 600, which would represent approximately 50 percent of the doctors graduating from Australian medical schools.

REFERENCES

1. Fabb WE, Heffernan MW, Phillips WA, et al: Focus on Learning in Family Practice. Melbourne, Family Medicine Programme, Royal Australian College of General Practitioners, 1976, pp 35–46.

The General Practice (Family Practice) Training in New Zealand*

J.G. Richards

Postgraduate general practice training has been somewhat slow in evolving in New Zealand. In 1977, the government formally recognized the need for an adequate program of education for general practitioners at the postgraduate level, and money was made available for the institution of what has become known as the Family Medicine Training Programme. Dr. Pat Hertnon of Tauranga was appointed to coordinate this throughout the country, and since then five programs have been established, of which the Auckland scheme is typical.

Training for General Practice Immediately after Graduation

As with other disciplines, all graduates are required to spend one year working in hospital to fulfill the requirements of the Medical Council for full registration. It is considered that for full registration, graduates should be required to spend approximately six months of their preregistration year in disciplines allied to surgery and six months in disciplines allied to medicine. Because of logistical constraints, it is seldom possible for physicians to obtain a series of posts which can be considered nonspecialized in their approach to both these main areas. Consequently, most graduates find that they have to spend at least one quarter in a highly specialized environment. Furthermore, there are certain runs, such as Accident and Emergency,

which are not uncommonly considered to be either medicine or surgery for the purposes of registration. It seems to be the case that some of the peripheral hospitals are able to cope with this problem more adequately than the more specialized base hospitals. For this reason it is often suggested, but certainly not required, that aspiring general practitioners should spend some time in a peripheral hospital.

The majority of graduates elect to spend a second year in hospital work. This addition to the statutory requirement enables them to broaden their experience, which has of necessity been somewhat specialized in the preregistration year.

The New Zealand College of General Practitioners, as a prerequisite for its membership, requires all candidates to complete a minimum of two years in hospital posts. It is assumed that this training will be as broad as possible. Fortunately, the concept of three-month rotating internships affords the opportunity to obtain experience in a diversity of medical and surgical disciplines.

Some hospitals (the Auckland group of hospitals among them) provide a system of streaming of hospital posts designed to provide specifically for the needs of physicians who are entering one or another of the specialist disciplines. Thus, in Auckland there are streams for medicine, surgery, and pediatrics, and a general stream which is of particular value to those people whose interests lie in the direction of family practice.

The so-called generalist stream is also used by physicians wishing to extend their hospital experience prior to entering a number of other specialties, such as anesthetics or dermatology.

* Reprinted by permission from *The Journal of Family Practice*, 8(6):1263–1264, 1979.

The present organization of the generalist stream in Auckland gives almost all entrants an opportunity to do six months at the National Women's Hospital. Thus, they gain experience in obstetrics and gynecology and are provided with the necessary practical training that enables them to take the examination for a diploma in obstetrics (which the postgraduate school attached to that hospital offers).

Registrar Training

Having completed two years of varied experience in one or more hospitals, the physician is eligible to apply for registrar posts. There is now a program of registrarships in general practice available for the intending general practitioner. This training is not obligatory but is highly recommended for those who intend to enter general practice. It is designed in such a way that the physician spends half the year in an approved general practice working under the supervision of experienced physicians and the other half of the year in hospitals filling out deficiencies in his earlier training. The year is divided into three-month segments so that experience in general practice alternates with experience in hospital. Part of the concept is that the physician-in-training identifies the deficiencies in his knowledge and experience in the general practice setting. On returning to the hospital, he then has an opportunity to remedy those deficiencies as far as this is possible in hospital inpatient and outpatient departments. Ultimately, it may be possible to do all the registrar training in general practice. However, many believe there is still something to be gained by the opportunity of returning to the hospital to learn techniques and skills which are best taught in that more specialized environment. In Auckland the hospital runs designated specifically for registrar training include general pediatrics, physical medicine, rheumatology, medical rehabilitation, otorhinolaryngology, with dermatology, accident and emergency, general medicine, geriatrics, and psychiatry.

Day Release

Throughout the year the general practice registrar is required to attend weekly seminars organized by the tutor in general practice. These seminars currently occupy the whole of Wednesday afternoon and are divided into several sections. Specifically, attention is given to clinical, behavioral, and organizational aspects of general practice. The registrars are encouraged to identify their own learning needs, and an attempt is made to pattern the program to meet their specific requirements. A physician who has completed the general practice registrar program should have the competence and confidence to enter general practice and practice high quality patient care. He is also eligible to take the written examination for membership in the College of General Practitioners.

It should be noted that this training program is not obligatory for candidates for the New Zealand College of General Practitioners' examination. Any physician who has completed two years of satisfactory and broad-based hospital training together with six months in general practice experience is entitled to take the written examination of the College.

Even successful completion of the College written examination does not in itself assure membership in the College. The College requires a final assessment five years after qualification and after a minimum of two years' hospital experience and a minimum of two years' general practice experience. The additional year may be spent either in general practice or in hospital or in a combination of both. Thus, the registrar year is a very appropriate way to spend this time.

The fact that the College requires a minimum of two years' general practice experience before awarding its membership is

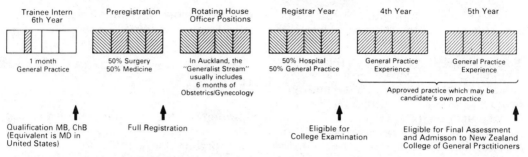

Fig. 1. General practice training scheme.

an indication that it believes there is no substitute for practical experience in the field. Without this, the situation would be comparable to a surgeon being Board Cer-tified in surgery without having ever per-formed an operation. An overview of the general practice training scheme is pre-sented in Figure 1.

A Network Model for Decentralized Family Practice Residency Training*

John P. Geyman, Thomas C. Brown

The organization of departments and divisions of family practice in a majority of medical schools in the United States has facilitated a recent trend toward increasing numbers of university affiliations with family practice residency programs in community hospitals. Many difficult issues arise when such affiliations are explored and developed. To date, the literature is meager on this important subject. This paper describes the elements of a network model for decentralized family practice residency training which has been in operation at the University of California Davis for over four years. Common issues are outlined, together with the various advantages of affiliation to the community hospital and the university. An active partnership between the medical school and community through a network of affiliated residency programs can effectively contribute to the quality of medical education and patient care on a regional basis and at the same time directly address the problem of physician maldistribution.

The last ten years have seen growing interest in several new directions in medical education, including increased emphasis on primary care education, increased involvement of community hospitals and practicing physicians in the educational process, and recognition of medical education as a continuum involving undergraduate, graduate, and postgraduate phases. There has been concurrent interest in addressing major problems of maldistribution of physician manpower, both by specialty and by geographic distribution. Medical schools have been expected by government at both state and federal levels to be more responsive to these issues than in the past. Major changes are occurring in medical education, including expanded responsibility for graduate education by medical schools[1] and the rapid and impressive development of family practice.

Since its inception as a specialty in 1969, there has been an impressive development of family practice residency programs throughout the country. Table 1 shows the rapid growth in the absolute number of programs and number of residents enrolled between 1970 and 1973. Since 1973,

while numbers of programs and residency positions have continued to increase, the rate of growth is somewhat less. The average number of residents per program has increased from 5.9 in 1970 to 17.2 in 1976. These data suggest that family practice residency programs are consolidating at or near their full complement of residents.

Initially, the large majority of family practice residency programs were in unaffiliated community hospitals. More recently, however, as departments/divisions of family practice have been organized in a majority of the nation's medical schools, the number of university-based and university-affiliated programs has steadily increased. Many medical schools are seriously exploring or starting development of additional affiliated relationships with outlying community hospitals, so that the number of university-affiliated programs can be expected to continue to increase.

A number of difficult issues present themselves as these affiliations are planned and implemented. To date there has been no report in the literature dealing specifically with this subject. Based on the experience at the University of California Davis in developing a regional network of affiliated family practice residency programs

* Reprinted by permission from *The Journal of Family Practice*, 3(6):621–627, 1976.

Table 1. *Growth of Family Practice Residencies**

Year	Number of Approved Programs	Number of Residents	Average Number of Residents per Program
1970	49	290	5.9
1971	87	534	6.1
1972	133	1015	7.6
1973	191	1771	9.3
1974	233	2671	11.4
1975	259	3720	14.4
1976	272	4675	17.2

* Information for this table was provided by the Division of Education, American Academy of Family Physicians, Kansas City, Missouri.

over the past four years, this paper will describe the elements of an operational network model for decentralized family practice residency training, outline some common issues involved, and list the various advantages to the community hospital and the university in developing affiliated relationships.

Rationale for Regional Network Approach

In recent years, a number of medical educators have called for an expanded role of the medical school on a regional basis.[2-6] The traditional role of the university medical center as a tertiary care center has been under pressure, not only through the development of excellent secondary and tertiary care capabilities in the larger community hospitals, but through the increasing pressure on university medical centers to provide primary care services as well. The relationship of the university medical center to the community now requires reassessment and the development of new linkages to the community, involving the extension of university resources to the adjacent region in a non-competitive and supportive way.

The spiraling costs of health care and medical education have brought serious reassessment of present funding methods, and major changes are in the legislative hopper at both state and federal levels. Funding to medical schools is increasingly in short supply for present and projected needs, and stipend support for residency training in some fields is being contracted or withdrawn altogether. It seems clear that we will have to fully utilize short resources in coming years if we are to address societal needs and maintain adequate quality in medical education. The sharing of teaching and evaluation resources on a network basis allows access by each affiliated program to substantial resources not otherwise available or affordable.

Legislative and societal interest in the problems of maldistribution of physicians by specialties and by geographic area has reached a high level and intense pressures have been placed on the medical education system to respond to such gaps. Based on the precept that family practice residency training should be patterned closely on the realities of the future family physician's practice, a well-developed network of affiliated programs should logically include educational models in urban, suburban, and rural settings. There is good evidence that physicians often locate their practices within 100 miles of the community where they completed residency training,[7,8] so that locating affiliated residencies in or near physician shortage areas can be expected to positively influence physician manpower in such areas.

The progressive extension of specialty

and subspecialty expertise and modern facilities to smaller communities throughout the country in recent years, together with the interest of many practicing physicians in teaching and the availability of excellent clinical facilities, allows for extension of residency training into new community settings. Many physicians recognize the teaching process as a stimulating and effective form of continuing medical education. Favorable experience has been reported during the past ten years with new approaches to decentralized medical education.[9,10]

Of all specialties within medicine, family practice lends itself most readily to residency training in decentralized settings. Instead of requiring exposure in depth to tertiary care problems, as is the need of most other specialty residency programs, a broad experience with primary and secondary care problems is essential in family practice, including emphasis on ambulatory care training. Reality-based learning settings are needed, including teaching by family physicians and consultants in other specialty disciplines. Smaller community hospitals can provide excellent teaching settings if support and interest within the medical community are high.

An Operational Network Model

The essential elements of an operational model can be briefly outlined for the University of California Davis Family Practice Residency Network Program, a decentralized regional program now in its fifth year of development. Some specifics of this program have been more fully described in a previous paper.[11] The intent, here, is to identify critical elements which particularly relate to network function. They are presented as one approach to the challenge of decentralizing resident training. Many of these approaches may be applicable elsewhere, although the details of implementing similar programs in other parts of the country must necessarily be

adapted to existing local and regional needs and available resources.

Overall Philosophy

The intent has been to develop a residency network in University of California Davis Affiliated Hospitals for Family Practice which provides a spectrum of teaching and learning settings in order to meet varied interests and needs of individual residents at geographically and culturally diverse locations. This network has been viewed as a dynamic system of closely interrelated programs, a "family" of programs, within which educational and clinical resources are shared to best provide excellent learning climates in each setting. Individual programs within the network are encouraged to develop specific strengths, and it is expected that curricular and teaching strategies may vary somewhat among the affiliated programs. At the same time, the network is integrated through various common approaches to general needs. The residency network is also seen as a basic structure upon which other teaching programs can be superimposed, both within the University Department of Family Practice and other clinical departments.

Varied Program Settings

There are 89 residents in five component programs within the network during the 1976–1977 year (Table 2). The University-based program is situated at Sacramento Medical Center, a 450-bed teaching hospital with a housestaff of 280 representing all major disciplines. A satellite family practice center is being developed in Davis, 14 miles from Sacramento, as an integral part of the University-based program. The affiliated program at San Joaquin General Hospital in Stockton, 65 miles south of Davis, is a full three-year program in a 249-bed hospital with a total housestaff of 52 (including residents in

Table 2. *Residents in Component Network Programs 1976–1977*

Component Program	Residents by Year*	Total Number of Residents†
University of California Davis		
Sacramento Medical Center	8–8–8	24
Davis satellite	4–4–0	8
First year for Merced and Redding	8–0–0	8
San Joaquin General Hospital, Stockton	5–6–5	16
Merced Community Medical Center	0–4–4	8
Shasta Cascade Program, Redding	0–4–3	7
Contra Costa County Hospital, Martinez	6–6–6	18
Total		89

* Figures indicate number of first, second, and third year residents.
† Total number of residents in network will ultimately be 96 (4–4–4 in the Davis satellite of the Sacramento program, 6–6–6 at Stockton and 0–4–4 at Redding).

family practice, internal medicine, surgery and obstetrics-gynecology). The affiliated program at Martinez, 60 miles southwest of Sacramento, is located at Contra Costa County Hospital, a 250-bed facility, without other housestaff. The affiliated programs in Merced and Redding are located 130 and 150 miles from Sacramento, respectively, in smaller community hospitals without other specialty residents. Each of these programs provides training for second and third-year residents who have completed their first year at Sacramento Medical Center.

There are currently 40 family practice residents in the University-based program at Sacramento Medical Center, including 24 (eight in each of three years) based there, eight in the Davis satellite part of the program, and eight categorical first-year family practice residents who will complete their training in Merced and Redding. The Davis-based residents relate to a family practice center and small community hospital in Davis, and serve inpatient clinical rotations on the major teaching services in Sacramento hospitals. There are 16 family practice residents (5-6-5) in the Stockton program, which also includes second and third-year inpatient rotations in the 300-bed St. Joseph's Hospital in Stockton. The Martinez program was converted to family practice last year from its previ-

ous structure as a general practice residency program, and is based in a hospital with a full-time staff of over 30 physicians serving a large urban-rural county. There are eight residents (0-4-4) in both the Merced and Redding programs, which are integrated with the University-based program for first-year training.

Merced and Redding represent the smallest communities within the network, each with a population in their immediate areas of approximately 50,000, and each involving the participation of at least 50 teaching physicians representing all major specialty disciplines. The Merced program involves one 160-bed hospital, while the Redding program involves two hospitals totalling 296 beds; the three-year integrated program for Merced and Redding residents also relates to the 450-bed Sacramento Medical Center for first-year and subsequent selective/elective experiences. The size of the teaching practice in the Family Practice Center of each of the component programs within the network varies with the size of each residency program.

Affiliation Agreements

Affiliation agreements have been concluded with each of the outlying community hospitals which define general responsibilities of the participating parties. Specific operational procedures subject to periodic revision are intentionally not spelled out in these agreements, but are verbally agreed upon between the university and community hospital before the affiliated relationship is initiated. Affiliation agreements which are now in force within the network call for joint responsibility between the university and community hospital for such functions as development, operation and evaluation of the family practice residency program, supervision of instruction, selection of residents and faculty, and malpractice liability. The dean of the medical school (through the director of the network program in the Department of Family Practice) is ultimately responsible for quality control of the educational program throughout the network, while residents in outlying affiliated hospitals are directly responsible to their base hospitals for performance of their everyday patient care responsibilities.

Program Administration

Monthly meetings are held at the University of California Davis, Sacramento Medical Center involving all program directors within the network. These sessions allow free interchange of ideas, coordination of common activities, troubleshooting of problem areas, and joint planning of educational and evaluational strategies.

The network base is responsible for all support mechanisms serving the network as well as overall coordination and quality control of the network. Application procedures are centralized so that resident applicants can arrange coordinated interview visits to any hospital and make application to the network as a whole, ranking individual preferences. Presently, three National Intern and Resident Matching Program (NIRMP) matching numbers are used, one for the Stockton program, one for the Martinez program, and one for Sacramento Medical Center and its integrated outlying programs, so that internal match-

ing is also required in the selection process. Resident contracts are signed by the three involved parties—the resident, the community hospital, and the university. All residents within the network are registered as graduate students of the university and are employees of their base hospital.

Curriculum Development

The initial design, development, evaluation and revision of the curriculum for the family practice residency is a collaborative effort involving the University and the affiliated community hospital. Initial and follow-up applications for accreditation by the Residency Review Committee in Family Practice are jointly prepared. Major changes of the curriculum in any affiliated program involve mutual agreement. The length and design of specific clinical rotations are adapted to the resources and needs of each affiliated hospital, and necessarily vary somewhat among hospitals within the network. Since both the Merced and Redding programs are integrated with the University-based program at Sacramento Medical Center for first-year resident training as well as later subspecialty selectives, careful coordination is required for scheduling of clinical rotations.

Visiting Professor Program

An active Visiting Professor Program, carried out for all affiliated programs, involves faculty from the various clinical departments in the School of Medicine. This program is conducted on a biweekly basis, the fields and subjects supplementing the educational resources available to each affiliated program. The format of the Visiting Professor Program varies with the consultant's field of interest and expertise but usually includes a didactic presentation as well as an informal seminar including case presentations by residents. Consultants may make rounds on hospitalized patients and audit selected charts as the basis of a teaching seminar. The presence of visiting professors from the university medical center in outlying affiliated hospitals allows productive exchange with practicing physicians and increases their awareness of consultation and referral services available through the medical school.

Visiting family practice faculty are also involved on a regular basis in supporting the teaching program in affiliated residency programs. They assist the affiliated program director with resident evaluation and teaching in the family practice center, troubleshoot problems in the training program, and coordinate the needs of the affiliated program for supplemental teaching through the Visiting Professor Program and self-instructional materials.

Network Teaching Bank

The program incorporates family practice self-teaching materials as integral supplements to the residency program. Through the support of a grant from the Kellogg Foundation, a Network Teaching Bank of self-instructional materials has been developed.[12] The Network Teaching Bank stresses the use of media which are portable and easily maintained and which facilitate individualized learning by the residents. Learning carrels are established in the family practice center of each affiliated residency site for the use of video cassettes, tape-slides, and other self-instructional media. Selected self-instructional units in the major clinical disciplines are rotated monthly to each affiliated program. In addition, residents, faculty, and local physician groups can request specific materials at any time from the Network Teaching Bank catalog. *Elective* usage of Network Teaching Bank materials involved 166 audiovisual units and over 4,500 days used during the 1974–1975 year, and 231 units and 10,110 days during the 1975–1976 year.

Network Self-Assessment Center

The Network Self-Assessment Center has developed several major components in an effort to monitor and improve the quality of resident training in all affiliated hospitals. These include a data bank of examination questions, an annual self-assessment examination, and performance files for each resident, including personality profiles and completed self-assessment and examination materials. Data collected on individual residents are considered confidential. The purpose of self-assessment is to provide individual feedback to each resident as well as to serve program directors by giving them overall information on resident characteristics for planning purposes.

The self-assessment examinations are geared to specific knowledge and skills considered by a criterion group of experienced family physicians and teachers as essential to the acce)table practice of family medicine. They are also used to facilitate continuing medical education for practicing family physicians in the region. The self-assessment examinations include two basic parts: a multiple-choice section and a section of slides which tests visual recognition of common clinical entities. Testing techniques include those used in the American Board of Family Practice examination. Confidential profiles of test results in each major clinical discipline assist each resident in identifying strengths and weaknesses, and question-specific feedback facilitates learning.[13]

Self-assessment procedures are closely related to other ongoing evaluation methods throughout the Network, including medical audit and data retrieval of resident experience. Criteria and results of audits in individual programs are shared throughout the Network. The Network Self-Assessment Center is also involved in ongoing longitudinal follow-up of residency graduates from all hospitals within the network. This effort provides feedback on such questions as the adequacy of their residency training for their practices, the spectrum and location of their practices, and their experience with certifying examinations of the American Board of Family Practice.

Teacher Development

An active teacher development program for members of the clinical faculty is considered vital to effective resident teaching. Periodic workshops are held in affiliated community hospitals for members of the network clinical faculty. Typical content areas include orientation to program objectives; overview of residency program curriculum and resident capability levels in each residency year; the ingredients of effective learning experiences; roles of the teacher and the resident in hospital and family practice center settings; use of the problem-oriented record as a teaching tool; audit of medical records; teaching techniques with emphasis on the critiquing approach; and resident and teacher use of self-instructional materials and self-assessment methods.

The teacher development program helps to increase the effectiveness of teaching by members of the clinical faculty in outlying communities, as well as increase the satisfaction from resident teaching derived by participating physicians. Teaching and learning activities are seen as dynamic opportunities for continuing medical education for the participating physicians.

Resident Exchange

An essential principle is that the Family Practice Center in each component program serves as home base for the residents assigned there. There are opportunities,

however, for a resident in any part of the University of California Davis Family Practice Residency Network Program to take electives in another part of the overall program, based upon individual needs and the particular strengths of the other parts of the program. For example, residents in affiliated programs in smaller communities can probably best meet their objectives in medical subspecialties and rehabilitation at the Sacramento Medical Center. Conversely, residents in larger hospitals may arrange for electives in smaller hospitals within the network for those experiences best offered there. Meanwhile, continuity of care for the resident's patients during these elective experiences away from home base is provided by other residents through a team approach.[14]

Locum Tenens Exchange

The preceptorship-locum tenens rotation is a required six-week rotation during the third resident year throughout the network. It is considered an important opportunity for an advanced resident to experience a real practice setting similar to that which he or she anticipates selecting on completion of training. The involved program director makes a site visit in advance to approve a potential locum tenens site as an effective learning setting. It is required that the resident have consultation readily available for outpatients and for any patients admitted to the hospital locally. The first two weeks of the six-week rotation are a preceptorship, during which the resident becomes acquainted with the practice, office staff, procedures, and local medical community. The practicing family physician may then return to the University of California Davis for two or four weeks of postgraduate training which includes self-assessment through the Network Self-Assessment Center, individualized learning through the Network Teaching Bank and individualized training using the resources of the Sacramento Medical Center or another university facility.

Family Practice Clerkships

Since the entire fourth year of the undergraduate curriculum in the School of Medicine at the University of California Davis is composed of elective courses, there is ample opportunity for students interested in family practice to participate in clerkships. Family practice clerkships, developed in conjunction with residency programs in the University of California Davis Affiliated Hospitals for Family Practice, are five to ten weeks in duration.

In a family practice clerkship, fourth-year medical students work under the supervision of faculty members and residents. They see and follow patients in the Family Practice Center, follow selected hospitalized patients, and assist with deliveries and other procedures. Students are expected to attend all teaching conferences, the Journal Club, meetings of the local chapter of the Academy of Family Physicians, and county medical society meetings.

Linkage with Family Nurse Practitioner Program

The Department of Family Practice at the University of California Davis conducts a regional family nurse practitioner program. This program is decentralized to teaching satellites conducted in conjunction with each residency site within the network. Efforts are made to facilitate the team approach to practice in each affiliated residency program. It is considered important that residents learn to share responsibility for patient care with other members of the health-care team, and the network residency system forms an ideal structure for collaborative training with family nurse practitioners.

Research

An annual conference is held involving residents from all affiliated programs to report the results of research and innovations from the various programs within the network. In addition, residents are given the opportunity of sharing particular strengths and weaknesses of various programs and becoming involved in problem resolution.

As the network matures past the usual initial organizational problems, research and original projects are being encouraged for the residents. Various research tools are implemented in each residency program, including the problem-oriented record, data retrieval systems, medical audit, and library search capabilities using Medline. Faculty from the university are available to outlying affiliated residency programs for assistance with research design, the conduct of projects and data analysis.

Funding

The concept of shared funding of program costs has been utilized from the outset of development of the network residency program. Participating hospitals generally are responsible for payment of their own resident salaries and costs of their related Family Practice Centers; patient-care revenue in turn reverts to each hospital. State funding has been instrumental in providing partial payment of starting costs of some programs within the network. The university shares equally with each community hospital in paying the salary of the program director and supports through grant funding the development and implementation of the various administrative, educational, and evaluation support mechanisms which have been outlined. The great majority of teaching physicians participate in the residency program as clinical faculty members on a volunteer basis without remuneration.

Common Issues Concerning Affiliation

As the University Department of Family Practice enters exploratory discussions with an outlying community hospital regarding a potential affiliated family practice residency program, a number of basic issues are usually raised. Some of the more important issues which we have encountered are likely to be applicable elsewhere.

The medical staff of a community hospital without previous experience with affiliated residency programs may well feel some degree of threat concerning possible excessive university involvement in medical care and existing operations of the hospital. Such fears are generally unfounded but must be dealt with through frank discussion of the goals and expectations of each party to the proposed affiliation.

Since family practice residency training, in contrast to many other specialty residencies, is usually based in large part (or even exclusively) in the participating hospitals and related family practice center, the curriculum and schedule of teaching rotations has maximum impact on the community hospital. In many cases, resident rotations are integral to a portion of patient care services provided by the hospital. Responsibility for curriculum design, evaluation, and revision must, therefore, be clearly understood and agreed upon by both parties to the affiliation.

It can be anticipated that questions will be raised as to responsibility for evaluation and quality control of the teaching program. Who is primarily responsible for this function? How are standards set and how is the experience and performance of each resident monitored? How are problems in resident performance to be dealt with?

Questions will certainly arise concerning the resident selection process—how are residents to be selected, by what criteria, by whom? Specific items requiring clarification and mutual agreement are NIRMP matching numbers, application forms, and resident contracts. Clarification of respon-

sibility in selection of teaching physicians likewise warrants discussion, including criteria for university teaching appointments.

A number of legal considerations must be considered in any proposed affiliation. An affiliation agreement must necessarily clarify responsibility for such matters as curriculum design, program evaluation, resident and faculty selection, malpractice liability of the residents and teaching physicians, employer-employee relationship of residents within the program, and appropriate procedures for research and publication.

Responsibility for funding various parts of the affiliated residency program inevitably needs careful definition. Who is to pay the resident salaries, faculty salaries, and expenses of the family practice center? How is billing for patient care services to be accomplished, and how is patient care revenue applied to program costs? How will grant proposals be initiated for extramural funding?

As the specifics of a proposed affiliated family practice residency program take shape, it is necessary to identify the specific administrative, educational, and evaluational support mechanisms required from the university to carry out the program. Once identified, questions must be raised concerning the availability of such resources and the logistics of extending these resources to the affiliated hospital, which may be located some distance from the university.

Advantages of the Network Approach

It is only natural that both parties to a possible affiliation take a hard look at "What's in it for us?" Clearly, any productive ongoing affiliated relationship between the university and the community hospital requires tangible gains to both parties.

The development and operation of a regional network of affiliated family practice residency programs requires a collaborative effort involving the university and outlying communities. Through formal affiliations in family practice with community hospitals, *participating hospitals* can realize a number of advantages:

1. Assistance in residency program development through the pooled experience of other affiliated programs.
2. Assistance with the establishment of educational objectives and evaluation of resident performance.
3. Expansion of teaching resources through visiting professor programs and self-instructional materials.
4. Augmented effectiveness of teaching through teacher development programs.
5. Increased potential to recruit well-qualified program directors and teaching physicians.
6. Enhanced potential for recruitment of residents of high caliber because of university affiliation and associated student clerkship programs.
7. Increased opportunities for resident electives, both at the university and elsewhere in the regional network program.
8. Access to allied health personnel being trained in other university programs, such as family nurse practitioners.
9. Potential for increased funding for some program costs through university and/or grant funds acquired for the network.

At the same time, the *university* will also realize a number of benefits, including:

1. Increased opportunity to contribute to the training of an appropriate number of well-qualified family physicians.
2. Extension of continuing medical education to a larger area beyond the medical school itself.
3. Increased clinical resources and learning opportunities for medical students, residents, and allied health personnel.
4. An augmented range of electives elsewhere in the network of affiliated hospitals for university-based family practice residents.
5. Opportunities to participate in the development of new models of education and health-care delivery.
6. Enhanced potential for collaborative research in family practice.
7. Facilitation of improved linkages between primary, secondary, and tertiary care on a regional basis.
8. Potential for increased utilization of the university for consultation and referral.

The ongoing operation of a regional network of family practice residency programs should increase the quality of education in family practice at all levels—undergraduate, graduate, and postgraduate. Such programs should also tend to increase the quality of care provided in outlying communities. In the long run, it is likely that these decentralized programs will favorably influence physician supply and expand primary care resources within the region.

Discussion

Initial experience with the network program as outlined has been excellent. Network support mechanisms are being well utilized and accepted. The network functions as a dynamic and evolving equilibrium among participating programs, each of which is encouraged to develop its own individual strengths. A cooperative spirit among affiliated programs has been developed and maintained, and has helped' to resolve operational problems as they have arisen.

Some examples of effective network functioning through cooperation of affiliated programs include the coordination of site selection for the locum tenens exchange of third-year residents; the involvement of all program directors in teacher development workshops being carried out at any one of the programs; effective planning by residents from all component programs of the annual research conference; sharing of audit criteria and results; and the joint development and testing of new network procedures, such as a manual system for data retrieval in family practice centers.

Despite the progress to date with the network program, continuing efforts are required to address several problem areas. There is a need for improved methods of recording of resident experience and evaluation of resident learning. There is considerable "down time" of faculty participating in the Visiting Professor program, and improved methods of communication within the network for consultation and teaching are needed. Separate NIRMP match numbers (not presently provided for integrated programs) would better facilitate matching firstyear residents to individual programs within the network. There is a continuing need for extramural funding to further consolidate network operation as it matures.

It is recognized that there is no single blueprint for development of a regional network residency program in family practice. Network approaches elsewhere must be adapted to particular regional needs and resources as they exist. It appears, however, that many of the concepts described here can be applied in other parts of the country and that such an approach can result in closer and more productive interaction between the medical school and its region. Such an active partnership with affiliated community hospitals can contribute to the quality of medical education and patient care on a regional basis, as well as provide a systematic approach to address the physician maldistribution problem.

Acknowledgments

The work reported in this paper was made possible by grants from the WK Kellogg Foundation and the Public Health Service, Department of Health, Education, and Welfare (Grant #09D 000478-02-0).

REFERENCES

1. Committee on Graduate Medical Education of the Association of American Medical Colleges: Guidelines for academic medical centers planning to assume institutional responsibility for graduate medical education. J Med Educ 48: 779–791, 1973
2. Cohen WJ: Medical education and physician manpower from the national level. J Med Educ 44:15–17, 1969
3. Dennis JL: Medical education, physician manpower, the state and community. J Med Educ 44:18–22, 1969
4. Jason H: The relevance of medical education to medical practice. JAMA 212:2093–2094, 1970
5. Evans RL: Use of community/private sector resources. J Med Educ 50(12) pt 2:49–56, 1975
6. Kowalewski EJ: Development of resources—toward real community involvement. J Med Educ 50(12) pt 2:57–61, 1975
7. Royce PC: Can rural health education centers influence physician distribution? JAMA 220:847–849, 1972
8. Bible BL: Physicians' views of medical practice in nonmetropolitan communities. Public Health Rep 85:11–17, 1970
9. Penrod KE: The Indiana program for comprehensive medical education. JAMA 210:868–870, 1969
10. Grove WJ: The University of Illinois plan for expanding medical education. JAMA 210:871–875, 1969
11. Geyman JP, Brown TC: A developing regional network residency program in family practice (Medical Education). West J Med 121:514–520, 1974
12. Geyman JP, Brown TC: A teaching bank of audiovisual materials for family practice. J Fam Pract 2:359–363, 1975
13. Geyman JP, Brown TC: An intraining examination for residents in family practice. J Fam Pract 3:409–413, 1976
14. Geyman JP: Implementing continuity in a family practice residency program. J Fam Pract 2:445–447, 1975

Developing an Objective Based Curriculum for a Family Practice Residency*

Carole J. Bland, Donald R. Houge, Harold J. Hofstrand,
Louis J. Filiatrault, John W. Gunkler

Although there is a preponderance of articles on behavioral objectives in education, few address the process by which objectives are developed and agreed upon in a residency training program. The process by which objectives are developed is critical to their eventual implementation. The development and implementation of objectives are particular concerns in family practice residencies which, because of their broad based content, are uniquely dependent on other departments for portions of the residency training program. This paper describes an approach for developing curriculum objectives in a Family Practice Residency Program which emphasized the personal involvement of individuals who would be instrumental in implementing the curriculum, such as program directors, coordinators of "other" specialty rotations, and resident representatives. This approach, although time-consuming, resulted in well-formulated objectives that could be implemented. Further, this approach allowed for intensive interaction among various faculty members representing many fields, resulting in increased mutual understanding and appreciation.

Many books and articles have been written on behavioral objectives in education.[1-5] The *Educational Index* alone references over 600 such publications for the last five years. However, only a small percentage of these publications address the role of behavioral objectives in medical education, and even fewer relate directly to residency training. The articles that do concentrate on objectives for medical education usually cover only an isolated area of undergraduate medical education,[6-19] and those which consider residency training relate largely to broad goals rather than defined objectives and ignore the process by which these goals were derived.[1,20-28] Thus, when beginning to write objectives for a residency training curriculum, the literature on objective writing provides little help in understanding the *process* of developing effective, agreed-upon objectives. The purpose of this paper is to describe such a process as it occurred in a newly developing department of a well-established

medical school. Some of the problems which arose may be unique to family practice because of its broad based content, its dependence on other departments, and its recent origin. The methods used in solving these problems, however, are likely to benefit many types of residency programs.

Setting

The Department of Family Practice and Community Health with an Affiliated Residency Training Program was established at the University of Minnesota in 1970. The Affiliated Residency Training Program has become the largest family practice residency in the country with 199 residents in nine programs. The rapid development of the department and its residency program, with wide responsibilities within an established University, contributed to the early recognition of the need for objectives. These same factors, however, presented some difficulties. How could objectives be established and implemented that would blend with the interests

* Reprinted by permission from *The Journal of Family Practice*, 4(1):103–110, 1977.

and resources of the University's other residency training programs and its medical school, while still meeting the specific needs of the residency programs in Family Practice and Community Health?

Why Write Objectives?

There are a number of generally recognized reasons why educational objectives are of value. Such reasons include better communication with colleagues and increased efficiency and effectiveness for both student and teacher as a result of understanding what is expected in the learning process. Many other reasons are discussed in the literature.[1-5]

The specific impetus for writing objectives in this situation came from persistent concerns within the department. The concerns fell into three categories: (1) program evaluation, (2) program delineation, and (3) faculty utilization. The need for evaluation was recognized early in the program's development. A norm-referenced, subjective evaluation system was instituted to provide continuous feedback to the program directors and department chairman about resident performance, teacher performance, and service or course effectiveness.[29] In addition to this subjective information, the faculty felt a need for defined criteria and for a more objective way to evaluate residents and learning experiences. It was the need for a clearer program delineation and faculty utilization, however, that finally crystallized the faculty's effort into a vigorous attempt to establish a set of minimum educational objectives. As the second and third years of the residency program developed and the number of residents increased, more learning experiences and more teachers were needed in family medicine and in the conventional specialties. Heavy reliance was placed upon the private practitioners of the community, the medical staff of the affiliated hospitals, and on the full-time academic faculty at the University Hospitals.

Subsequently, the family practice teachers felt the pressure of overextension and the chairmen of several other departments in the medical school voiced their concern over the extent of their departments' involvement in the family practice educational program. A clearer description of the program's curriculum was needed to make more efficient use of all faculty and to identify the role of conventional specialties in family practice resident training.

Who Writes the Objectives?

As a result, several departments of the medical school were asked to participate in the development of core curriculum objectives and in the planning of educational strategies for family practice residents. Representatives from these departments became involved and they, along with the family practice program directors and other persons from the affiliated hospitals, constituted core curriculum committees whose responsibility it was to outline the curriculum and establish or maintain learning experiences to meet curriculum goals. Each core curriculum committee was responsible for the delineation of a major subdivision, such as surgery, of the residency training program.

The educational psychologists in the Department of Family Practice and Community Health joined with the members of the core curriculum committees in the spring of 1974 to write educational objectives for the residency program. By the fall of 1974 a set of objectives had been written covering the minimum competencies expected of family practice residents in the area of surgery. Even though a draft of the surgical objectives had been completed by working with the entire surgery core curriculum committee, it was decided to implement a program of objective writing which did not require the involvement of all the core curriculum committee members. This was done to make more efficient use of faculty time and to establish a smaller group which was more able, among other things, to schedule meetings and hold discussions.

Volunteers from the core curriculum committees as well as other interested family practice faculty became a working task group and began to develop skills of curriculum design and objective writing. The task group included the family practice program directors, educational psychologists, representatives from each conventional specialty and behavioral science, and other family practice faculty who were particularly interested in curriculum development. The original core curriculum committees were maintained to handle immediate curriculum needs and to screen the behavioral objectives written by the task group. Although the task group was to do the majority of the actual objective writing, it was important to maintain the input of the core curriculum committees as they were an invaluable resource representing the specialties touched by family practice. Perhaps, even more important, they needed to share in the development of the objectives since they and their departments would be asked to help accomplish the stated objectives and their contributions would be evaluated in terms of the objectives. This effort, to share the responsibility for developing the objectives, was a cornerstone throughout the objective writing process, a process which involved family practice faculty, other specialty faculty, and residents. It was thought that only through such personal involvement and commitment in the development of the objectives would they become a useful statement of the curriculum instead of a dusty book on a shelf.

Stages Involved in Writing the Objectives

The process of writing the objectives was broken down into four stages as follows: Stage 1: Training in objective writing, Stage 2: Writing objectives for specific areas, Stage 3: Organizing the objectives, and Stage 4: Review, revision, and approval of objectives.

Table 1. *Proposed Uses of Curriculum Objectives*

A. Instructional purposes
  1. To provide a guide for resident expectations
  2. To define expected residency competencies for:
      a. Residents
      b. Teachers
      c. Evaluators
  3. To provide guidelines for developing learning strategies
  4. To provide a delineation of generally stated goals
  5. To provide guidelines for developing teacher competence
B. Evaluation purposes
  1. To provide a basis for developing instruments which will evaluate:
      a. Resident competencies
      b. Teaching effectiveness
      c. Effectiveness of learning experiences
      d. The program as a whole
      e. Program units
      f. The appropriateness of the objectives
C. Communication purposes
  1. To provide a description of the family physician for interested persons, such as,
      a. Patients
      b. Medical students
      c. Other specialties
  2. To illustrate the interrelation of the family physician to other medical specialties and disciplines
D. General purposes*
  1. To provide guidelines for other residency programs
  2. To provide guidelines for residency review committees or other groups establishing standards
  3. To provide guidelines for continuing education programs
  4. To provide guidelines for practicing physicians in self-education and self-assessments

* The general purposes are adapted from the 1974 draft of the "Foundations for Evaluating the Competency of Pediatricians," from the American Board of Pediatrics, Chicago.

Stage 1: Training in Objective Writing

Two workshops were held for the task group during this stage. The first workshop presented the potential uses of the curriculum objectives (Table 1), the role of objectives as an integral part of the curriculum, and a short course on the mechanics of writing objectives.[30]

The second workshop was concerned with establishing a framework or organization for the objectives and with increasing the objective writing skills of the task-group members. There are many ways to outline the curriculum of family practice. The core curriculum outline from the Society of Teachers of Family Medicine[31] and the Educational Objectives from the Family Medicine Residency Training Program at Regina, Saskatchewan,[26] are examples of the different organizations that were considered in developing an outline. It was decided, however, that in this residency program it would be most practical to organize the objectives around the traditional specialty areas such as pediatrics and internal medicine.

During the second workshop, a video tape was presented to demonstrate a strategy for objective writing and the process of give and take involved in writing with others. In addition to outlining a step-by-step procedure for objective writing, the video tape served as a modeling device. It illustrated a method of questioning, working, and writing with others which was unfamiliar to many family physicians who commonly work alone. Since a family practice residency consists of many disciplines besides medicine, the tape showed a physician and an educational psychologist working together, capitalizing on their complementary assets as they developed objectives. The actual steps for objective writing as they were outlined in the tape are diagrammatically presented in Figure 1.

The model presented in Figure 1 illustrates the steps in the objective writing pro-

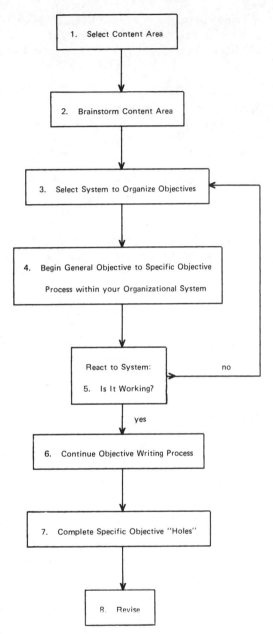

Fig. 1. Model for objective writing process.

cess, which begins with the selection of a content area about which one wishes to write behavioral objectives. The content areas which were identified as core areas in the curriculum were Ob/Gyn, Pediatrics, Internal Medicine, Surgery, Family Medicine, Behavioral Science, Community Health, and Health-Care Coordination.

Stage 2: Writing Objectives for Specific Areas

Stage 2 began with a meeting at which the various core areas were assigned to members, who became subgroups of the task group. Each of these subgroups sketched a breakdown of the area, and took as a "homework" task the job of individually brainstorming a part of the core area (step 2 in the model). The brainstorming process meant simply outlining very loosely and in any format the core area chosen. This brainstorming usually took the form of a dictated collection of somewhat disconnected sentences and thoughts.

During a second set of meetings in stage 2, each subgroup considered various methods of organizing the core area which had been brainstormed (for example, a patient age sequence or a sequence of patient organ systems involved). The next step was to take the brainstormed comments and write actual objectives within the system or organization. Both general and specific objectives were created. The general objectives consisted of phrases like, "the resident will understand. . . . " The specific objectives were the measurable behaviors that characterize a resident who "understands." The specific objectives were usually only a representative sample of information, skills, and attitudes to be learned, and were not an exhaustive list. The specific objectives used words like, "the resident will discuss . . ." or "the resident will perform. . .," or "the resident will identify . . ."* (steps 3 and 4 in the model).

* This format of general and specific objectives is adapted from "Stating Behavioral Objectives for Classroom Instruction," by Norman E. Gronland. London, Macmillan Company, Collier-Macmillan Limited, 1970.

As the subgroups wrote the general and specific objectives, the original organization (for example, chronological or by organ systems) at times seemed cumbersome, and it was occasionally necessary to reorganize and begin again. However, once the system was working, objective writing continued until the core area was complete and defined. Frequently it was easier to write the general objectives, with only a few specific objectives added, leaving "holes" to be filled later by additional specific objectives. Stage 2 proceeded with each subgroup writing and revising their objectives with the assistance of the Department's educational psychologists (steps 5 to 8 in the model).

Stage 3: Organizing the Objectives

During this stage the educational psychologists, with the assistance of various faculty members, began the process of organizing the objectives from all the core areas into a usable package. This consisted of filling in "holes," editing, and organizing the objectives into several more practically useful packages depending on the audience, such as residents, program directors, core coordinators, or preceptors. It was thought that each of these groups had different purposes for the objectives and that different packaging and introductory material would, therefore, help in their understanding and use of the objectives.

Stage 4: Review, Revision, and Approval of Objectives

During this stage each of the nine affiliated program directors, the faculty of the Department of Family Practice, and the members of the core curriculum committees reviewed the objectives. This stage is still being implemented. Final review and approval rests with the faculty of the Department of Family Practice and Community Health, but it was thought important

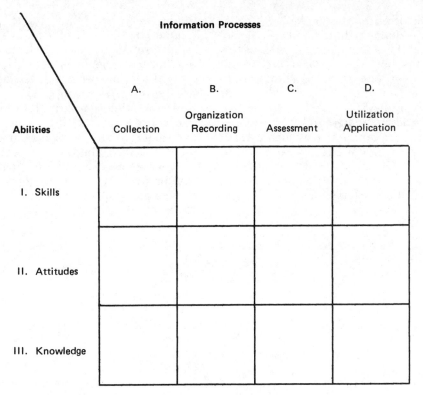

Fig. 2. Grid format. This concept is similar to that used by the American Board of Pediatrics in developing the "Foundations for Evaluating the Competencies of Pediatricians," Chicago, American Board of Pediatrics, 1974.

that each department and hospital which would be asked to implement these objectives continue to have a role in their development and final form.

What Do the Objectives Look Like?

The core curriculum objectives that have resulted from this process define the competencies a family physician should possess when he/she has completed the University of Minnesota Affiliated Residency Training Program in Family Practice and Community Health. One way of conceptualizing the family physician is to view him/her as an information processor for problem solving and health maintenance. The role of the information processor can be viewed as: (A) collecting information, (B)

organizing and recording information, (C) assessing information, and (D) using information to solve problems or direct health maintenance. The core curriculum objectives were organized around this concept of the family physician as an information processor—a "cold" but functional definition for a hopefully very "warm" process.

Thus, the core curriculum objectives are the skills, attitudes, and knowledge a family physician needs in each of the four general areas of information processing. These physician abilities and information processes are woven into an organizational grid with delineated competency areas as shown in Figure 2. The reader may wish to refer to Figure 2 and Figure 3 while reading the following description of the core curriculum objectives.

The core curriculum objectives found in

the Family Practice Master Grid (Figure 3) outline the domain of the family physician. In each of the 12 competency areas of this Family Practice Master Grid are found three types of objectives: (1) common objectives, (2) integrative objectives, and (3) generic objectives.

Common objectives describe basic competencies that are common to all medical specialties and include such things as basic history-taking, basic physical examination techniques, basic investigatory testing, basic recording systems, or basic attitudes towards patients.

The *integrative objectives* describe the unique combination of competencies the family physician possesses that enable him/her to merge or bridge different specialty disciplines when addressing patient situations. These competencies may include such things as attitudes which facilitate use of several disciplines together, knowledge of the domain of many disciplines, or recording systems which easily incorporate a variety of information from various disciplines. Other specialties may possess parts of the integrative objectives. However, the family physician who pos-

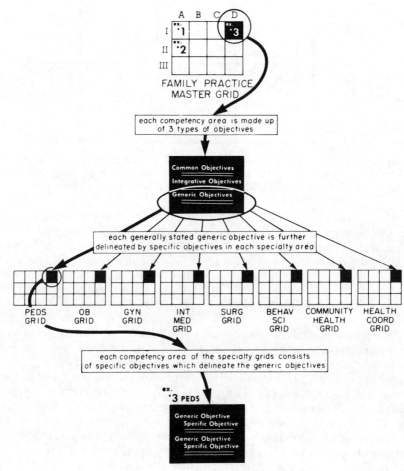

Fig. 3. Family practice master grid.

sesses all the integrative objectives has a unique combination of abilities that allows him/her to effectively interact, merge, and bridge medical specialties as well as other disciplines when problem solving.

The *generic objectives* refer to competencies the family physician uses from other specialty disciplines and applies to specific problems or situations within his/her patient population. For example, the family physician uses specific pediatric abilities in intubating a newborn or specific behavioral science abilities in interpretation of certain psychological test results.

These three types of objectives in the Family Practice Master Grid enjoy different levels of specificity. Common and integrative objectives are stated very specifically, whereas generic objectives are only broadly stated. It is the common and integrative objectives that are primarily addressed by the Family Practice Center or its associated programs, conferences, and seminars. The generic objectives are most likely *first* accomplished on the resident's specialty rotations.

To further delineate the competencies needed within other specialty areas, eight additional grids were derived. Each additional grid has its own specialty designation. Within each of these specialty grids are the specifically stated objectives which further define the broadly stated generic objectives of the Family Practice Master Grid. This spells out for the family practice resident and specialty preceptor(s) the specific competencies the resident should master while on that specialty rotation. The preceptor is thus better able to tailor the experience and teaching strategies.

The above discussion has described the organization and components of the core curriculum objectives. In order to better understand the three types of objectives and how they exist in the various grids, the following examples are given.

Example 1 (See Figure 3.)—The following is an example of a common objective from the Family Practice Master Grid com-

petency area of skill(s) in information collection.

The resident is able to identify and to demonstrate skills designed to establish rapport, such as,

Open-ended questions
Silence
Reflection of feeling
Genuineness
Specificity of expression

Example 2 (See Figure 2.)—The following is an example of an integrative objective from the Family Practice Master Grid competency area of attitude(s) in information collection.

The resident shows concern for the effect of information collected and the manner or means of its collection on the patient and others by, for example,

Getting family's opinions regarding client's health situation;
Sensitively avoiding making statements which elicit fear, hostility, withdrawal, inaction or overstatement from the client;
Providing a gown and appropriate dressing area for teenage patient;
Examining frightened toddler on mother's lap;
Taking the danger and cost of an arteriogram into account before ordering the study;
Using person-to-person, rather than mass media methods for collecting information about an epidemic to avoid causing panic in the community;
Understanding possible effects that a teenage pregnancy could have on the spectrum of family dynamics; and
Taking into account the factors of danger, effectiveness, cost and information gain on patient's entire life of any investigatory work-up or procedure.

Example 3 (See Figure 3.)—The following is an example of a generic objective from the Family Practice Master Grid competency area of skill(s) in information utilization/application.

The resident is able to implement various modalities of intervention for the remediation of patient problems clarified or identified in assessment.

Since this objective is only generally stated in the Family Practice Master Grid, it is more specifically delineated in each specialty grid competency area of skill(s) in information utilization/application. The following is an example taken from the Pediatric Grid to illustrate how this particular generic objective is specified in pediatrics:

Example 3 (See Figure 3.)—The following is an example of a specific objective from the Pediatric Grid competency area of skill(s) in information utilization/application.

The resident is able to implement various pediatric modalities of intervention, such as the following, for the remediation of problems clarified or identified in assessment of the pediatric patient.

Injections
  subcutaneous
  intramuscular
  intravenous
Tracheal intubation
Suctioning
Emergency tracheotomy
Cardiac defibrillation
Closed cardiac massage
Mouth-to-mouth resuscitation
Ventilation with bag respirator
Cardiac monitoring
Intravenous line
  scalp vein on scalp
  peripheral vein
  transcutaneous catheter placement (subclavian vein)
  cutdown
Umbilical catheter placement (both vein and artery)
Set up and administration of blood

Regulation of incubator
Proper breast suckling technique
Administration of any oral medicine
Thoracentesis
Abdominal paracentesis
Unique office procedures
  eg, remove gum in hair
    remove foreign body from any orifice
Nasal packing
Clip frenulum on tongue
Remove labial adhesions
Remove skin tags
Remove umbilical granuloma
Myringotomy
Immobilization procedures of joints or extremities
Preparation of newborn for transport

In the OB Grid, there would be a similar objective to Example 3 generated from the same generic objective in the Family Practice Master Grid; however, it would address itself to interventions for remediation of obstetric problems. The other specialty grids also fit into this same flow.

The merging of competencies drawn from each of these specialty areas along with the common and integrative competencies, into a family physician can be visualized by examining the Family Physician Daisy (Figure 4). The area within the dotted inner circle represents the Master Grid objectives. The family physician portion of the petals represents the specialty specific objectives.

This organization of the core curriculum objectives is particularly useful as it clearly shows the unique perspective of the family physician working within a variety of disciplines while also expressing his/her dependence upon other disciplines. In addition, this organization of the core curriculum objectives is useful in that the specialty objectives can stand alone as those competencies a resident is expected to acquire in a particular specialty that are unique to that specialty. Thus, specialty preceptors may wish only to read their respective set of specialty objectives.

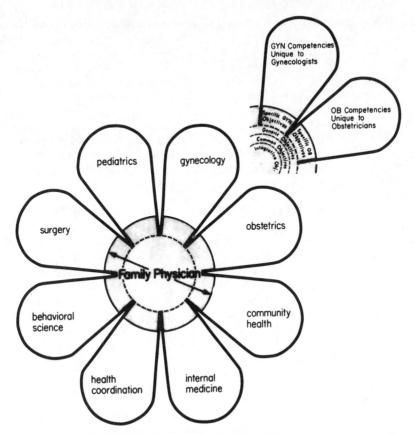

Fig. 4. Family physician daisy.

Discussion

The University of Minnesota Affiliated Residency Training Program in Family Practice is not the first medical area or residency to attempt to define its program in behavioral objectives. However, the method for writing objectives and the resultant objectives at Minnesota differ from other residency programs.[21-24,26,28]

The Minnesota program chose to derive its objectives through the group involvement approach described in this paper because, in developing specific program objectives, it has advantages over the commonly used survey approach. The survey approach employs a small, self-selected group which writes the objectives and mails them to staff physicians, practicing physicians, or students to change, add, delete, or rate.[10,13,32] Schwab, in his article on problems in curriculum development, addresses the advantages of the group involvement approach when he points out that there are "meanings" impossible to encompass in a written statement of objectives that are understood only when one is privy to the initial deliberations.[33] For this reason it is important to include the people who will be involved in the implementation of the curriculum in the initial writing of the objectives. By their inclusion, they gain a full understanding of the final objectives and have a vested interest in seeing them implemented in the full spirit intended.[34] The establishment of the core curriculum committees which linked the Family Practice Residency Program to the many departments and hospitals it touches and the direct involvement of at least one member of each of these committees in the writing of the family practice objectives allowed the program to benefit from the vast resources of a complex university/community system. Just as important, it allowed other departments to assess their role in the Family Practice Residency and to have a direct input into that program.

The involvement of so many people does make the objective writing process slow. However, it results in well-formulated objectives that are likely to be fully implemented, since many people in the various departments who are involved in the family practice training program have an interest in seeing that the objectives that they helped formulate are utilized. Furthermore, within the Family Practice Department, it was important for each program director and faculty member to have a personal interest in the objectives, since their residents and the training program itself would be evaluated by these objectives.

The final form of the Minnesota objectives differs from other residency objectives.[21,24,26-28] Because of the proposed use of these objectives, it was thought that a listing of topic areas or broad goal statements would not be adequate. Although both broad goal statements and lists were helpful in the early stages of writing, it was felt that a measurable performance statement was eventually needed.

The method used at Minnesota for deriving objectives was not, however, without its disadvantages and difficulties. Curriculum planning always involves a long-term reward. The effort put into curriculum planning is made in the hope that the learner, as well as the teacher and the program, will eventually benefit. Certainly, the potential to affect the learning of many residents through joint planning of a uniform curriculum exceeds the effect that teachers can have individually. Individual teaching, however, brings with it immediate rewards while the reward for sitting long hours trying to compose objectives are more distant. Therefore, one needs to be aware of the problems an educator faces when given the choice of writing objectives or spending time teaching residents. Both the objective writers and the educational consultants recognized this difficulty and used many tactics to maintain motivation. Weeks in advance, hours would be blocked off on appointment calendars for sitting and writing. Meetings were arranged where writers were given food and drink and simply went to opposite corners and worked.

This objective writing process not only allowed for the completion of a curriculum defined by objectives, but also resulted in some unexpected byproducts. As a result of learning and writing about objectives, many of the faculty have increased their understanding of the curriculum, instruction, and evaluation. They now feel more comfortable as teachers and managers of an educational program. Perhaps more important, this total program effort, which included much give and take, served to bring the members of the affiliated programs together. They grew to know each other and to understand each other better as they shared in developing and defining the objective based curriculum which defines the Affiliated Family Practice Training Programs at the University of Minnesota.

Acknowledgment

The process and product described in this paper are the result of the combined efforts of the unit directors of the affiliated program, core curriculum committee members, and other interested faculty. Thus, this paper represents the efforts of many more people than the authors listed.

Authors' Update

In the three years since this article appeared, we have changed our approach to curriculum development, evolved a different framework for organizing our curricular objectives, and developed related in-training assessment instruments.

We believe these changes solve two enduring problems in developing objectives: (1) lack of consensus among faculty about the competencies expected of a resident graduate; and (2) need for a simple system of organizing the many competencies that a graduate resident should possess. We used our early experiences in tackling these difficulties to develop a slightly different strategy for writing objectives and a very different system for organizing them.

Single Unit, Not "All-Program" Writing Group

The objective writing task group described in the above paper was drawn from interested persons across the entire Affiliated Program. It was difficult, however, to arrange meetings for this program-wide group. Thus, task groups writing objectives for the remaining content areas consisted primarily of faculty members from only one residency training unit which served as a pilot site. This change built on established relationships among faculty at that site. After one residency training unit had developed objectives for a content area, the five other units in the Affiliated Program reviewed them to be sure that the objectives truly represented a consensus of the competencies to be achieved by a resident graduate.

Revised Framework for Developing Objectives

A simpler framework for generating objectives has evolved. Now only skill objectives are written, and related knowledge and attitude objectives are omitted. We agreed that the attitudes and knowledge portions of each objective could be addressed by simply stating the necessary skill, and alerting preceptors and residents that each stated skill objective assumes all the related attitudes and knowledge. Thus, everyone knows that all three—knowledge, skill, and attitude—are expected to be taught and accomplished.

As the above article describes, objectives in all content areas seem to fall into four categories: (1) collecting information, (2) organizing information and recording it, (3) assessing information, and (4) using the information to plan and carry out a treatment. As we worked with these categories in the various content areas, the same types of competencies kept appearing, regardless of the content area. For example, in category 1, collecting information, all preceptors wanted residents to be able to (1) perform a complete interview, (2) conduct a physical exam, and so forth. We realized that what differs from content area to content area is the specific demonstration of these general abilities. The way a resident performs a complete pediatric interview, for instance, is different from the method in an adult medicine interview. Thus, more of the framework of rewriting objectives evolved. Now the objectives for each core curriculum area are organized as shown in the figure. First, each content area is divided into the four information categories. Then, in each respective category, whatever the content area, the same general objectives appear. Finally, under the general objectives the specific objectives or statements of competencies resident graduates must possess are denoted. It is the specific objectives that vary from content area to content area.

Further Developments

1. Core curriculum objectives in each content area have been written and ap-

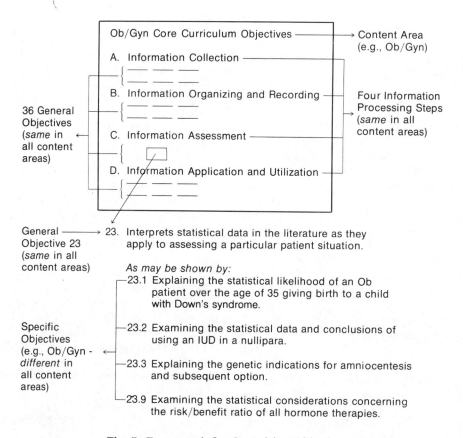

Fig. 5. Framework for Organizing Objectives.

proved by faculty for the entire Affiliated Program.

2. Evaluation checklists which match the rotation structure at each residency site are being constructed.

3. A program-wide computerized exam based on the objectives is being developed.

4. Several articles have been published which discuss in detail various aspects of the changes briefly summarized here.[1,2,3,4]

REFERENCES

(for Update)

1. Holloway RL, Bland CJ, Asp DS, Prestwood SR: Some issues surrounding the implementation of objectives-based education in family medicine. In-house document, Department of Family Practice and Community Health, University of Minnesota, 1980

2. Holloway RL, Bland CJ: An objectives-based curriculum for instruction and evaluation in family practice residency training. Fam Med Teacher, 12:6, 12–14, 1980

3. Holloway RL: Some processes for designing objectives-based instruction and assessment in family practice education. Paper presented at the annual meeting of the Society of Teachers of Family Medicine, Boston, May 1980

4. Holloway RL, Asp DS: Some suggestions for implementing family medicine curriculum objectives. J Med Educ 55:800, 1980

REFERENCES

1. Mager RF: Goal Analysis. Belmont, CA, Feron Publishers, 1972

2. Mager RF: Preparing Instructional Objectives, ed 2. Belmont, CA, Feron Publishers, 1975
3. Baker EL, Popham J: Expanding Dimensions of Instructional Objectives. Englewood Cliffs, NJ, Prentice-Hall, 1973
4. Popham J, Baker EL: Establishing Instructional Goals. Englewood Cliffs, NJ, Prentice-Hall, 1970
5. Gronlund NE: Stating Behavioral Objectives for Classroom Instruction. London, The Macmillan Company, 1970
6. Moreland EF, Provenza DV, Barry SC: Development of operational objectives for a dental curriculum: The anatomies. J Dent Educ 36:39–41, 1972
7. Rous SN, Teitelbaum H: To determine educational objectives for undergraduate urologic teaching: Results of a comprehensive study. Urology 3:107–111, 1974
8. Varagunam T: Student awareness of behavioral objectives: The effect on learning. Br J Med Educ 5:213–216, 1971
9. Arsham GM, Colenbrander A, Spivey BE: A prototype for curriculum development in medical education. J Med Educ 48:78–84, 1973
10. Arsham GM, Good N: Determination of internship objectives. J Med Educ 49:446–448, 1974
11. Depalma RG, Izant RJ, Jordon A, et al: Objectives and methods in undergraduate surgical education. Surgery 75:915–924, 1974
12. Everts JV, Marsh I, Nairn R: The GP's task: Educational objectives. NZ Med J 78:491–493, 1973
13. Braddom RL, Johnson EW, Trzebiatowski G: Curriculum objectives in rehabilitation medicine: Results of a survey. Arch Phys Med Rehabil 55:289–293, 1974
14. Ghai OP: Instructional objectives for training in pediatrics—a paradigm. Indian Pediatr 10:199–201, 1973
15. Schuck RF, Watson CG, Shapiro AP, et al: The use of behavioral objectives in the development and evaluation of a third-year surgical clerkship. J Med Educ 49:604–607, 1974
16. Spivey BE: Developing objectives in ophthalmologic education. Am J Ophthalmol 68:439–445, 1969
17. Spivey, BE: Ophthalmology for medical students: Content and comment. Arch Ophthalmol 84:368–375, 1970
18. Vontner LA: A use of instructional objectives to increase learning efficiency. J Med Educ 49:453–454, 1974
19. Bieszad JM, Lawlor MA Sr: The development and use of level objectives in a diploma program. J Nurs Educ 12(4):30–38, 1973
20. Olsen C: A systems approach to a postgraduate course based on behavioral objectives. Br J Educ Technol 4:204–215, 1973
21. Bacchus H: Preparing educational objectives in internal medicine. J Med Educ 47:708–711, 1972
22. Hiss RG, Peirce JC: A strategy for developing educational objectives in medicine: Problem-solving skills. J Med Educ 49:660–665, 1974
23. Hiss RG, Vanselow NA: Objectives of a residency in internal medicine. Assoc for Hosp Med Educ J 4(1):11–52, 1971
24. College of Family Physicians of Canada: Canadian Family Medicine: Educational Objectives for Certification in Family Medicine. Willowdale, Ontario, College of Family Physicians of Canada, 1974
25. Foundations for Evaluating the Competency of Pediatricians. Chicago, American Board of Pediatrics, 1974
26. Family Medicine Residency Training Program: Educational Objectives. Plains Health Centre, 4500 Wascana Parkway, Regina, Saskatchewan, Canada, 1973
27. Committee on Objectives in Graduate Medical Education for Family Practice: Outline of Residency Objectives. Miami, Florida, University of Miami Department of Family Medicine, 1974
28. Baker RM, Gordon MJ: Competency-based objectives for the family physician. Assoc for Hosp Med Educ J 7:2–16, Summer 1974
29. Bland CJ, Houge DR, Filiatrault LJ, et al: Normative Evaluation in a Residency Training Program. Minneapolis, Minn, University of Minnesota, Department of Family Practice and Community Health, 1974
30. Harris IB: Workbook: Objectives. Minneapolis, Minn, Office of Current Affairs: Evaluation and Research. University of Minnesota Medical School, 1974
31. Spivey BE: A technique to determine curriculum content. J Med Educ 46:269–274, 1971
32. Schwab JJ: The practical 3: Translation into curriculum. School Review 81:501–522, 1973
33. Lighthall FF: Multiple realities and organizational nonsolution. An essay on anatomy of educational innovation. School Review 81:255–294, 1973

Continuity of Care in a Family Practice Residency Program*

Peter Curtis, John Rogers

Continuity of care, one of the basic characteristics of family medicine, was studied over a 12-month period in a family practice residency program. Continuity was measured in three contact areas; office hours, after hours, and on the inpatient service. The intensity of continuity was defined at three levels, from encounters with the personal physician to those with physicians on other medical teams. Continuity was further assessed in relation to family encounters.

Third year residents averaged 83 percent continuity with their individual patients and 70 percent with their assigned families. Residents from other years were noted to have lower levels of continuity. Similar figures were noted for family practice inpatients. Continuity of care in private practice occurs in about 80 percent of patient encounters and it seems reasonable and feasible to expect residency training programs to come close to this figure.

Continuity of care has been identified as one of the important characteristics of primary care.[1-3] The discipline of family medicine has played a leading role in defining the concept of continuity and underlining its importance in educational programs.[4] To achieve accreditation, family practice residency programs are expected to provide, among many factors, evidence that strong efforts are made on both inpatient and outpatient services to ensure continuity of care for patients by their personal physicians. This evidence, in general, consists of the assignment of a physician to a specific group of patients or families, the provision of regular office hours for that physician through the three-year training period, and arrangements for following the patients on the family practice inpatient service. Critics of these attempts to provide continuity suggest that it is in fact not achieved, in spite of the organization of other supporting mechanisms such as physician teams and nurses.

This report investigates the nature of continuity of care in the Family Practice Residency Program at the University of North Carolina over a one-year period.

During this time, a population of 5,020 active patients was served by 17 residents and four faculty physicians divided into three medical teams.

Methods

Continuity of care was studied in three areas of patient contact; office hours contacts, after-hours contacts, and inpatient contacts on the family practice inpatient service. Continuity was classified into three levels. The most intense or first level occurred when the patient interacted only with his or her personal physician over the study period. The second level occurred when the patient made contact with another physician on the same medical team, and the third level was noted when the patient interacted with a physician from another team.

In addition to the study of continuity for the individual, office hours contacts were investigated further in order to ascertain the continuity provided for the families assigned to each physician. Levels of continuity were judged using the same categories as described earlier. Over a period of a year, 11,482 visits were made during office hours and 2,213 contacts were made after hours (both face-to-face and by tele-

* Reprinted by permission from *The Journal of Family Practice*, 8(5): 975–980, 1979.

phone). The average office consultation rate was 2.7 visits per year. Seventy-five percent of the illness episodes only required a single visit and only 12 percent of patients made two visits.

Each patient encounter was documented using an encounter form on which was coded the identification numbers of the patient's personal physician and the contact physician seeing the patient. These, of course, could be one and the same number. The data were punched and stored on computer tape. Inpatient data were obtained by reviewing the medical records and identifying the admitting, discharging, and personal physicians.

Results

Office Hours Contacts—Individual Patient Continuity

Only one half-day was spent per week by first year residents in the Family Practice Center. These physicians therefore saw a

relatively small group of patients. Figure 1 shows that, on average, 187 patients were seen by each first year resident over the 12-month period. First level continuity of care was provided for between 68 percent and 80 percent of their patients. On the average, 17 percent of the first year residents' patients were seen by another physician from the same team. Continuity given by the second year residents is shown in Figure 2. On average, 80 percent of patients saw only their personal physician over the 12-month study period. Figure 3 demonstrates that first level continuity provided by 6 third year residents, who had an average of 901 patient contacts during the study, averaged 83 percent; the faculty physicians averaged 85 percent.

Family Continuity

When the members of a family were seen only by their personal physician over the 12-month period, continuity was regarded

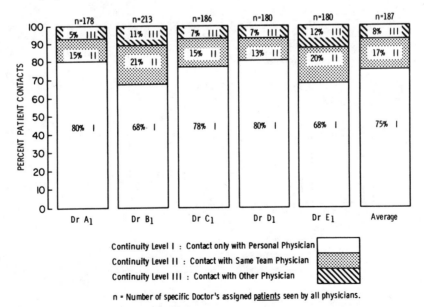

Continuity Level I : Contact only with Personal Physician
Continuity Level II : Contact with Same Team Physician
Continuity Level III : Contact with Other Physician

n = Number of specific Doctor's assigned patients seen by all physicians.

Fig. 1. Continuity of care in a university family medicine program. Office hour contacts: levels of continuity between individual patients and physicians, first year resident physicians.

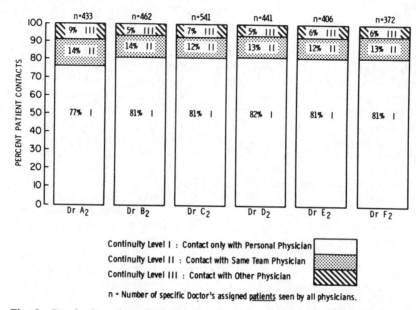

Fig. 2. Continuity of care in a university family medicine program. Office hour contacts: levels of continuity between individual patients and physicians, second year resident physicians.

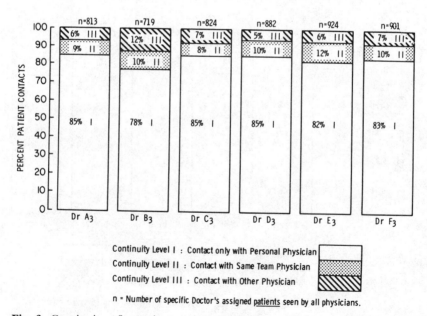

Fig. 3. Continuity of care in a university family medicine program. Office hour contacts: levels of continuity between individual patients and physicians, third year resident physicians.

as being at the first level. Second and third levels of continuity were lumped together for ease of analysis. Any family receiving care from a physician who was not their personal physician was regarded as having received second or third level continuity of care. However, in 90 percent of this latter group the family still saw their personal physician for all contacts except for one encounter. Family continuity of care provided by third year residents is shown in Figure 4. These physicians served 60 percent of the total practice population. First level continuity was provided for 66 to 76 percent of all families seeking care over the 12-month period. Similar figures were obtained for faculty physicians (74 percent on average) but were lower for second year residents (70 percent average) and first year residents (53 percent).

After-Hours Contacts

The major portion of care after office hours was provided by third year residents and the remainder by second year residents. As shown in Figure 5, the first level of continuity, in which the patient consulted with his or her own personal physician, was low for third year residents (9 to 19 percent of each physician's contacts) and even lower for second year residents, averaging six percent of contacts. In general, only a third of the patients made after-hours contact with a physician from their own medical team during the study, so that the lowest level of continuity was provided to patients after hours for approximately two thirds of all the contacts.

Inpatient Services

Over the period of 12 months, 168 patients were admitted to the family practice inpatient service. Continuity of care was presumed to occur if the personal physician was involved in either admitting or discharging his or her patient, or both. Social visits by the personal physician on the wards were difficult to ascertain from the

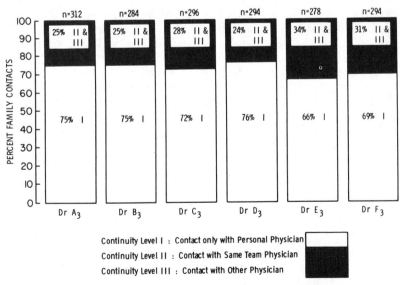

Continuity Level I : Contact only with Personal Physician
Continuity Level II : Contact with Same Team Physician
Continuity Level III : Contact with Other Physician

n = Number of specific Doctor's assigned families seen by all physicians.

Fig. 4. Continuity of care in a university family medicine program. Office hour contacts: levels of continuity between nuclear families and physicians, third year residents.

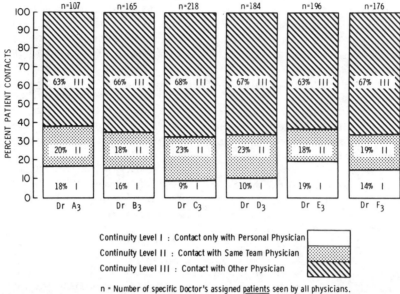

Continuity Level I : Contact only with Personal Physician

Continuity Level II : Contact with Same Team Physician

Continuity Level III : Contact with Other Physician

n = Number of specific Doctor's assigned <u>patients</u> seen by all physicians.

Fig. 5. Continuity of care in a university family medicine program. After-hours contacts: levels of continuity between individual patients and physicians, third year residents.

records and no attempt was made to document these. The percentage of patients receiving continuity of care from their physicians on the inpatient service is shown in Table 1. In all, 68 percent of all patients were involved in some continuity of care by their personal physician. This continuity of care was provided for 92 percent of the patients assigned to third year residents, 77 percent of patients assigned to second year residents, and 50 percent of the patients assigned to faculty physicians.

Discussion

Continuity of care has been characterized into five theoretical dimensions by Hennen: chronological, geographic, interdisciplinary, interpersonal, and informational.[5] It is not possible to adequately measure all of these characteristics, but Hansen has detailed variables of continuity that are measurable.[6] The continuity of care in the present study was provided mainly in the chronological dimension over a 12-month

Table 1. *Inpatient Continuity*

Personal Physician Activity	Third Year Patients	Second Year Patients	First Year Patients	Faculty Patients	Patients
Admitted and discharged	68	15	0	6	89
Admitted only	4	2	1	0	7
Discharged only	10	6	0	3	19
No contact	7	7	2	25	41
Total number of patients	89	30	3	34	
Physician unidentified					12

period; and in the geographical dimension in the Family Practice Center and on the inpatient service.

The analysis was based on single contacts between patients and their families and physicians. Consequently, continuity over illness episodes was not studied. The investigation of illness episodes might reflect more accurately the implementation of continuity of care but is probably not so significant in the present study since 75 percent of the illness episodes required only one visit.

Little is known about continuity in private practice, but it is presumed to be high. In England, with relatively static populations compared to the United States, continuity of care given by family physicians occurs in 80 percent of all contacts, and in Canada the figure is 83 percent.[7,8] In a US private pediatric practice, the percentage of continuity was 84 percent, but this figure dropped to 64 percent after the practice became a university training program.[9]

It seems reasonable to expect a figure of 70 to 80 percent first level continuity for individual patients and 60 to 70 percent for families in the family practice residency training program. Similarly, one should expect continuity of care (characterized by some administrative and medical contact with the personal physician) in 65 percent of inpatients on the family practice service. Although these figures probably do not replicate exactly those of private practice, it is likely that they represent enough continuity of care to engender the necessary feeling of responsibility in young physicians in training.

In spite of the presumption of its long standing value, continuity of care has only recently been shown to have valid benefits in medical care, particularly in the areas of reducing health costs, improving patient and physician satisfaction, increasing efficient utilization of health care services, and reducing hospitalization rates.[10,11] Unfortunately the mobility of both patients and

physicians in industrial society tends to detract from the principle of continuity of care, which therefore may be difficult for the family to attain over long periods of time.[12]

REFERENCES

1. McWhinney IR: Continuity of care in family practice: Implications of continuity. J Fam Pract 2:373, 1975
2. The Royal College of General Practitioners: The Future General Practitioner: Learning and Teaching. London, British Medical Journal, 1974
3. American Academy of Family Physicians: Official Definition of Primary Care. AAFP reprint No. 302, 1975
4. Carmichael LP: Social and educational factors affecting development of the health care system. In Bryan TE (ed): Academic Missions of Family Medicine, Proceedings No. 38 of the National Institutes of Health (Bethesda, Md): Fogarty International Center Series. DHEW publication No. (NIH) 77-1062. Government Printing Office, 1977, p 84
5. Hennen BK: Continuity of care in family practice: Dimensions of continuity. J Fam Pract 2:371, 1975
6. Hansen MF: Continuity of care in family practice: Measurement and evaluation. J Fam Pract 2:439, 1975
7. Cobb JS, Baldwin JA: Consultation patterns in a general practice. J R Coll Gen Pract 26:599, 1976
8. Hill M, McAuley RG, Spaulding WB, et al: Validity of the term "family doctor.": A limited study in Hamilton, Ontario. Can Med Assoc J 98:734, 1968
9. Breslau N, Reeb KG: Continuity of care in a university-based practice. J Med Educ 50:965, 1975
10. Becker MH, Drauchman RH, Kirscht JP: A field experiment to evaluate outcomes of continuity of physician care. Am J Public Health 64:1062, 1974
11. Haggerty MC, Robertson LS, Kosa J, et al: Some comparative costs in comprehensive versus fragmented pediatric care. Pediatrics 46:596, 1970
12. Boyle RM: An analysis of returning patients in family practice. Presented at the Sixth Annual Meeting of the North American Primary Care Research Group, Toronto, Ontario, April 12–15, 1978

A Family Practice Residency Inpatient Service: A Review of 631 Admissions*

E. Scott Medley, Michael L. Halstead

This study reports a review of 631 admissions by family practice residents and staff over a 12-month period to an autonomous family practice service in a large U.S. Army medical center. The diagnoses, number, and types of consultations requested, types of patients cared for by residents in various levels of training, and other pertinent data are reviewed. The study indicates that an inpatient family practice service can be very successful in terms of physician and patient satisfaction.

Up to now much of the emphasis on education in the rapidly emerging field of family practice has been on outpatient care. This is a reasonable educational concept, as the majority of the family physician's time will be spent in an ambulatory care setting. The experience in the Department of Family Practice at Dwight David Eisenhower Army Medical Center is in keeping with this concept, as shown by the large number of outpatient visits. There are 4,500 patient visits per month among the 3,500 families enrolled in the family practice clinic. There are several studies[1,2] detailing the most common types of outpatient diseases seen by family physicians in practice and in residency programs. One educator has even had the audacity to suggest that family physicians are "outpatient doctors."[3,4]

In contrast, there are few studies[5] on inpatient services provided in family practice residency programs, though many authors[6-8] have pointed out the need for family physicians to provide inpatient care. Many programs, especially in large centers, are struggling with the idea of forming a family practice inpatient service. One problem is logistical in nature, ie, where should the patient be admitted? Establishing completely separate and autonomous family practice wards would prove very difficult from nursing and supply perspectives because of the varying ages and multiplicity of problems dealt with by family physicians. On the other hand, if a patient is admitted to a specialty ward he/she may have his care assumed by the specialty (thus, losing the benefits of family medicine), or there may be confusion as to who is responsible for the patient. The Millis[9] report states that family practice patients should be "admitted to services not separate from other specialty services."

The purpose of this paper is to outline the operation of the family practice inpatient service at the Dwight David Eisenhower Army Medical Center and to review all admissions to this service for a period of one year. The number and types of consultations obtained, most common diagnoses, and levels of training of admitting physicians will be reviewed. This study does not address such commonly audited items as length of hospital stay, infection rates, and other quality control parameters. Family practice care is audited at this hospital by the same criteria applied to other specialties for the problem reviewed.

Methods

A retrospective chart audit was made of all patients admitted to the family practice

* Reprinted by permission from *The Journal of Family Practice*, 6(4):817–822, 1978.

service from February 1, 1976 to January 31, 1977. Information obtained directly from the charts included primary discharge diagnosis, level of training of primary physician, and number and types of consultations obtained on each patient. "Consultations" included informal notes written by consultants in the progress notes as well as formal consultations written on consultation forms. Only consultations to the other physicians were included, although consultations to such ancillary services as physical therapy, occupational therapy, social work services, and dietetics were numerous and invaluable.

Only primary discharge diagnoses are listed, though many of the patients, especially in the internal medicine category, had multiple complicating problems.

During the time of most of this study, there were 12 first year residents, eight second year residents, five third year residents, and seven board certified or eligible staff family physicians in the program. The physicians were divided into four teams, each team consisting of three first year residents, and one third year resident, and one or two staff physicians. Any patient admitted to the family practice service was seen first by his primary family physician and then by the staff physician heading that team. The patient was followed throughout hospitalization by all the members of the team to which the primary physician belonged. Admissions at night and on weekends were seen and evaluated by the first or third year family practice resident on call immediately following which the family practice attending physician obtained an independent history and physical and discussed the assessment and plan with the house officer. If the patient's primary family physician was available, he was responsible for the evaluation of the patient. Decisions regarding consultations to other services were made jointly by the primary physician and the family practice staff physician heading that team. Patients were housed on the ward appropriate to their problems throughout the 643-bed

hospital, including the medical intensive care and coronary care units, but care was rendered by family practice physicians unless a consultation was requested.

Results

There were 631 admissions over the 12-month review period. Tables 1A–1D outline the most common discharge diagnoses grouped by specialty categories. Also included in these tables is the level of training of the physicians who rendered the primary care for the patients. In the "other" diagnoses in the medicine category were many interesting and complicated patients. Diagnoses here included: psoriatic arthritis, pancreatitis, leukemia, lymphoma, hypersensitivity vasculitis, ulcerative colitis, several types of malignant tumors, and many more.

Table 2 lists the number of patients admitted in each specialty category and the number of patients seen in consultation by other specialists. Some patients were seen by more than one consultant as reflected by the total number of consultations. Of the 631 admissions, 38.1 percent had medical problems, 28.5 percent were admitted to the pediatrics ward, 21.5 percent to obstetrics-gynecology wards, and 12 percent to other wards. Two hundred and ten patients or 33.3 percent of the total were seen by consultants. The types of consultations obtained are listed in Table 3.

The groups of patients admitted to specialty wards other than medicine, pediatrics, and obstetrics-gynecology received the most consultations, 57.9 percent. The reasons for this are primarily the large number of patients with possible or actual herniated nucleus pulposes who were evaluated by neurosurgery for possible myelograms; the patients seen by psychiatry after overdoses; and the patients with trauma seen in consultation by orthopedics, neurosurgery, or general surgery.

Of the patients admitted to the medical wards, 46.5 percent were seen in consulta-

Table 1A. *Most Common Diagnoses (medicine)*

Diagnosis	Number of Cases	Level of Training of Physicians*			
		Staff	*R3*	*R2*	*R1*
Chest pain, possible MI	26	12	5	8	1
Arteriosclerotic heart disease, acute MI	16	6	1	6	3
Arteriosclerotic heart disease, not specified	14	4	2	7	1
Arteriosclerotic heart disease, congestive failure	13	4	2	6	1
Gastroenteritis	13	8	1	2	2
Diabetes mellitus	10	4	3	1	1
Abdominal pain	9	2	6	0	1
Thrombophlebitis	8	2	1	3	2
Hypertension	8	5	2	0	1
Urinary tract infection	8	5	2	1	0
Chronic obstructive pulmonary disease	6	2	2	1	1
Bronchitis, acute	6	3	0	2	1
Pneumonia	5	3	0	2	0
Asthma	4	4	0	0	0
Leg pain	4	2	0	2	0
Cellulitis	4	2	1	1	0
Supraventricular tachycardia	4	3	1	0	0
Reflux esophagitis	3	3	0	0	0
Other	80	40	14	20	6
Total	241	114	43	63	21
Percentage	(100)	(47)	(18)	(26)	(9)

* R3—3rd year resident, R2—2nd year resident, R1—1st year resident.

Table 1B. *Most Common Diagnoses (pediatrics)*

Diagnosis	Number of Cases	Level of Training of Physicians*			
		Staff	*R3*	*R2*	*R1*
Newborns (uncomplicated)	90	22	22	32	14
Newborn (complicated)†	26	9	7	8	2
Asthma	11	3	2	4	2
Pneumonia	7	3	1	2	1
Seizures	4	3	0	1	0
Gastroenteritis	4	2	1	0	1
Croup	4	3	0	0	1
Viral illnesses	4	2	0	1	1
Juvenile onset diabetes mellitus	3	2	0	0	1
Other	27	7	3	13	4
Total	180	56	36	61	27
Percentage	(100)	(32)	(20)	(33)	(15)

* R3—3rd year resident, R2—2nd year resident, R1—1st year resident.
† Includes all newborns with jaundice requiring phototherapy, as well as respiratory distress syndrome, congenital defects, and other specific problems.

Table 1C. *Most Common Diagnoses (obstetrics-gynecology)*

Diagnosis	Number of Cases	Level of Training of Physicians*			
		Staff	R3	R2	R1
Intrauterine pregnancy (uncomplicated)	96	30	22	32	12
Intrauterine pregnancy (complicated)	13	8	2	2	1
Pelvic inflammatory disease—					
tubo-ovarian abscess	6	0	2	3	1
Spontaneous abortion	4	0	0	2	2
Excessive weight gain	2	0	1	0	1
Pyelonephritis	2	0	0	1	1
Other	12	4	2	3	3
Total	135	42	29	43	21
Percentage	(100)	(31)	(21)	(32)	(16)

* R3—3rd year resident, R2—2nd year resident, R1—1st year resident.

Table 1D. *Most Common Diagnoses (other categories)*

Diagnosis	Number of Cases	Level of Training of Physicians*			
		Staff	R3	R2	R1
Low back pain other than					
herniated nucleus pulposes	13	4	2	5	2
Drug overdoses	11	6	3	2	0
Concussion	10	4	3	1	2
Soft tissue trauma	10	2	5	3	0
Herniated nucleus pulposus	7	4	2	1	0
Bony trauma	6	3	1	1	1
Depression	3	1	1	1	0
Ureteral colic	3	1	1	1	0
Conversion reaction	2	1	0	1	0
Situational stress reaction	2	1	0	1	0
Epididymitis	2	0	1	0	1
Other	7	2	1	2	2
Total	76	29	20	19	8
Percentage	(100)	(38)	(26)	(25)	(11)

* R3—3rd year resident, R2—2nd year resident, R1—1st year resident.

Table 2. *Category of Admissions and Percentage of Consultations*

Category	Medicine	Pediatrics	Obstetrics-Gynecology	Other	Total
Number of admissions	241	180	135	76	631
Percentage of admissions	38.2	28.5	21.4	12	100
Number of patients seen in consultation (total number of consultations)	112 (131)	29 (35)	25 (26)	44 (51)	210 (241)
Percentage of patients seen in consultation	46.5	16.1	18.5	57.9	33.3

Table 3. *Number of Consultations by Subspecialty*

Cardiology	49
General surgery	22
Obstetrics	20
Neurosurgery	19
Neurology	18
Pediatrics	18
Psychiatry	14
Urology	13
Orthopedics	12
Pulmonary	10
Gastroenterology	10
Otolaryngology	7
Vascular surgery	6
Gynecology	5
Other	19

tion. A large part of this percentage was accounted for by cardiology consults, usually involving patients admitted to Intensive Care-Coronary Care Units (ICU-CCU) with myocardial infarctions, congestive heart failure, or other problems related to arteriosclerotic heart disease. Pulmonary and gastroenterology specialists were often consulted to perform bronchoscopies, esophagogastroscopies, and other endoscopic procedures.

Only 16.1 percent of pediatric patients were seen in consultation, ten percent being seen by pediatricians and 6.1 percent by other subspecialists. In addition to many common pediatric diagnoses listed, children were hospitalized for Crohn disease, systemic lupus erythematosus, congestive heart disease with failure to thrive, Rocky Mountain spotted fever, and duodenal ulcer. Of the obstetrics-gynecology patients, 18.5 percent were seen in consultation. These primarily involved complicated deliveries and cesarean sections, but other patients requiring consultation had diagnoses such as pelvic vein thrombophlebitis, tubo-ovarian abscess, and premature labor.

As can be seen in Table 1, residents at all levels of training were admitting patients with varying problems. It should be reemphasized that all residents' patients were also seen on admission by a family practice staff physician. Also, when a staff physician admitted a patient, that patient was followed by a team consisting of six residents along with the primary staff physician, so that residents were learning about the inhospital care of patients other than their own. Most first year residents had few admissions because of the small number of families (25) in their panels. These residents, however, were receiving a great deal of inpatient training while rotating through inpatient specialty services. Residents at all levels rotated through various specialty services throughout their training, with first year residents spending one half-day per week, second year residents three half-days per week, and third year residents five half-days per week, in the family practice clinic.

Conclusions

This review shows that a family practice residency program can provide a great deal of inpatient experience for its residents while at the same time maintaining a busy outpatient service. It also demonstrates that family practitioners can manage most of their patients' inhospital care. Two thirds of the total patients, over half of the medical patients, and over 80 percent of pediatric and obstetrics-gynecology inpatients were managed without consultation. When consultations were obtained, they were done appropriately with the consultant lending his/her expertise to the care of the patient, but with the family practitioner maintaining his role as primary physician.

This study also shows that family practice attending physicians and residents in residency programs can care for large numbers of patients of all ages with a variety of major health problems. Physicians at all levels of postgraduate training were involved in the inpatient care of their patients, with appropriate back-up by staff physicians and consultants.

Comment

The opportunity for inpatient care may be somewhat unique at the Dwight David Eisenhower Army Medical Center because there is a very large family practice patient population enrolled and (other than a psychiatry residency) there are no other residency programs in this large medical center. There is no reason, however, why this same degree of inpatient responsibility could not apply either to other military residencies or to civilian programs in university medical centers or community hospitals where other specialty residents undergo training. The strategic location of the family practice clinic on the seventh floor of the medical center facilitates the ease with which inpatient care can be accomplished, but with the disadvantages of having to share the medical records department and x-ray and laboratory facilities with the other services in the hospital. Many family practice ambulatory care centers are located more distant from their inpatient services. Nevertheless, there is no reason why this slight increase in distance from the inpatient services should significantly hinder the inpatient services offered by clinic physicians.

Patient satisfaction seems to be at a maximum in this system as evidenced by the large numbers of patients applying to the program and the very low drop-out rate for enrolled families. Part of the reason for this patient satisfaction may be that the patient and family already are acquainted with the resident or staff physician who admits and cares for them during hospitalization and after discharge. Physician satisfaction is also great.

The family practice attending physicians and residents maintain their skills in inpatient medicine and do not lose contact with their hospitalized patients. The other specialists have an opportunity to teach the family practice residents, to act truly as consultants rather than as primary physicians, and to be continually stimulated by the residents.

The "team" concept for following inpatients seems particularly appealing because the entire team of family practice physicians becomes familiar with the patients and vice versa, providing a smooth transition and familiar faces when a patient must be hospitalized in the occasional absence of the patient's primary family physician. This same concept extends to outpatient services, since the teams operate in the family practice outpatient clinic also, in some ways simulating a group practice.

In short, the opportunity and demonstrated ability of the family practice physician to care for his own patient allow him to maintain continuity of care while providing the best possible inpatient management, including appropriate specialty consultation, while heightening patient and physician satisfaction.

Author's Update (E.S.M.)

During the 3½-year interval since this paper was prepared, I have had the pleasure of being affiliated with two more Family Practice Residency Programs with busy inpatient services, first at the Medical University of South Carolina and now at Alachua General Hospital and the University of Florida. The average number of hospital admissions for each of these programs is approximately 50 to 75 patients per month for a combined total of at least 2000 patient admissions over the past 3½-years. The tenets which we put forward in the above article still prevail and have been further reinforced as I have observed these numerous patient admissions. I remain convinced that family practice residents can manage large numbers of patients on a family practice inpatient service; that patients of all ages with a wide variety of problems, simple and complex, can be cared for in a quality manner on such a service; and that at the same time a quality educational experience can be provided to the residents. In fact, it is my belief that more family practice educators are finding it very beneficial, if not necessary, that an exclusively family-practice directed inpatient service be an integral part of a Family Practice residency training experience.

A further observation is that the types of patients admitted, the types of consultation obtained, and the need (or lack of need) for consultation from other specialists and subspecialists has not changed appreciably over the past 3½-years. As stated in the original abstract of this paper, "an inpatient family practice service can be very successful in terms of physician and patient satisfaction."

REFERENCES

1. Johnson AH, Wimberly W: Comparative profiles of residency training and family practice. J Fam Pract 1(3/4):28, 1974

2. Marsland DW, Wood M, Mayo F: A data bank for patient care, curriculum, and research in family practice: 526,196 patient problems. J Fam Pract 3:25, 1976

3. Petersdorf RG: Issues in primary care: The academic perspective. J Med Educ 50:5, 1975

4. Petersdorf RG: Internal medicine and family practice: Controversies, conflict, and compromise. N Engl J Med 293:326, 1975

5. Diener IL: Establishing a separate family practice inpatient service. Del Med J 28:585, 1976

6. Alpert JJ: Graduate education for primary care: Problems and issues. J Med Educ 50:123, 1975

7. Rakel RE: Training of family physicians. J Med Educ 50:145, 1975

8. Rogers DE: Medical academe and the problems of primary care. J Med Educ 50:171, 1975

9. Millis JS (Chairman): The graduate education of physicians: Report of the Citizens Commission on Graduate Medical Education. Chicago, American Medical Association, 1966

Obstetrics in Family Practice: A Model for Residency Training*

David A. Lynch

Family physicians have a unique service to offer families at the time of their reproduction, and have a role to play that cannot be duplicated by an obstetrician-gynecologist or pediatrician. The process of a family integrating a new member is a natural concept to family practice and lends itself to a family-centered model of care seldom seen in medicine. Practicing obstetrics has a positive effect on a family physician's practice, for without obstetrics a practice largely of episodic adult internal medicine develops. Obstetrical care provided by a family physician is a natural answer to the currently articulated public need for personalized, sensitive, family-centered, and expert childbirth care. Obstetrical training in the family practice residency needs to include a longitudinal pregnancy care experience in addition to block rotation on hospital services to teach residents skills of good obstetrical practice and to develop an attitude of family-centered health-care advocacy. A detailed program of family-centered patient education classes practical for a private group practice has been developed to extend throughout the entire course of pregnancy and includes classes after delivery.

Family practice provides comprehensive care for the whole family and views each person as a member of the family unit. In actual practice, however, many training programs and physicians in private practice approach family practice as a mixture of internal medicine, pediatrics, obstetrics-gynecology, surgery, and behavioral science. There often has been little to distinguish care given by family physicians from that delivered by another specialist except that the family physician is able to offer the patient services that cut across the traditional "specialties" which may so often fragment the delivery of health care.

Recently, attention has been focused on obstetrical care in family practice as the best example of longitudinal *health* care, involving the family, with an opportunity for unique contributions by the family physician.[1-3] This stems from the fact that the family physician is a member of the only specialty that deals with the entire process of individual development through embryo, fetus, infant, adolescent, and adult. Due to the family physician's broad base of training in behavioral science and family therapy, pediatrics and neonatal medicine, internal medicine and surgery, he or she is uniquely able to deal with the family as a whole during what is naturally a family-centered event—the care and guidance of the pregnant woman and her husband during the gestation, delivery, and subsequent nurturing of their offspring. This process of a family integrating a new member lends itself to a family-centered model of care as does no other process in medicine.

Family physicians are able to initiate pediatric care before delivery through anticipatory guidance of parenting problems, and discussion of circumcision, breast-feeding, immunizations, and use of infant auto safety seats. A partnership is established between the physician and the family during the course of the pregnancy that does not end abruptly at the time of delivery, but instead can extend into the subsequent years of care rendered to the family. Instead of the physician getting to know family members through episodic illness care, he or she is able to use the months of pregnancy to get to know the family better and to begin effective health education

* Reprinted by permission from *The Journal of Family Practice*, 7(4):723–730, 1978.

dealing with labor, delivery, problems of sexual adjustment, changes in family dynamics, and issues of early childrearing.

Enhancing the birth experience for the pregnant woman and her family is another area for which the family physician is uniquely suited. Consumers of health care are asking for a style of childbirth that emphasizes the interpersonal, family-centered nature of the event, while preserving the advantages of skilled medical observation and capacities for needed intervention. Le-Boyer has described modifications of the birthing process designed to minimize psychological trauma to the infant.[4] The process of labor is increasingly being recognized as an important social process, while at the same time the medical community is recognizing the importance of early parent-child interaction as a determining factor of later parenting success.[5-7]

The family physician has a special opportunity to modify the interactional and environmental influences surrounding the birth of the child because of his unique position as caretaker of all family members. Unlike the obstetrician-gynecologist, the family physician can sit down with the parents following the delivery and examine their newborn infant with them. There is no waiting to see the pediatrician, no hiatus in care, no chance for fears or misconceptions to build in the minds of anxious parents. The family's questions are answered by the trusted health-care provider they have worked with through all of their pregnancy, and not by a new, unfamiliar face.

One of the most valuable needs that can be filled by the family physician is using his position as a trusted confidant to smooth the way if specialized obstetrical or perinatal care is needed. Klein and Papageorgiou[8] have described effective mechanisms to reconcile the technical advances of perinatology with family-centered maternity care, minimizing the trauma entailed by transfer of the mother or compromised neonate to the perinatal unit. The family practice specialist, as the only physician

who bridges the perinatal period, is in a unique position to deal with the anxieties of the family while facilitating the introduction of the new physician to the family at its time of crisis.

Positive Effects of Obstetrics on Family Practice

Practicing obstetrics has several positive effects upon family practice as a specialty. Mehl et al studied four physician group practices, two of which did include obstetrics and two which did not.[2] Those without obstetrics were found to do very little pediatrics or gynecology, but focused primarily on acute care of episodic problems and long-term-care internal medicine. Those including obstetrics in their practice did significantly more pediatrics, gynecology, minor surgery, and psychotherapy. Most importantly, those practicing obstetrics saw five times as many family members for continuous comprehensive care at the same location.

By not practicing obstetrics, the family physician effectively eliminates from his practice two clearly recognizable points of entry into the medical care system—the woman seeking prenatal care and the woman seeking care for her newborn child. The established health care delivery system functions to direct patients away from the family physician who does not use the natural entry of the family into his practice at the time of childbirth. If care is obtained from the obstetrician-gynecologist and the pediatrician, the family has learned a model of health care delivery that traditionally tends toward fragmentation. The family physician then becomes the physician who sees members of the family for the care that is "left over" when the patient cannot identify another physician who might handle his problem. Therefore, when a physician decides to include or exclude obstetrics from his practice, he may actually be determining whether or not he will practice family-centered health-care delivery.

Obstetrics in Family Practice Residency Training

Family practice residency programs in university and community hospitals have differing situations that affect the experience of their residents.[9,10] There is no reason, however, why there cannot be a common concept about the family-centered nature of the birthing process and the value of the family physician. Recently, consensus has been achieved between the American Academy of Family Physicians and the American College of Obstetricians and Gynecologists regarding a core curriculum for obstetric-gynecological skills and knowledge for family practice residents (Table 1).[11,12] Candib has identified three major objectives of the family practice movement that recognize the unique contribution of family practice in the delivery of obstetrical care and which can serve to unify the approach of various residency programs, regardless of the level of obstetrical training. These objectives are: "(1) to develop an alternative strategy to the delivery of maternity care which provides a family-centered experience for all members of the family; (2) to provide access to training [in] . . . childbirth to family practitioners at different levels of training; and (3) to assure the growth and development of family practice as a discipline by offering care to families entering the health care system at the moment of pregnancy."[3]

Traditional training within family practice residency programs has been largely borrowed from obstetrics and gynecology. The focus has been on the abnormal, and family-centered interpersonal relations have been ignored. Block rotations in obstetrics under the supervision of obstetrician-gynecologists have not been able to provide family practice residents with the experience and insight necessary to meet the family's needs for longitudinal care

during health, with appropriate emphasis on changing family dynamics, nutrition, and patient preparation and education. As Candib observes, "the longitudinal experience of knowing patients before they are pregnant, being the provider of the news that they are pregnant, dealing with the patient's fears and hope about the process, following the changes and the patient's state at different stages of pregnancy, observing changing family dynamics with the expectation of the new baby, being present during the labor process, mediating that process to both mother and father and extended family, participating with the family in the delivery, assuring the family of normalcy or explaining the event of any abnormality in either mother or baby or the process itself, and, of course, following mother, baby, and family back into the home setting—*this by nature longitudinal process is at the center of the experience of family practice.* This process is obscured by training in block rotations in the hospital setting under the supervision of specialists."[3]

At Family Medicine Spokane the author has participated in the design of an approach to obstetrical training that tries to combine the intense inhospital experience necessary to develop technical competence with the longitudinal experience and family-centered approach necessary to develop the concept of family-centered health care advocacy. The traditional aspects of obstetrical training are highlighted by six months of inhospital delivery service experience, two months in each of the three resident years (Figures 1 and 2). On the inhospital delivery service the first year family practice resident is supervised and taught by his/her second or third year family practice resident teammate and the various attending physicians. The second year resident, in a more supervisory role, provides his first year teammate with an introduction to procedures and approach to the patient. In addition, the second year resident assumes night call where he continues to gain new experience and patient exposure. The third year resident acts as

Table 1. *ACOG-AAFP Recommended Core Curriculum**

Core Curriculum	Maternal and Perinatal Health Regional Planning

I. Cognitive knowledge†
  A. Normal growth and development, and variants
 	
  B. Gynecology
    Physiology of menstruation
    Abnormal uterine bleeding
    Diagnosis of pediatric gynecologic problems
    Infections of the female reproductive tract and urinary systems
    Sexual assault
    Trauma
    Benign and malignant neoplasms of the female reproductive tract
    Pelvic tissue injury
    Menopause and geriatric gynecology
    Assessment of surgical needs
 	
  C. Obstetrics
    Antepartum care
    Labor and delivery
    Postpartum care
    Care of the newborn
    Obstetrics complications: diagnosis and management, including emergency breech delivery and postpartum hemorrhage
    Pregnancy risk assessment systems and their implementation
 	
  D. Family life education
    Family planning and fertility problems
    Interconceptional care
    Family and sexual counseling
 	
  E. Process and examination
    Pediatric female reproductive examination
    Adult female reproductive examination
 	
  F. Consultation and referral
    Individual patient consultation and referral
    Women's health care delivery systems
	II. Skills: Emotional preparation and performance of the gynecologic examination at all ages
	  A. Gynecology
	    Obtaining vaginal and cervical cytology
	    Endometrial biopsy
	    Cervical biopsy and polypectomy
	    Culdocentesis
	    Cryosurgery/cautery for benign disease
	    Microscopic diagnosis of urine and vaginal smears
	    Bartholin cysts drainage or marsupialization
	    D and C
	    Conization (II)
	
	  B. Conception control
	    Oral contraceptive counseling
	    IUD insertion and removal, and counseling
	    Diaphragm fitting and counseling
	    Voluntary interruption of pregnancy to ten weeks gestation
	
	  C. Pregnancy
	    First examination—evaluation of pelvic adequacy
	    Use of risk assessment protocols
	    Evaluation of fetal maturity and feto-placental adequacy
	    Normal cephalic delivery including outlet forceps
	    Exploration of vagina, cervix, uterus
	    Manual removal of placenta
	    Episiotomy and repair
	    Pudendal and paracervical block anesthesia
	    Fetal monitoring
	    Induction of labor (II)
	    Third degree perineal repair
	    Cesarean section (II)
	
	  D. Surgery
	    Assist at common major surgical procedures
	    Tubal ligation with cesarean section (II)

* (Developed by a joint ad hoc committee of the American Academy of Family Physicians, the American College of Obstetricians and Gynecologists, and the Council on Resident Education in Obstetrics and Gynecology). Condensed from AAFP reprint 261. Used by permission.

† Core cognitive ability and skill should require a minimum of three months experience in a structured obstetric-gynecologic educational program, with supervised management of at least 30 vaginal deliveries. Substantial additional obstetric-gynecologic experience will be obtained during the three years of their experience in family practice centers. Residents will return to the family practice centers for their scheduled times even during the obstetric-gynecologic rotation.

For those electing additional training, particularly those who are planning to practice in communities without readily available specialist consultation, an additional minimum of three months experience in a structured obstetric-gynecologic educational program is strongly recommended. This program should include experience in induction of labor, cesarean section (a minimum of ten procedures), and tubal ligation if appropriate to physicians beliefs, and gynecologic procedures such as conization. These advanced skills are identified by (II).

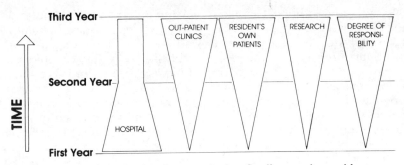

Fig. 1. Time distribution by year during family practice residency.

the chief resident on the obstetrical service, supervising the first year family practice resident, teaching the introductory obstetrical syllabus and procedures, and concentrating on the American College of Obstetrics-Gynecology—American Academy of Family Physicians (ACOG-AAFP) essential goals of training outlined for family practice residents[12] (Table 1). Traditional aspects of training include outpatient obstetric-gynecological experience in private physicians' offices, and ongoing experience in public family planning centers and in a college health center. In addition, residents are required to submit an individual research project on some aspect of family medical care during their third year.

Family-Centered Training

Today most family practice residency programs are providing residents with some experience intended to enhance the physician's ability to provide family-centered obstetrical care, even though obstetrical training may not be emphasized in the residency itself (Figure 2). As at Family Medicine Spokane, the knowledge a resident gains in formal behavioral science training helps in developing expertise with personality diagnosis, family dynamics, and individual stress factors. Familiarity with community resources also helps the physician aid his patient. Pediatrics and neonatal nursery experience not only provide the opportunity to learn medical care for chil-

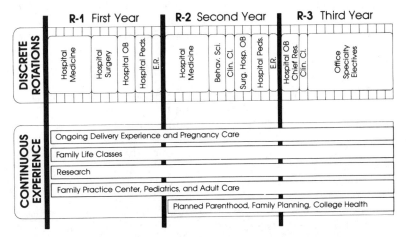

Fig. 2. Family-centered resident education at Family Medicine Spokane.

dren, but also provide additional experience with the family at times of stress. The opportunity to deal with the parents of an ill newborn infant often equips the resident with a sensitivity and depth of experience that helps immeasurably when counseling his pregnant patient concerning the fears she has about her unborn child. The ability to bridge the gap between pregnancy and newborn care provides a unique opportunity to work with patient families in a manner not possible for physicians in other specialties. General medical and surgical experience obtained by the residents during their training also enhances the family-centered nature of care by providing an excellent background for dealing with unexpected medical or surgical problems encountered by the patient. Often, instead of needing to refer a patient during the critical time of pregnancy, the resident is able to provide care himself and strengthen the bond between patient and physician. When another specialist does need to be consulted the resident is able to maintain the role of patient advocate in continuing to participate in her care.

At the heart of teaching family-centered obstetrics in the family practice residency is the ongoing patient care experience over the three years. Obstetrical care is probably the best example of the family's need for longitudinal care during *health*. Certainly isolated block rotations in obstetrics under the supervision of obstetrician-gynecologists can in no way provide family practice residents with experience in continuity of care. During the ongoing experience of pregnancy care at the family practice center, the family practice resident soon learns that he or she is a unique health-care provider offering a service that cannot be duplicated by any other medical specialist.

When another family member becomes ill or is affected by or as a result of the woman's pregnancy (eg, Couvade syndrome), the family physician is able to intervene directly and use previously gained knowledge of the family to best advantage.

When the illness of a child or other family member might have potentially serious effects on the pregnant woman, (eg, Rubella), the family physician again is uniquely able to initiate proper measures. The resident soon learns that problems previously categorized in medical school as falling into the domain of narrow specialties are no longer so easily placed. Does working with a pregnant woman incapacitated by fear about her unborn offspring fall into the domain of obstetrics, psychiatry, or pediatrics? Here lies the value of family practice! Brazelton notes that pediatricians who want to be effective guardians of their patients' well-being "are pressed into a role equivalent to the old 'family doctor'" since they are implying "a familiarity with the child's environment and participation with the parents in rendering it as favorable as possible to his well-being."[13] It seems obvious there is no one in a better position to render this anticipatory guidance to parents regarding their children than the family practice specialist of today.

Designing the Ongoing Patient Care Experience

A practical problem faced by residency programs is how to assure an adequate patient population for ongoing family-centered pregnancy care experience. "Patients have been educated to expect obstetrical care from obstetricians and new-baby care from pediatricians. Bringing obstetrics back into family practice is crucial to reversing this trend toward fragmentation of family care which became the leading dynamic of access to care in the 1960s. During that time, many family physicians stopped doing obstetrics as a means of limiting the growth of their practices."[3]

At Family Medicine Spokane, the problem of exposing the residents to an adequate family obstetrical experience has been approached mainly in two ways. First, all second and third year residents are required to take a one-month rotation with rural family physicians who practice obstetrics. During this time they are exposed to a role model and to patients in rural communities where medical care has not yet developed the fragmentation usually seen in the larger cities where training programs must locate.

Secondly, childbirth educators together with some of the family practice residents have designed a unique family-centered approach to patient care and education. This program is attracting increasing numbers of pregnant women and their husbands to the residency practice. The keystones of this program are the family life classes (Table 2). Unlike traditional childbirth classes which meet only in the third trimester of pregnancy, the family life classes begin in the first trimester when the patient first learns she is pregnant. The classes attempt to focus on the changing concerns and motivation of the couple as pregnancy progresses. For example, during the first trimester class, discussion centers around changing physiology, fetal development, prenatal exercises, nutrition and weight gain, mood changes of pregnancy, strains on the couple's relationship, and the dangers of drugs, smoking, and alcohol use. A short series of classes during the second trimester comprise the mid pregnancy series. Discomforts of pregnancy are usually becoming more important to the pregnant woman at this time, and these are discussed along with an exercise program. Family changes, sexuality, preparation for the baby, and anticipation of parenting problems are other topics that are discussed in an informal and relaxed atmosphere. Classes during the third trimester focus primarily on the techniques of prepared childbirth, relaxation, and understanding of the birthing process. A unique feature of the classes is that the last session occurs after delivery. Parents are encouraged to share with others their experience with the new offspring, and this serves as an introduction into infant development and feeding problems. Issues of parenting effectiveness are covered and important milestones in the newborn and infant medical care are discussed.

The classes at Family Medicine Spokane are coordinated and taught by childbirth educators and other qualified health care professionals. Residents do not have primary responsibility for teaching in the classes, but are able to attend and participate as desired, often acting as a medical

Table 2. *Family Life Classes: Family Education*

First Trimester: One 3-Hour Class	Second Trimester: Four 2-Hour Classes	Third Trimester: Four 2-Hour Classes	Parenting
1. Physiology	1. Physiology	1. Physiology	1. Infant development and feeding
2. Fetal development	2. Discomfort of pregnancy	2. Exercise and relaxation	2. Newborn and infant medical care
3. Prenatal exercise and relaxation	3. Exercise	3. Breathing techniques	3. Mothering, fathering, and parenting
4. Nutrition and weight gain	4. Family changes	4. Signs of labor and stages	4. Individual and family-centered care
5. Psychology	5. Sexuality	5. Variations in labor	
6. Drugs, smoking, and alcohol	6. Preparation for baby	6. Bonding to the newborn (family integration)	
7. Discussion	7. Parenting—adjusting to the newborn	7. Physical changes after delivery	
	8. Discussion	8. Sexuality	
		9. Dealing with relatives	

resource. Residents attending the classes find that they not only learn from the course offering but also from the concerns of their patient families who attend and participate. The family-centered nature of the classes and the fact that they extend throughout pregnancy into the postpartum period do not allow couples to concentrate on the delivery experience itself as the determination of the success of their class participation. Instead, pregnancy and childrearing are presented as a continuum, with the delivery an important part of the process. The patient experience in the classes nicely complements the family-centered care provided by the resident.

Patient enthusiasm for the family life classes is now resulting in a steady increase in families coming to the residency program for pregnancy care since the classes were instituted one year ago. Many family physicians in the area also encourage their patient families to attend the classes. Couples opting for this approach to pregnancy care and education enthusiastically voice the opinion that the obstetrical care delivered by the family practice resident is fulfilling their need for a personalized, sensitive, family-centered birthing experience. Currently, each resident delivers approximately 10 to 15 of his or her own patients per year.

Importantly, the classes conducted at Family Medicine Spokane are also practical and financially realistic for physicians in private practice. As presently conducted, the classes are financially self-supporting with approximately 120 deliveries per year, allowing easy incorporation into a two, three, or four physician family practice. The entire series is offered to the patient and family for $22. The childbirth educators are paid $5 per hour of instruction time and $2.50 for preclass preparation, for a total cost of $130 per series. There is no charge for a meeting room, since classes are held at the residency. If a minimum of eight couples are registered and pay the $22 fee, $176 is available to pay instructors, purchase some light re-

freshments, and amortize the cost of reading materials and teaching aids. Classes can start whenever the required number of couples are registered for that particular section, preventing overcrowding but insuring that costs will be met.

In order to begin similar classes, an interested residency or group practice should plan on investing approximately $500 to cover the cost of basic teaching aids needed. A considerably larger sum is required to provide the classes with a reference library. Often local public service groups can be approached to endow classes with needed materials when the classes are conducted on a nonprofit basis and accept all registrants.

It may be stated in conclusion that obstetrics is a vital part of delivering comprehensive health care to families in the Family Medicine Spokane residency practice because of the unique opportunities of the family physician for effectiveness and the positive effects upon family practice as a specialty.

Acknowledgments

This paper is based in part on a display which was prepared in collaboration with James A. Ross, MD, and Robert K. Maudlin, PharmD, and presented at the 30th Annual Scientific Assembly of the American Academy of Family Physicians in Las Vegas, Nevada, October 1977.

The Family Life Classes were begun with a grant from Spokane County Chapter March of Dimes, and coordinated by Jeanne Brotherton, RN.

REFERENCES

1. Price JG: Obstetrics in family practice. Med Dig 6:9, 1976
2. Mehl LE, Bruce C, Renner JH: Importance of obstetrics in a comprehensive family practice. J Fam Pract 3:385, 1976
3. Candib L: Obstetrics in family practice: A per-

sonal and political perspective. J Fam Pract 3:391, 1976

4. LeBoyer F: Birth Without Violence. New York, Alfred A Knopf, 1976

5. Klaus MH, Kennell JH: Mothers separated from their newborn infants. Pediatr Clin North Am 17:1015, 1970

6. Klaus MH, Kennell JH: Human maternal behavior at the first contact with her young. Pediatrics 46:187, 1970

7. Klaus MH, Jerauld R: Importance of the first postpartum days. N Engl J Med 286:460, 1972

8. Klein MC, Papageorgiou AN: Can perinatal regionalization be reconciled with family centered maternal care? J Fam Pract 5:969, 1977

9. Lynch DA: Different but equal medical practice. N Engl J Med 293:204, 1975

10. Lynch DA, Gavareski DJ: Internists and family practice. N Engl J Med 293:1268, 1975

11. Layton RH: The future of obstetrics and gynecology training for family physicians. Wash Acad Fam Physicians J 4(2):13, 1977

12. ACOG-AAFP Recommended Core Curriculum and Hospital Practice Privileges in Obstetrics-Gynecology for Family Physicians. Developed by a joint ad hoc committee of the American Academy of Family Physicians, the American College of Obstetricians and Gynecologists, and the Council on Resident Education in Obstetrics and Gynecology. Kansas City, Mo, 1977

13. Brazelton TB: Anticipatory guidance. Pediatr Clin North Am 22:533, 1975

The Residency Assistance Program in Family Practice*

Thomas L. Stern, G. Maureen Chaisson

The Residency Assistance Program in family practice was inaugurated in September 1975 as a plan to mobilze and finance the matching of consultant expertise in family practice residency education with program directors desiring to improve the quality of their residency programs through consultative assistance. The Residency Assistance Program is administered by a Project Board composed of representatives of four national family practice organizations. A panel of 30 consultants, carefully selected by the Project Board, are prepared for rendering effective consultative services through intensive training in consultative skills. They operate under the guidance of consensually developed standards for quality graduate education in family practice. Consultations are only scheduled at the written request of a residency program director. The confidential, nonpunitive, and voluntary nature of a Residency Assistancy Program consultation is carefully guarded, because it is felt that these qualities enhance the information-sharing, collaborative problem-solving nature of the consultative process. This paper describes the development, features, and operational process of this Program.

The Residency Assistance Program (RAP) in family practice was developed to improve the quality of graduate medical education in family practice through the provision of consultative services to program directors at their request. The consultations are available to all family practice residency programs that have been approved by the Liaison Committee for Graduate Medical Education. This service is not offered to newly developing residency programs in family practice. Such programs can obtain assistance from a list of consultants appointed by the Commission on Education of the American Academy of Family Physicians.

Residency Assistance Program consultations are provided by a panel of approximately 30 family practice educators who have been carefully selected by the RAP Project Board for their expertise in the field. The panel of consultants includes representatives from community, university, and military milieus. These consultants serve for a one-year term, with the option for reappointment.

The concept for the Residency Assistance Program was initially formulated by the Director of the Division of Education of the AAFP in 1974 as a plan to respond to the heavy demands for consultative services received by the AAFP from residency program directors eager to upgrade the quality of their programs. During the period from 1970 to the inception of RAP in 1975, requests for such consultative services were handled by the medical staff of the Academy's Division of Education and through educators identified as consultants by the AAFP's Commission on Education. As the specialty of family practice expanded, with an accompanying accretion of approved residency programs nationwide (30 in 1969 to 310 in March 1977), the demand for these consultative services became too great for this limited system to provide. The need for a panel of consultants to respond to the requests for consultative assistance soon became apparent. Since there was a growing pool of experienced and successful educators in family practice who were capable and willing to provide such services, a plan was developed to mobilize their expertise and make it available upon request. The Resi-

* Reprinted by permission from *The Journal of Family Practice*, 5(3):379–381, 1977.

dency Assistance Program was developed as a vehicle to facilitate, administer, and finance the matching of consultant expertise with programs in need of such expert assistance.

Development and Organization

The plans for such a Program were initially presented at the Program Directors' Workshop of the American Academy of Family Physicians in June 1974. The proposal was subsequently presented for endorsement to each of the organizations representing family practice and their members. Initial responses were encouraging. By spring 1975, the three national family practice organizations—the American Academy of Family Physicians (AAFP), the American Board of Family Practice (ABFP), and the Society of Teachers of Family Medicine (STFM—had committed themselves to the project as sponsoring organizations. Funds were awarded by the W. K. Kellogg Foundation in August 1975. The first fiscal year of the project began in September 1975 under a grant to the Family Health Foundation of America (FHFA), a nonprofit organization.

The terms of the Kellogg grant call for funds to subsidize the first three years of the Residency Assistance Program with an understanding that the Program will eventually become self-supportive. After the first three developmental years, it is anticipated that the cost of the Program will be amortized among the institutions requesting assistance. If necessary, the parent family practice organizations may continue to subsidize the Program to a limited degree, but major support for the continued operation of the Program will be expected to come from those institutions who receive RAP services.

As overseer of the grant, the Family Health Foundation of America is charged with the responsibility of assuring that the objectives of the grant are met. The

FHFA, in turn, delegates the responsibility for making overall policy decisions regarding the administration of the Program to a Project Board consisting of nine members —two representatives from each of the four sponsoring organizations (AAFP, ABFP, STFM, and FHFA) and the project director, as illustrated in Figure 1.

The RAP Project Board members are expected to represent the interests of the specialty of family practice and to act as liaison agents between RAP and their respective sponsoring organization. The RAP project director manages the day by day decision-making regarding the development and maintenance of the Program. The project director also acts as a link between the Project Board and the project staff whom he supervises at AAFP headquarters in Kansas City, Missouri. All RAP consultants are appointed by the RAP Project Board for a one-year renewable term and are responsible to the Project Board in the performance of their role as RAP consultants.

Early in the development of the project it was felt that family practice residents ought to participate in the formulation of the criteria for evaluation of the residency programs. For this reason, five residents were selected to participate in the developmental and renewal stages of the RAP project. They do not, however, participate as members of a consultative team.

Unique Features of RAP

Two unique features of the Residency Assistance Program that differentiate it from other similar consultative services are: (1) All of the consultants have participated in training designed to perfect their consultative skills, and (2) The guidelines used by each consultant in evaluating a residency program were consensually developed by the total panel of RAP consultants in the fall of 1975, subsequently revised in the fall of 1976, and will be revised annually during the project. With the RAP guide-

Communication, Decision-Making, and Responsibility

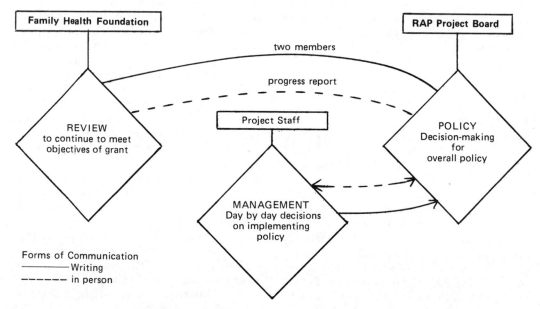

Fig. 1. RAP administrative/management flow sheet.

lines as a resource, each consultant is capable of providing assistance to programs based upon national standards rather than upon subjective evaluation derived from individual experiences and biases.

From its inception, the keynote of RAP has been its confidential and nonpunitive nature. The confidentiality of the Program is carefully guarded, requiring that all information flowing among the program director, the RAP consultants, and staff will be held in strict confidence. Only the requesting program director has the prerogative of disseminating the consultation report in a judicious fashion. At no time are consultations offered to a third party who wishes to obtain an external evaluation of a family practice residency program.

The original developers of RAP felt that the voluntary, nonpunitive nature of the Program would enhance its effectiveness and result in greater participation. The developers believed that family practice educators with concerns about improving the quality of their residency programs would welcome the opportunity for an external evaluation designed to help them diagnose and address problems in their programs that might hamper the quality of the educational experience offered to residents. RAP sponsors also felt that a residency program's participation in a RAP consultation could effectively demonstrate to students that their faculty is interested in continually upgrading the quality of the students' training experience.

The RAP Consultative Process

The Residency Assistance Program consultations are arranged through the RAP staff at the AAFP headquarters in Kansas City. The consultant and the program director confer in planning the events of the two-day consultative visit. On-site preparation for the visit is the responsibility of the requesting program, while responsibility for external arrangments is assumed by the staff at RAP headquarters. During the first year of the project, consultants made site visits in pairs as part of the training process. Since September 1, 1976, consultations have been performed singly.

The Pre-Site-Visit Questionnaire

In order to provide a consultant with some essential background information about the residency program prior to his/her arrival on location, the residency program director is asked to complete a pre-site-visit questionnaire. This questionnaire is simple and brief, requesting only basic elements of information about the residency program that can be reported with relative accuracy. Also, each program is asked to have the following documents on hand for the consultant's use in evaluating the residency program:

1. Copy of the budget and funding sources;
2. Evaluational forms and/or written explanation of evaluational procedures in current use; and
3. Pertinent written materials which are descriptive of the program.

Collaborative Problem-Solving Process

The two days of a RAP consultative visit are a period of intense, concentrated, collaborative problem solving. The RAP consultant needs to become informed quickly about the essential aspects of the residency program, from an understanding of its organizational and economic foundation to the essentials of the curriculum and details of patient care services. Usually a RAP consultant will spend the first day of the consultation collecting information about the program through interviews with faculty, staff, and residents as well as observing on-site the ambulatory care in the Family Practice Center and the in-patient experiences of the residents.

In understanding and diagnosing a residency training program, the RAP consultant depends upon the residency program director as a primary source of information. The information provided by him or her is considered in relation to data obtained from other sources, both within and without the program, in order to arrive at an equitable judgment of the program's strengths and weaknesses. The collaborative information-sharing relationship between the RAP consultant and the program director provides an ideal combination of internal and external perspectives about the program. The external stance of the RAP consultant allows him/her to apply a degree of objectivity not available to the program director. On the other hand, the program director can supply an important awareness of the internal dynamics of the residency program. This combined insight shared in a nonthreatening, helping relationship promotes a thorough analysis of the residency program and its particular needs for change and renewal.

The RAP Consultant's Checklist

To assist the RAP consultant in thoroughly reviewing all the significant aspects of the residency program, as determined by the RAP guidelines, a checklist of areas to observe on-site has been developed. The questionnaire and the checklist are inclusive data collection instruments which assure the acquisition of all program information that needs to be evaluated in light of the RAP guidelines. The checklist focuses on accounting for complex information that requires on-site observation and interviewing to acquire, ie, information that is difficult or impossible to collect exclusively by means of a self-report questionnaire.

The Consultation Report

When the consultative visit is completed, the pre-site-visit questionnaire and the RAP consultant's checklist provide ready references for the consultant in compiling the final consultation report. The report summarizes the material discussed by the RAP consultant and the program director in the "wrap-up" session. The report stresses both positive and negative aspects of the residency program. The recommendations are classified according to priorities given in RAP guidelines and are keyed as "crucial" or "enrichment" to the quality of the residency program. When appropriate, the consultant suggests strategies for implementing proposed changes. Many programs may be of such high caliber that they will merely need encouragement to continue their present plans.

Only two copies of the final consultation report are issued. The first copy is sent to the program director to be used at his/her discretion. The second copy, retained at RAP headquarters, is never released to a third party. Both copies are water-marked to identify their source.

Evaluation

The RAP Project Board has identified two methods of evaluating its own Program. The first of these is the evaluation of the consultant's immediate effectiveness and his/her personal skills as a consultant. This instrument is mailed to the residency program director as soon as the consultation is completed. Immediate feedback is given to the consultant regarding his/her personal effectiveness. The second instrument is mailed four to six months following the consultation and seeks to evaluate what changes have occurred in the residency program as a result of the RAP evaluation and consultation.

Annual Renewal and Update

In order to maintain the dynamism of the Program and relevancy of the RAP standards, an annual renewal session for all RAP consultants has been adopted. The first renewal session was held at the end of August 1976. At that time, the first four months of implementation of the Program were thoroughly evaluated with an eye toward refining written materials, updating guidelines, and improving the overall Program, based upon the experiences of the consultants in the field. The first four months had been planned as a trial period for testing the capabilities of the Program as originally designed. Anecdotal reports from residency program directors who have received a RAP consultation indicate that through its consultants, the Residency Assistance Program is making a valuable contribution to family practice education in this country.

Authors' Update

Since the publication of the first article on the Residency Assistance Program (RAP), 240 consultations have been performed. The program has successfully completed five years of operation. Currently, a research project is in progress to determine the effectiveness of RAP, as well as to do confidential correlations between RAP evaluations and Residency Review Committee letters of transmittal and stated deficiencies.

In addition to its original purpose to provide consultation to existing graduate medical education programs in family practice toward the maintenance or development of programs of excellence, RAP is now doing developing program consultations as well as target consultations where specific areas of need are identified by the program director.

Graduate Education in Family Practice: A Ten-Year View*

John P. Geyman

Assessment of the progress of graduate education in family practice after ten years shows that the original goals established for residency training in this specialty are being effectively met. There are now more than 360 approved family practice residencies in the United States with over 6,000 residents in training. Student interest in these programs has remained at a high level, and attrition has been low. Graduates of these programs have favored partnership and group family practice, and are well distributed in rural, suburban, and metropolitan areas. Heavy emphasis has been placed upon quality control mechanisms for both internal and external review of family practice residency programs. This paper outlines some concerns regarding the present status of family practice residencies, and suggests some directions for future development of these programs.

It has been just ten years since family practice was recognized as the 20th specialty in US medicine with the formation of the American Board of Family Practice in 1969. The past decade has been marked by vigorous activity within the new specialty, particularly in terms of organizational and educational development.

The evolution of graduate education in family practice during the 1970s reflects much of the essence of the specialty's development to date, since the planning and operation of residency training programs required coming to grips with such basic questions as the anticipated role of the future family physician and definition of the goals and curricular content of the emerging residency programs. In 1970, there was just a handful of operational family practice residency programs in the country. At the close of the 1970s, there are now over 360 approved family practice residencies with more than 6,000 residents in training.

Much has been learned from the last ten years in graduate education for family practice. The purpose of this paper is five-fold: (1) to outline the dimensions of progress from this experience; (2) to discuss briefly some of the important lessons

that have been learned; (3) to summarize how graduate education in family practice relates to other changes in graduate medical education; (4) to identify some concerns with respect to today's family practice residency training; and (5) to present some challenges with regard to the future development of graduate education in the field.

Entry to the 1970s: The Beginnings

Since family practice had no formal place in medical education in the United States prior to 1969, some fundamental questions needed to be addressed by the pioneering educators in the field. Some of these included the following: Can viable residency programs be organized and maintained at a high level of quality? What are the special requirements for residency programs in various settings ranging from university medical centers to unaffiliated community hospitals? How can appropriate curricula be defined and organized in order to prepare graduate family physicians for their needed roles in a changing health care system of the 1980s and beyond? To what extent and in what ways are linkages between university and community hospital programs desirable? What

* Reprinted by permission from *The Journal of Family Practice*, 9(5):859–871, 1979.

disciplines should be represented on the faculties of the developing programs? Can interest among medical students in specialty training in this field be developed and sustained? Will graduates of family practice residencies locate their practices in areas of need?

Most of the founding directors of family practice residency programs left active practice as family physicians to enter full-time teaching. They usually left their practice communities and moved to a "foreign" environment of a teaching hospital or medical school. They immediately found a world of new surroundings, including expectant residents, hard-nosed administrators, sharks and alligators. The identity of some of these inhabitants was often unclear to the uninitiated and a new language had to be learned, including that of educational objectives and grantsmanship.

The only signpost available to these beginning family practice educators was provided by a two-page document, the *Essentials for Graduate Training in Family Practice.* Jointly developed by the American Academy of Family Physicians, the American Board of Family Practice, the Section on General/Family Practice of the American Medical Association, and the AMA Council in Medical Education, this document called for three-year, coordinated family practice residency programs involving a broad and balanced clinical training in

family practice and its related disciplines. Emphasis was placed upon the importance of the Family Practice Center as the clinical and teaching base of the program, and the hallmark of the curriculum was flexibility. From these uncharted beginnings, the success of the early pioneers and of those to follow during the next ten years is quite apparent by the remarkable progress which has been made during these years.

Entry to the 1980s: Bench Marks of Progress

Growth of Residency Programs

Perhaps the most remarkable dimension of progress during the last ten years in family practice is the growth in the number of family practice residency programs. Table 1 shows the increase since 1970 in the total number of approved family practice residency programs in the United States together with the number of residents in training.

That this growth is qualitative, not just quantitative, is suggested by persistently high levels of student interest in family practice residency training and relatively low levels of attrition of residents from family practice residency programs. These programs have been consistently oversubscribed; more than 2,600 graduates of US

Table 1. *Growth of Family Practice Residencies**

Year	Number of Approved Programs	Number of Residents	Average Number of Residents per Program
1970	49	290	5.9
1971	87	534	6.1
1972	133	1,015	7.6
1973	191	1,771	9.3
1974	233	2,671	11.4
1975	259	3,720	14.4
1976	272	4,675	17.2
1977	325	5,421	16.6
1978	358	6,033	16.8

* Information for this table was provided by the Division of Education, American Academy of Family Physicians, Kansas City, Missouri.

Table 2. *Attrition in US Family Practice Residency Programs*—First and Second Year Residents, 1977*

	Number	Percentage of 1977 First Year Residents	Number	Percentage of 1977 Second Year Residents
Research	1	0.1	0	0.0
Teaching	0	0.0	0	0.0
Administration	0	0.0	0	0.0
Further training†	96	5.2	18	1.1
Practice	69	3.7	20	1.3
Other	80	4.3	21	1.3
Totals	246	13.2	59	3.7

* Information for this table was provided by the Division of Education, American Academy of Family Physicians, Kansas City, Missouri.
† Other than family practice.

medical schools applied for the 2,200 available first-year positions in family practice residencies in 1978. Table 2 shows the reasons for attrition of first and second year residents in 1977. About one third of the residents leaving family practice residencies in 1977 continued on in other family practice residency programs. Of the 5,421 family practice residents in training in 1978, there was an overall attrition rate of only 2.9 percent.

Diversity of Settings

Since family physicians are needed in a wide variety of urban, suburban, and rural settings, and since the nature of family practice varies somewhat by geographic setting, it is most appropriate that a spectrum of settings be represented by operational family practice residency programs. That this is the case is suggested by Figure 1, which reflects the breakdown in 1978 of family practice residency programs by type and setting. It can be noted that about one half of the programs are in university affiliated community hospitals. The proportion of university affiliated programs continues to increase. Geographic settings vary from large teaching hospitals in metropolitan areas to 200-bed general hospitals in communities as small as 40,000 in population.

In a classic paper on medical education in 1970, Jason stressed the importance of relevance of medical students' and residents' learning experiences to their future

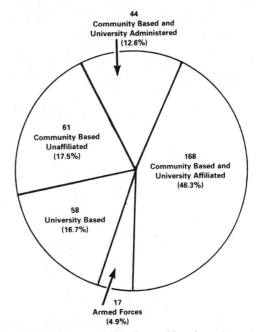

Fig. 1. Types of family residencies, August 1978. Twelve of the 348 operational programs utilize one location for the first year and another location for the last two years. (Based on information provided by the Division of Education, American Academy of Family Physicians, Kansas City, Missouri.)

practice needs.[1] There is some evidence that the clinical experience of family practice residency training rather closely approximates the clinical spectrum of family practice in the community. The statewide Virginia Study, for example, demonstrated comparable clinical content of teaching and nonteaching family practices as illustrated in Figure 2.[2]

Organizational Approaches

Various types of organizational approaches have accompanied the development of family practice residency programs in diverse settings. Whether in the medical school or community hospital, the department of family practice has provided an essential base for these efforts. Over two thirds of US medical schools have established departments of family practice; an additional 17 percent of the nation's medical schools have divisions of family practice or other programs under development. In the community hospital, a growing number of *clinical* departments of family practice have been formed which

are increasingly active in educational activities, in monitoring of the quality of care provided by family physicians, and in the delineation of their hospital privileges conjointly with other departments.

A growing number of university based departments of family practice have established networks of affiliated family practice residency programs for such purposes as sharing of clinical and educational resources, collaborative problem solving, faculty development, and related common needs. These networks have supported a variety of organizational patterns adapted to particular institutional and/or regional needs. One such example is the "one-and-two" program; the resident spends the first year related to a large teaching hospital in a metropolitan area and the final two years based in a family practice center in an outlying community involved with one or more smaller community hospitals.[3]

Faculty Recruitment

Substantial progress has been made in faculty recruitment. By 1977 there were

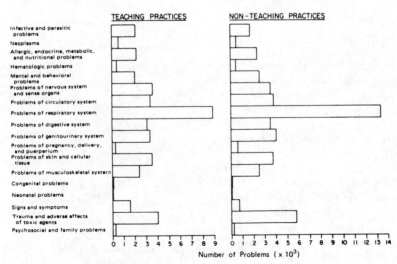

Fig. 2. Content by diagnostic category: Teaching vs. non-teaching practices. (Source: Marsland DW, Wood M, Mayo F: A data bank for patient care, curriculum and research in family practice: 526,196 patient problems. J Fam Pract 3:25-28, 36-68, 1976.)

about 400 full-time family practice faculty in US medical schools, plus a much larger number of full-time faculty in community based family practice residencies. Many thousands of additional family physicians have become involved in part-time residency teaching, usually on a voluntary basis.

A national study of 240 full-time family practice faculty in 1975 showed their average age to be 45 years; two thirds of this group had completed two or more years of graduate training, usually in general/family practice residencies and had at least ten years of practice experience. Almost all were board certified, usually in family practice.[4]

Most family practice residencies have included other disciplines on their faculties on either a full-time or part-time basis. In the behavioral science area, for example, psychiatrists, clinical psychologists, and social workers are most frequently involved in family practice teaching.[5]

Faculty development efforts have been increasingly active during the 1970s toward augmenting the teaching and research skills of family practice faculty. The Society of Teachers of Family Medicine and the American Academy of Family Physicians have sponsored many regional and national workshops for family practice faculty. There are now over 30 federally funded faculty development programs in the country ranging from short-term experiences to formal, one-year fellowship programs. Two-year Family Medicine Fellowship programs have been established in five medical schools through funding provided by the Robert Wood Johnson Foundation.

Sustained Student Interest

Since the advent of family practice as a specialty and the organization of family practice residency programs, a growing number of US medical graduates are opting for careers in family practice. Between 1975 and 1977 the proportion of graduates opting for family practice residencies increased from 12.7 percent in 1975 to 15 percent in 1977.[6] Many medical schools report 20 to 35 percent of their graduates entering family practice residency training. A positive correlation has been demonstrated between the proportion of graduating classes selecting family practice and the presence of departments of family practice in medical schools, as shown in Table 3.[7]

There is considerable evidence documenting the high caliber of medical graduates entering family practice residencies. One study, for example, compared family practice residents with residents in four other major specialties on the basis of cognitive and noncognitive measures. Family practice residents were found to equal the highest scoring group in cognitive tests and to score higher on affiliation need and

Table 3. *Type of Administrative Unit and Proportion of Students Choosing Family Practice Residencies*

Administrative Unit	Percentage Choosing Family Practice				
	0–10	11–20	21–30	34–40	N
Department	10.6	51.1	27.7	10.6	47
Division	66.7	22.2	11.1	0.0	9
Other	50.0	50.0	0.0	0.0	6
N	14	29	14	5	62

Source: Beck JD, Stewart WL, Graham R, et al: The effect of the organization and status of family practice undergraduate programs on residency selection. J Fam Pract 4:663, 1977.

lower on aggression and materialism than the other groups.[8]

Curriculum Development

Perceptions were somewhat vague and undefined in 1970 concerning the scope and depth of desirable curricula in family practice residencies. This uncertainty has been largely resolved in recent years. Although the curricula of US family practice residency programs are by no means standardized, a general pattern has emerged of curriculum content focused on the various stages of comprehensive care—prevention, early diagnosis of asymptomatic disease, care of symptomatic disease, rehabilitation, and care of terminal illness. Emphasis is directed to the family as the object of care and to individual and family development from the perspective of growth over a life cycle. Teaching objectives are oriented toward three distinct capability levels.[9]

1. *Definitive capability* (ie, management of most common clinical and behavioral problems of families and life threatening emergencies).
2. *Partial capability* (eg, initiation of appropriate diagnostic and/or therapeutic measures for more complex problems requiring consultation and/or referral).
3. *Limited capability* (eg, recognition or suspicion of rare or complex problems for referral).

The resident's experience and training is derived from the ongoing care of his/her patients in the Family Practice Center and in the hospital or on the Family Practice Service, as well as that derived from inpatient and ambulatory rotations on other specialty services and in other community settings. The typical family practice residency involves teaching rotations of about one year in internal medicine and medical subspecialties (including cardiology, neurology, and dermatology); five or six months of pediatrics; three to six months of obstetrics-gynecology; six months of surgery and its subspecialties (including ophthalmology, otolaryngology, orthopedics, and urology); and two months of emergency medicine. A strong thread of behavioral science is presented longitudinally over the three-year program, usually including a short rotation on psychiatry. The resident's time in the Family Practice Center generally increases from one to two half-days per week in the first year to three to five half-days per week in the third year.

It is beyond the scope of this paper to describe in detail the curricular content of family practice residencies. Several examples, however, are representative of the levels of proficiency acquired by graduates of the typical three-year residency in family practice. Graduates of these programs are experienced in the diagnosis and management of most medical problems of adults and children, including proficiency in such procedural skills as liver biopsy, thoracentesis, lumbar puncture, bone marrow aspiration, cutdown, circumcision, and endotracheal intubation. In obstetrics-gynecology, the graduates of most programs are experienced in prenatal care, normal delivery, postpartum care, recognition of obstetric emergencies, and office gynecology; many graduates have developed proficiency with such procedural skills as dilatation and curettage, termination of pregnancy, tubal ligation, and cold conization of the cervix. Some gradutes have elected extra obstetric training to include cesarean sections. In surgery and emergency care, many graduates have acquired proficiency with such procedural skills as vasectomy and other minor surgery procedures, closed reduction of common fractures, tube thoracostomy, and tracheostomy.

Curriculum development in family practice residencies has frequently involved an interdepartmental planning process. An excellent example of such an effort on the national level is the core curriculum in obstetrics-gynecology jointly developed by the American Academy of Family Physicians and the American College of Obstetricians and Gynecologists. This curriculum defines the recommended content of cognitive knowledge and skills for both basic and advanced competency levels.[10]

Evaluation Methods

The development of effective evaluation methods has received strong emphasis in US family practice residency training at three levels: (1) at the overall program level; (2) at the level of individual parts of the program (eg, an inpatient teaching rotation); and (3) at the level of the experience and performance of the individual resident. At the program level, external review has been carried out within networks of affiliated residency programs. On the national level the Residency Assistance Program (RAP)[11] provides consultation and assistance at the request of individual programs. These approaches have helped to identify strengths and weaknesses within a residency program in such a way that problem solving is encouraged.

On the levels of the individual teaching rotation and of the individual resident's experience and performance, a variety of approaches have been developed. Monitoring of resident experience has been accomplished by use of a problem category index[12] and by practice profiles using a diagnostic index, the E-book.[13,14] Resident performance has been assessed by chart review and patient profiles.[15,16] In-training examinations have been used by many programs,[17,18] and evaluation of faculty performance has likewise been addressed.[19]

Impact of Residency Programs

There is already abundant evidence that graduate education in family practice is effectively addressing the nation's problems of specialty and geographic maldistribution of physicians. As previously noted, attrition from US family practice residency programs has been minimal. The great majority of graduates of these programs enter family practice in the community, and are well distributed geographically. Table 4 shows that 8.4 percent of 1978 graduates located in rural communities with less than 2,500 population and over 50 percent located in communities less than 25,000 in population, while 27.1 percent located in large communities with populations over 100,000 people.

The problems of solo practice clearly played a role in the attrition of physicians from general practice in previous times. Table 5 shows that about 60 percent of graduates of family practice residencies in 1978 entered partnership and group family practice, with only 13.6 percent opting for solo practice.

With regard to the quality of care provided by family physicians, several studies have demonstrated comparable performance levels relative to that of other specialties.[20-22]

Some Lessons from the Last Ten Years

The following points, in my view, stand out as important lessons from the last ten years' experience in graduate education for family practice.

1. Viability and Quality of Family Practice Residencies

The 1970s have amply demonstrated that excellent family practice residency programs can be developed and maintained with the capability to attract sustained student interest and to produce well-trained graduate family physicians to meet public needs. Quality control mechanisms have been developed which will assure the future viability of these programs.

Table 4. *Distribution of Graduating Residents by Community Size**

Character and Population of Community	Number of Reporting Grads	1978 Graduating Residents	
		Percentage of Total Reporting Grads	*Cumulative Percentage of Total Reporting Grads*
Rural area or town (less than 2,500) not within 25 miles of large cities	91	8.4	8.4
Rural area or town (less than 2,500) within 25 miles of large city	34	3.1	11.5
Small town (2,500–25,000) not within 25 miles of large city	257	23.8	35.3
Small town (2,500–25,000) within 25 miles of large city	183	16.9	52.2
Small city (25,000–100,000)	186	17.2	69.4
Suburb of small metropolitan area	38	3.5	72.9
Small metropolitan area (100,000–500,000)	90	8.3	81.2
Suburb of large metropolitan area	103	9.5	90.7
Large metropolitan area (500,000 or more)	72	6.7	97.4
Inner city/low income area (500,000 or more)	28	2.6	100.0
Total	1,082	100.0	

* Information for this table was provided by the Division of Education, American Academy of Family Physicians, Kansas City, Missouri.

2. Need for Flexible Approaches

First-rate family practice residency programs can and should be developed in varied settings ranging from university medical centers to 200-bed general hospitals in smaller outlying communities. The organizational approaches and structure, however, of programs in such diverse settings must necessarily be flexible and adapted to

Table 5. *Practice Arrangements of Graduating Residents**

Type of Practice Arrangement	1978 Graduating Residents	
	Number of Reporting Grads	*Percentage of Total Reporting Grads*
Family practice group	411	30.2
Multispecialty group	138	10.2
Two-person family practice group (partnership)	262	19.3
Solo	185	13.6
Military	130	9.6
Teaching	70	5.1
USPHS	61	4.5
Emergency room	12	0.9
Hospital staff (fulltime)	51	3.8
None of the above	39	2.8
Total	1,359	100.0

* Information for this table was provided by the Division of Education, American Academy of Family Physicians, Kansas City, Missouri.

local and institutional needs and resources. There is no single or fixed blueprint for a successful family practice residency. The quality and value of learning experiences for residents depend on such factors as the characteristics of the learning setting, clinical volume, level of resident responsibility, availability and competence of teaching faculty, and the motivation and capability levels of individual residents.

3. Value of University Affiliation

The increasing trend toward university affiliation of community hospital based family practice residencies reflects a growing awareness that more can be accomplished through the cooperative efforts of groups of programs than by isolated individual programs. The partnership between medical school departments of family practice and affiliated family practice residencies within a network provides many benefits to all parties, including sharing of clinical and educational resources, joint planning and problem solving, enhanced linkages with predoctoral and continuing medical education activities, and the potential for collaborative research.[23]

4. Hazard of Overcommitment

Regardless of the setting of a newly established family practice residency, there are invariably many more expectations of the potential service and teaching roles of the program than can reasonably or effectively be met. The quality and integrity of the teaching program itself must be the guiding factor in deciding whether or not a program will accept clinical or teaching roles in other facilities or programs, such as Emergency Rooms, family planning clinics, other health department programs, and satellite clinics.

5. Need for "Critical Mass" of Residents

Especially during the early years, some family practice residencies were estab-lished with as few as two or three residents in each year of the three-year program. It has become clear, however, that a larger group of residents is required to meet the needs for continuity of care and coverage of the Family Practice Center and the major teaching rotations, and to meet other necessary commitments of the program. It is the general consensus today that the smallest effective "critical mass" for a family practice residency is 12 residents (4-4-4).

6. Importance of Shared Funding Sources

There are four major sources of funding to support family practice residency programs: (1) patient care revenue; (2) contributions from participating hospitals; (3) state funding, often on a capitation basis; and (4) other grants (eg, federal, foundations). Many primary care services are inadequately compensated under current third-party reimbursement policies, and extensive teaching commitments necessarily limit the service capability of a program. It is, therefore, not possible for a program to generate much more than one half of its total costs from patient care services. The continued support of participating hospitals is vital, together with ongoing supplemental funding by government.

7. Clear Identity of Family Practice Residents

Since the first year of most family practice residencies is largely hospital based for block rotations on the major teaching services not unlike the traditional rotating internship, many first year family practice residents have experienced difficulty in establishing their identity in family medicine. This problem can be effectively addressed by means of an orientational family practice rotation early in the first year and by other focused experiences in family medicine during that year.[24]

8. Importance of Structured Third Residency Year

Some of the early family practice residencies were relatively unstructured, particularly during the third year, even to the extent of a totally elective third year. It was found that such loose curricula often led to inadequate breadth and depth of curriculum over the three-year program, and some programs experienced attrition of residents due to the relative lack of curricular structure. Today's family practice residency curricula are more carefully structured over the three-year program, usually including greater use of *selectives* (especially in the medical and surgical subspecialties) during the third year.

9. Value of Concurrent Learning Experiences

The customary organizational approach to many learning experiences in medical education is to establish block rotations on hospital and/or ambulatory teaching services for periods of one or more months. This approach is both awkward and wasteful of time for many curricular needs in family practice residencies. Many curricular areas can be effectively organized as concurrent rotations (eg, two half-days per week) in combination with other teaching rotations. Examples of this approach include dermatology, otolaryngology, ophthalmology, allergy, and other subspecialty areas.

10. Integration of Behavioral Science

Considerable effort has been directed to behavioral science teaching in most family practice residencies. At times, this teaching has been insufficiently related to the resident's everyday management of common clinical problems. To the extent that this disparity exists, behavioral science teaching may be viewed as ineffective and off-target. The goals of behavioral science teaching in terms of knowledge, skills, and attitudes must be intimately related to the resident's daily role in patient care along the lines of Engel's psychobiomedical model,[25] which combines psychosocial and biomedical factors into a single, integrated approach to patient care.

Family Practice and Specialty Redistribution

The last few years have seen increasing recognition by health planners and policy makers that there is no longer a shortage in the aggregate number of physicians, and that the real problems of physician supply involve specialty and geographic maldistribution of physicians. Two key elements of current health manpower policy involve the termination of expansion in the total output of graduates of US medical schools and redistribution of the "mix" of graduate medical education (GME) positions by specialty.

There is mounting evidence that a growing number of the nonprimary care specialties are already in surplus. Although there was a reduction of 8.4 percent in the total number of general/family physicians, internists, and pediatricians between 1965 and 1972, there was an increase of 19.6 percent in the number of surgical specialists and an increase of 33.6 percent in the number of other specialists during that same period.[26]

Current federal health manpower policy calls for a minimum of 50 percent of graduate medical education (GME) positions to be in the three primary care fields (family practice, general internal medicine, and general pediatrics), with 25 percent of all positions in family practice. This kind of redistribution will involve reduction in the size and number of residency programs in many of the other specialties. The American College of Surgeons has already called for a reduction in the number of residency graduates in the surgical specialties from

2,600 per year to between 1,600 and 2,000 per year.[27]

It is quite likely that some form of national health insurance will be enacted during the 1980s. Table 6 represents current federal projections for demand-based requirements for primary care physicians in the United States in 1980 and 1990 based upon three estimated rates of utilization of services, any one of which will require a major increase in the number of practicing family physicians.[28]

Only time will tell whether the currently accepted target of 50 percent (for the proportion of the three primary care disciplines of total GME positions) will meet the nation's needs. This may fall short of the mark, particularly since a substantial number of graduates from residencies in general internal medicine and general pediatrics later subspecialize in practice.[29] In any event, more family practice residency programs are still needed, together with expansion of many existing programs, and the long-term need for family physicians may even require an increase in the presently accepted goal of 25 percent of US medical graduates opting for careers in family practice.

Major Concerns Today

The progress of graduate education in family practice during the last decade has been quite remarkable, but present chal-lenges are great and much remains to be done. I have four major concerns with respect to the current status of family practice residency training:

1. High-Risk Diseases of Curriculum

With regard to predoctoral medical education, Abrahamson has recently described several important diseases of the curriculum (Table 7).[30] These same diseases occur in graduate medical education, and family practice education is at full risk for these endemic problems.

Several examples of these problems bear mention. First, with regard to *curricular hypertrophy,* there is constant pressure in this direction. New additions to the curriculum are conceived and developed, together with expansions of existing curriculum, and the tendency is to implement these additions without contraction of existing curriculum. This tendency can become pathologic if it progresses to decompensation on the downslope of Starling's curve. Two specific examples of common curricular deficiencies in many family practice residencies today are orthopedics (especially the care of common fractures) and problems of aging. It is inevitable that other areas will need to be incorporated into future curricula, and methods of inclusion must be developed which avoid "congestive failure of the curriculum."

There is already some evidence of *curric-*

Table 6. *Demand Based Requirements for Primary Care Physicians Under National Health Insurance*[28]

	1980			1990		
Primary Care Physicians	1975 Utilization Rate	30 Percent Increase	75 Percent Increase	1975 Utilization Rate	30 Percent Increase	75 Percent Increase
Totals	97,990	127,390	171,480	107,910	140,280	188,840
General and family practice	64,900	84,370	113,580	71,400	92,820	124,950
Pediatrics	14,300	18,590	25,030	15,910	20,680	27,840
Internal medicine	18,790	24,430	32,880	20,600	26,780	36,050

Calculations based on 1975 utilization rates and specified increases in those rates.

Table 7. *Diseases of the Curriculum*[30]

Disease	Underlying Problems
1. Curriculosclerosis	Hardening of the categories
2. Carcinoma of the curriculum	Uncontrollable growth of one segment of curriculum
3. Curriculoarthritis	Dysfunction of articulations and communications between related segments of curriculum
4. Iatrogenic curriculitis	Excessive tampering and meddling with curriculum
5. Curriculum hypertrophy	Progressive increase in didactic teaching requirements
6. Idiopathic curriculitis	Mask for poor teaching
7. Curriculum ossification	Casting in concrete; often epidemic

ulosclerosis of the curriculum of family practice residencies. The natural result of the accreditation process over time is "hardening of the categories." For example, there is a tendency by some today to regard four or five half-days per week in the Family Practice Center for second and third year residents as absolutely essential for the teaching of continuity of care. While the importance of continuity of care in family practice cannot be disputed, there is no evidence to date that this amount of time spent in the Family Practice Center—rather than two and three half-days per week in the second and third residency years, respectively—leads to improved learning outcomes compared to lesser amounts of time. A recent study of the continuity of care in a family practice residency program showed that continuity of care for individual patients averaged 75 percent for first year residents scheduled in the Family Practice Center only one half-day per week, with continuity of care provided by another resident on the team for an additional 17 percent of visits.[31] Two additional reasons to avoid excessive time commitments in the Family Practice Center are the need to preserve sufficient flexibility to accommodate revisions and additions to the curriculum (particularly through concurrent learning experiences during other scheduled rotations), and the importance of preparing residents to share patient care responsibilities with their colleagues as members of a group practice.

Curriculoarthritis must be prevented by maintaining a high index of suspicion. An example of this problem, involving loss of freely mobile articulation between curricular elements, is the relative lack of integration of behavioral science teaching with common clinical management in some programs.

2. Study of Clinical Experience in Family Practice

The organizational, educational, and logistic aspects of family practice residency training have necessarily received the most attention by family practice faculty to date. Most family practice residencies already have implemented the basic tools needed to monitor and study the clinical experience within their teaching practices, including the use of the problem oriented medical record, practice profiles, age-sex registers, classification, and data retrieval systems. Few programs, however, have yet developed an adequate priority for critical study and review of the process and outcomes of care in family practice. A milieu of critical inquiry among family practice faculty and residents is vital to the long-term success of these programs and to the development of family medicine as an academic discipline. The dividends of this process include expansion of the body of knowledge which family physicians will teach, increased practice satisfaction, and, most importantly, improved patient care.

3. Complacency Toward Future Development

Because of the successful development of family practice residencies to date, it would be easy to become complacent concerning the need for future improvements and further development. In addition, since the ongoing management of family practice residency programs is totally absorbing, it would also be easy to become complacent about the need to expand the output of family practice residency programs to meet societal needs.

The 1980s will require improvement of existing family practice residencies, the expansion of some programs and initial development of others, the refinement of teaching methods and skills, the maintenance of effective quality control efforts, and the expansion of the content areas taught by family physicians.

4. Instability of Long-Term Funding

Present funding of family practice residency programs is an unstable patchwork of federal, state, and local support. Under existing reimbursement policies, revenue from patient care will not support more than one half of the total costs of these programs. Participating hospitals find themselves caught by the constraints of hospital rates commissions, and federal support of family practice residencies has favored start-up and "last-dollar" funding, not supplemental support of ongoing operational costs. In order to stabilize the funding of family practice residency training and to allow expansions of the output of programs to meet the public need, ongoing state and federal support is urgently needed as well as revision of reim-bursement policies to more adequately cover the range of services provided by family physicians.

Challenges for Future Development

Based on the foregoing and by way of summary, the following challenges relate to the future development of graduate education in family practice.

1. The patient is the reason for teaching, and clinical excellence represents the foundation of any good teaching program.
2. A spirit of critical inquiry is the basis for learning and improved patient care.
3. Balance and integration of curriculum content must be sought through a continual process of curriculum review and development.
4. The feedback loop from residency graduates must be carefully considered in future curricular changes.
5. Ossification of accreditation requirements must be avoided, and sufficient flexibility preserved to facilitate future improvements of residency programs.
6. The core content in obstetrics-gynecology jointly developed by AAFP and ACOG is an exemplary model for inter-specialty curriculum development in other areas.
7. Family practice residency programs have both the opportunity and the responsibility to become involved with predoctoral and postgraduate education in family medicine.
8. The potential role of family practice residencies in scholarly activity, development and testing of innovations in patient care, and teaching should not be underestimated.
9. An ongoing emphasis on quality control should accompany the expansion of family practice residency training to meet the public need in the 1980s.

REFERENCES

1. Jason H: The relevance of medical education to medical practice. JAMA 212:2093, 1970
2. Marsland DW, Wood M, Mayo F: A data bank for patient care, curriculum, and research in family practice: 526,196 patient problems. J Fam Pract 3:25, 1976
3. Geyman JP: The "one-and-two" program: A new direction in family practice residency training. J Med Educ 52:999, 1977
4. Longenecker DP, Wright JC, Gillin JC: Profile of full-time family practice educators. J Fam Pract 4:111, 1977
5. Hornsby JL, Kerr RM: Behavioral science and family practice: A status report. J Fam Pract 8:299, 1979
6. Willard WA, Ruhe CHW: The challenge of family practice reconsidered. JAMA 240:454, 1978
7. Beck JD, Stewart WL, Graham R, et al: The effect of the organization and status of family practice undergraduate programs on residency selection. J Fam Pract 4:663, 1977
8. Collins F, Roessler R: Intellectual and attitudinal characteristics of medical students selecting family practice. J Fam Pract 2:431, 1975
9. Geyman JP: A competency-based curriculum as an organizing framework in family practice residencies. J Fam Pract 1(1):34, 1974
10. Stern TL: A landmark in interspecialty cooperation. J Fam Pract 5:523, 1977
11. Stern TL, Chaisson GM: The Residency Assistance Program in family practice. J Fam Pract 5:379, 1977
12. Tindall HL, Henderson RA, Cole AF: Evaluating family practice residents with a problem category index. J Fam Pract 2:353, 1975
13. Boisseau V, Froom J: Practice profiles in evaluating the clinical experience of family medicine trainees. J Fam Pract 6:801, 1978
14. Terrell HP: Documentation of resident exposure to disease entities. J Fam Pract 6:317, 1978
15. Kane RL, Leigh EH, Feigel DW, et al: A method for evaluating patient care and auditing skills of family practice residents. J Fam Pract 2:205, 1975
16. Given CW, Simoni L, Gallin RS, et al: The use of computer generated patient profiles to evaluate resident performance in patient care. J Fam Pract 5:831, 1977
17. Donnelly JE, Yankaskas B, Gjerde C, et al: An in-training assessment examination in family medicine: Report of a pilot project. J Fam Pract 5:987, 1977
18. Geyman JP, Brown TC: An in-training examination for residents in family practice. J Fam Pract 3:409, 1976
19. Kelly J, Woiwode D: Faculty evaluation by residents in a family medicine residency program. J Fam Pract 4:693, 1977
20. Garg ML, Mulligan JL, Gliebe WA, et al: Physician specialty, quality and cost of inpatient care. Soc Sci Med, in press
21. Ely JW, Ueland K, Gordon MJ: An audit of obstetric care in a university family medicine department and an obstetrics-gynecology department. J Fam Pract 3:397, 1976
22. Phillips WR, Rice GA, Layton RH: Audit of obstetrical care and outcome in family medicine, obstetrics, and general practice. J Fam Pract 6:1209, 1978
23. Geyman JP, Brown TC: A network model for decentralized family practice residency training. J Fam Pract 3:621, 1976
24. Burr BD: The first-year family practice resident: An identity crisis. J Fam Pract 2:111, 1975
25. Engel G: The need for a new medical model: A challenge for biomedicine. Science 196:129, 1977
26. Holden WD: Attitudes of the Coordinating Council on Medical Education toward physician manpower. Bull NY Acad Med 52:1078, 1976
27. American College of Surgeons and American Surgical Association: Surgery in the United States: A Summary Report of the Study on Surgical Services for the United States. Baltimore, American College of Surgeons and American Surgical Association, 1975
28. Physician manpower requirements. Prepared for the Graduate Medical Education National Advisory Committee. In Bureau of Health Manpower (Rockville, Md): Health Manpower References; also in Bureau of Health Manpower (Rockville, Md): GMENAC Staff Papers, No. 1. DHEW publication No. (HRA) 78-10. Government Printing Office, 1978, p 34
29. Wechsler H, Dorsey JL, Bovey JD: A follow-up study of residents in internal medicine, pediatrics and obstetrics-gynecology training programs in Massachusetts: Implications for primary care physicians. N Engl J Med 298:15, 1978
30. Abrahamson S: Diseases of the curriculum. J Med Educ 53:951, 1978
31. Curtis P, Rogers J: Continuity of care in a family practice residency program. J Fam Pract 8:975, 1979

ABSTRACTS

Geyman JP: Conversion of the general practice residency to family practice. JAMA 215:11, 1802–1807, 1971

The purpose of this article is threefold: (1) to outline the ways in which the general practice residency does and does not prepare the family physician for practice, (2) to enumerate some of the advantages of family practice residencies, and (3) to describe methods of conversion of the general practice residency to family practice, together with some initial results.

An approved residency program in general practice was in continuous operation at Community Hospital of Sonoma County in Santa Rosa, California, from 1938 to 1970. In this 230-bed general hospital, a two-year residency program was the only graduate training program. This residency was organized as a series of block rotations on traditional specialty services, both for outpatient and inpatient care. The emphasis of the program was on episodic care of acute illness. General practice training was more crisis oriented for the management of individual patients than oriented to continuity of care of the patient as a member of a family.

Valuable training and experience may be provided by a general practice residency program of this kind. It may afford excellent preparation for the competent management of over 90 percent of acute clinical problems across a wide spectrum of medical and surgical problems of families. It may also allow one not only to expand his or her clinical capabilities, but also to learn his or her own limitations, and when consultation should be obtained.

There were, however, certain areas in which this general practice program did not fully prepare the resident for practice as a family physician:

1. No training in outpatient psychiatry. Psychiatry experience was limited to the evaluation and management of acute psychiatric patients requiring 72-hour hold. There was no exposure to office counseling techniques or family dynamics.
2. Minimal emphasis on preventive medicine and comprehensive care.
3. Little training in techniques of rehabilitation.
4. Minimal emphasis on community resources and the roles of allied health services in health care.
5. Weak emphasis on practice organization and management.

Although the conversion of any general practice residency to a family practice program involves an individualized approach, many of the steps taken in this program would be applicable to others; in this instance, ten major changes were implemented in January 1970:

1. Planning of a three-year family practice residency.
2. Reorganization of the Outpatient Clinic into a Family Practice Center.
3. Modified block rotations on inpatient services whereby residents can admit their own patients to any inpatient area of the hospital throughout their residency.
4. Revision of consultant coverage with the addition of more family physicians on the teaching faculty.
5. Addition of outpatient psychiatry.
6. Diversification and coordination of conferences to include additional

areas, such as common office problems and behavioral science.
7. Addition of experience in community medicine.
8. New emphasis on preventive medicine.
9. Addition of electives.
10. Initiation of evaluation conferences.

Among the important observations evident from the initial ten months of the family practice residency program are the following:

1. Increased patient satisfaction due to improved continuity of care under one family practice resident.
2. Increased resident satisfaction with outpatient work, with greater interest being shown in continuity of care.
3. Increase in total outpatient clinic volume by 30 percent, with the majority of this increase reflecting greater utilization of the family practice clinic.

4. A shift in the proportions of patient volume in individual clinics; 80 percent of all outpatients are now being seen in family practice clinic, while most other specialty clinics have a decreased volume which is more oriented to complex problems and cases of particular teaching value.
5. Greater awareness by the resident staff of the importance of functional illness and interest in techniques of office psychiatry.
6. Improved detection of asymptomatic disease by provision of more comprehensive health care.
7. Increased interest in the family practice residency by medical students and interns. Conversion of the general practice residency to family practice has resulted in an increase in the ratio of the number of inquiries to available positions from 3:1 to 8:1, and a similar increase in the ratio of applicants to positions from 1.5:1 to 6:1.

Hannay DR: Postgraduate training in family medicine: McMaster University and West Scotland. Can Fam Physician 26:448–452, 1980

This study compares the experience of residents in family medicine at McMaster University in Hamiton, Ontario, with that of vocational trainees at Glasgow University in the West of Scotland.

The main difference between the two centers is that in Canada, postgraduate training in family medicine is primarily the responsibility of the university departments, whereas in Scotland the vocational training schemes depend on general practitioners in the community. The postgraduate adviser for general practice in Glasgow is attached to the medical faculty, but is not a member of the university department of general practice, which is mainly concerned with undergraduate teaching. In contrast, about 90 percent of family

medicine residencies in Ontario are run by university departments, which are consequently much larger than those in Scotland with staff members running practices for the purpose of training residents.

Although the McMaster undergraduate course is unique in many ways, the postgraduate training follows a similar pattern to other family medicine residencies in Canada. The core program lasts for two years, beginning with a three month block of family medicine in the first year, with a further six month block in the second year, interspersed with appropriate hospital rotations of two or three months each. During these hospital rotations the residents spend half a day per week with their family medicine team, thus insuring a continuity of patient care over the whole two years. There are also seminars in behavioral science for half a day per week throughout the two years, and electives may be spent in clinical specialities or in an academic program such as epidemiology. There is also a three month block elective in the second year which can be spent in something like family therapy or a rural practice in northwestern Ontario. The residency program therefore has considerable flexibility at McMaster, and this is enhanced by an optional third year for some, which may be spent in remedying deficiencies or acquiring additional skills.

In order to become vocationally trained for general practice in the United Kingdom, it is necessary to do two years of appropriate hospital jobs after the preregistration year in hospital, as well as spending a year as a trainee in practice with an approved trainer. Postgraduates may arrange their own hospital jobs, usually for six months at a time, and then apply directly to trainers who advertise for trainees in the medical press. Alternatively, after the preregistration year, a doctor may apply to join a training scheme for three years, as in the West of Scotland. In such schemes the hospital jobs are linked with the year in general practice, usually with provision for half day release courses. The postgraduate office at Glasgow University coordinates schemes based on ten different hospital groups in western Scotland. For six of these the last year is spent in general practice, but in two of the schemes centered on Glasgow hospitals, 18 months are in hospital rotations and 18 months in two different practices. In another scheme the second year is spent in practice, and in one the general practice training takes place for six months at the beginning and end of the three years.

This paper compares the experience of residents in family medicine at McMaster University with that of vocational trainees in the West of Scotland by means of a time-log diary used for two weeks toward the end of their fulltime attachment in family

Table 1. *Preference for Residency Program or Vocational Training Scheme**

Alternatives for GP Training	Average Score	
	McMaster	*West of Scotland*
1 year hospital/1 year practice	2.5	1.8
2 years hospital/1 year practice	4.0	4.0
1 year hospital/2 years practice	3.4	1.7
1½ years hospital/1½ years practice	4.0	3.8

Reprinted by permission from Hannay: Can Fam Physician, 26:448, 1980.
* Preference graded from 5 for "Most appropriate" to 1 for "Very inappropriate."

practice. Trainees in the West of Scotland see far more patients, but have much less supervision than their counterparts at McMaster. The findings are discussed in the context of postgraduate training for family medicine in Canada and the United Kingdom.

Both groups were asked to rank various combinations of hospital experience and family medicine as being most appropriate for vocational training, and the results are compared in Table 1.

Vocational training is much longer in Scotland, and both the hospital and general practice components are more oriented toward a service commitment than primarily being concerned with training. As such, these training schemes are essentially apprenticeships, and the lack of specific educational input is further reflected by the fact that university departments of general practice in the United Kingdom have no formal responsibility for postgraduate training. As family medicine strengthens its academic base as a discipline in its own right, so the potential contribution of university departments will increase. The challenge for the future of vocational training in family medicine will be to strike the right balance between academic input and clinical experience.

Gray DJP: A system of training for general practice. Occasional Paper 4. J R Coll Gen Pract, September, 1977

This Occasional Paper of the *Journal of the Royal College of General Practitioners* represents a monograph on today's postgraduate (vocational) training in general practice in England. Topics covered include the historical evolution of vocational training (equivalent to residency training in the U.S.), educational theory, aims and objectives, methods, and assessment of vocational training.

As an example of educational objectives for vocational (residency) training now being used in England, the following list has been developed by the Exeter Department of General Practice. The trainee shall demonstrate his/her ability to:

1. Know what it feels like to be a patient.
2. Maintain the dignity of the patient(s) in all consultations.
3. Practice patient-centred medicine.
4. Identify his or her learning needs.
5. Remedy his or her own learning needs.
6. Assess himself/herself objectively after learning.
7. Analyse accurately his/her own doctor/patient relationships.
8. Understand illness as deeply as possible in terms of the patient's pathology.
9. Assess accurately the capacity of a home/household to care for one of its sick members.
10. Offer, in more than half of an unselected series of consultations in general practice, practical preventive medical advice to his/her patients.
11. Regard general practice as a branch of medicine in its own right with its own body of knowledge, skills, and attitudes.
12. Tolerate uncertainty.
13. Promote the patient's autonomy.
14. Read and analyse critically the literature of general practice.
15. Regard his/her list of patients as a population at risk for which the doctor is responsible, whether or not they happen to be consulting.
16. Analyse a problem in medical care, devise a research project to investigate it, gather data, interpret these, and present a report of the study.

For the first time in medical history family practice is beginning to overcome its long-standing educational deprivation; for the first time it has the chance, through its College and through its new university departments, of training postgraduates in personal, primary, and continuing medical care outside hospital.

The results so far have been electric. A whole new generation of outstanding graduates is choosing general practice as its first-choice career; some of the best of young British doctors are now entering practice in the community, bringing to it great intellectual abilities, energy, and enthusiasm.

Lincoln JA: The three-year paired residency program: A solution to a teaching dilemma. J Fam Pract 1(1):31–33, 1974

A basic premise of a family practice residency program requires continuing ambulatory training in a Model Family Practice Unit as well as hospital experience. This dual requirement often leads to a teaching problem: How can family practice residents be assigned real responsibility for inpatients and at the same time be periodically relieved of these assignments so that they can care for their patients in a continuing practice? This article describes the approach to this problem developed in the Family Practice Residency Program at the University of Washington School of Medicine.

The members composing each pair are from the same year of training, i.e., two first year residents are bracketed together and for practical purposes can be looked upon as one person. An inpatient service (e.g., internal medicine) is asked to provide a position for one house officer. A pair of family practice residents is assigned to fill the position. The pair meets the other residents and the attending staff on the ward each morning. They make rounds together and attend the teaching activities and conferences together. After lunch they separate. One remains on the ward to see new patients, perform procedures, and do ward tasks while the other goes to the Family Medical Center to see outpatients. The next day the two residents reverse

roles. In this way, the ward patients are always covered while one of the pair is available each afternoon in the model practice where they are each assigned to the same multidisciplinary team. Each team includes a pair of residents from each of the three years of the program, two faculty physicians, a nurse, and a secretary. A medical social worker functions with three teams.

After one year's experience, the pairing system has functioned well. Various advantages have been cited by particpating residents for the paired system. The point made most often was that pairing facilitated cooperation and provided a model for working with other physicians in one's own practice. Others stressed that "we have been learning to communicate with one another." Still other comments brought out the fact that the system has given them a chance to spend a reasonable amount of time with outpatients, that it made it possible to take time for conferences, that it allowed them wider clinical experience than they would otherwise have had (with both inpatients and outpatients), and that it has provided patterning of important behavior. Finally, two residents pinpointed what we had really hoped for when we first inaugurated the paired residency system: it has given them a chance to fulfill multiple commitments—"to do two things at once—literally."

Geyman JP: The "one-and-two" program: A new direction in family practice residency training. J Med Educ 52:999–1001, 1977

As increasing experience has been gained with graduate education in family practice, it has been recognized that programs of high quality can be developed in varied settings and through different ap-

proaches. An important new concept in family practice residency training is the affiliated program involving two separate communities.

This paper describes a prototype of a

"one-and-two" family practice residency program within a regional network for family practice residency training involving a medical school and affiliated community hospitals. In the past several years a number of additional one-and-two programs have been developed in California, Washington, Colorado, Iowa, and other states. In each instance, the first year of training is conducted in a larger community involving a sizable teaching hospital, and the last two years of the three-year family practice residency are conducted in a smaller community setting.

Although these programs vary somewhat according to the needs and resources of each setting, the following description of a curriculum will illustrate the organization of a typical program. The first year is entirely based in the larger teaching hospital, with the exception of a one-month family practice rotation in the affiliated smaller community setting. This rotation stresses the principles of family medicine and provides an introduction to the resident's future base which helps to facilitate the resident's transition at the end of the first year. The remaining 11 months of the first year are devoted to teaching rotations in internal medicine, pediatrics, obstetrics-gynecology, surgery, and emergency medicine. Additional teaching rotations in these fields are conducted in the affiliated smaller community hospital during the second and third years of the program, together with other teaching rotations in ambulatory settings in the community. The typical three-year curriculum includes the following: general internal medicine and

medical subspecialties, 6 months; emergency medicine, 2 months; psychiatry, 1 month; and electives, 3 to 7 months. Additional training in behavioral science is provided as a longitudinal experience throughout the second and third years of the program.

First-year family practice residents in a one-and-two program may be involved in a family practice center (for example, one half day per week) if the larger teaching hospital has its own family practice residency program. The major continuity of care experience, however, will be in the family practice center related to the affiliated community hospital.

Organization of a family practice residency program on a one-and-two basis has the following advantages:

1. Creates an attractive blend of residency training for those family practice residents desiring a combination of experiences in larger and smaller community settings.
2. Affords "reality-based" educational experiences in smaller community settings without the resources needed for a full three-year program.
3. Utilizes the potential teaching resources increasingly available in smaller communities in all specialties.
4. Facilitates new regional linkages between primary, secondary, and tertiary care resources.
5. Provides an effective approach to help meet physician manpower needs in areas distant from the medical school.

Rabinowitz HK, Hervada AR: Pediatric training in family medicine residency programs. J Fam Pract 11(4):575–579, 1980

Because it is of prime importance that the increasing number of family physicians be competent in child health care, and in

order to help plan and evaluate child health care training for family physicians a survey was performed to obtain information regarding various aspects of pediatric training in current family medicine residency programs in the United States. While there are numerous parameters which are important in this area, this paper represents a descriptive analysis of the duration, types of rotations, and program attitudes regarding the child health care component of current residency programs.

A questionnaire was sent to the program directors of all 236 family medicine residency programs which had graduated residents by July, 1978. Eighty-two percent returned the questionnaire.

The mean duration of child health care training in the three year residency was 9.0 months. This included 3.4 pediatric equivalent months in the ambulatory Model Family Practice Unit (MFPU) and 5.6 months on pediatric rotations in the following areas: normal newborn nursery (1.0 months), intensive care nursery (0.6 months), inpatient (2.3 months), outpatient-general (1.5 months), and outpatient-subspecialty (0.2 months). Forty-six percent of programs have one or more fulltime, board certified pediatricians on the family medicine staff.

Respondents believed that family physicians should be competent to provide total care for normal newborns (93 percent), general inpatient care (79 percent), and general ambulatory care (99 percent). Pediatric training in family medicine residency programs, which constitutes 25 percent of curriculum time, is accomplished by utilizing the MFPU as well as pediatric rotations. Significant variations exist among programs, however, and the quality of training still needs to be evaluated.

Thompson B, Richardson CJ: Use of kittens in teaching neonatal resuscitation to family medicine residents. J Fam Pract 9(1):128–129, 1979

Neonatal resuscitation and delivery room care of the meconium-stained infant are two problems that the resident must learn to manage, but it is often difficult for all residents to learn these important procedures.

In order to teach neonatal endotracheal intubation, some programs have used anesthetized kittens as a teaching model. The pharyngeal anatomy of the four- to six-week-old kitten is similar to that of the human neonate and thus serves as a readily accessible and realistic model for teaching endotracheal intubation.

The Department of Family Medicine at The University of Texas Medical Branch at Galveston provided a special practical experience in neonatal resuscitation to their first year residents during the orientation period in July. The 10 first year family medicine residents were divided into two groups. Each group received a 45-minute lecture followed by a 90-minute practical experience. The pathophysiology of perinatal asphyxia was presented in the lecture, followed by presentation of a case, in which the step-by-step management of an asphyxiated neonate was outlined. The special case of the meconium-stained infant was discussed as an exception to the recommended practice of bag and mask ventilation as the initial maneuver in neonatal resuscitation.

The practical experience was divided into two parts: first, bag and mask ventilation and second, endotracheal intubation. A dummy infant model was used to demonstrate the technique of bag and mask ventilation. Emphasis was given to the principle that after the secretions are cleared away, most neonates can be resuscitated with bag and mask ventilation.

Live kittens, four- to six-weeks-old, were anesthetized with ketamine, administered intramuscularly, in a dose of 15 mg/lb, 10 to 15 minutes before the exercise. The kittens maintained muscle tone, and the presence of secretions and a cough reflex made the experience realistic. The kittens remained anesthetized for at least 60 minutes and tolerated repeated intubations. The same kittens were used again the following week. The kittens were used no more often than once a week in order to avoid excessive trauma and edema to their vocal cords.

Rubber models lack the intact laryngeal reflexes, vocal cord spasms, cough reflexes, and secretions that complicate intubation and resuscitation in infants. Anesthetized live kittens offer all of these features and provide a realistic experience for teaching neonatal endotracheal intubation to first year family medicine residents.

Harris BA Jr, Scutchfield F: Obstetrical and gynecological teaching in family practice residency programs. J Fam Pract 4(4):749–750, 1977

In order to assess the extent of training in obstetrics-gynecology, a study was conducted of U.S. residency training programs in family medicine. During 1975, the 227 family practice residency programs then listed in the American Academy of Family Physicians Directory were surveyed. A total of 190 programs (84 percent) replied.

Respondents were asked to estimate the number of deliveries that a family practice resident would accomplish during a three-year residency. This includes not only the deliveries performed as a result of a formal obstetrical and gynecological rotation, but also deliveries of the resident's family practice patients. Programs were also asked to estimate the number of major gynecological procedures and the number of hysterectomies performed by residents during their three-year experience.

The mean number of procedures performed by family practice residents was as follows: normal deliveries, 148; complicated deliveries, 17; cesarean sections, four (with 45 percent of programs doing no sections); minor GYN procedures, 21; major GYN procedures, four; and hysterectomies, two. The average program devoted 12 weeks to an OB/GYN rotation. Fifteen

Table 1. *Normal Deliveries*

Number of Normal Deliveries	Number of Residencies	Percent
0– 49	33	19.0
50– 99	56	32.3
100–149	46	26.4
150–199	28	16.1
200–249	9	5.1
250–299	0	0.0
Total	**174**	**100.0**

Reprinted by permission from Harris, Scutchfield: J Fam Pract, 4(4):749, 1977.

Table 2. *Complicated Deliveries*

Number of Complicated Deliveries	Number of Residencies	Percent
0	35	20.2
1– 5	20	11.5
6–10	31	17.9
11–15	24	13.9
16–20	19	11.0
21–25	13	7.5
26–50	25	14.5
50	6	3.5
Total	**173**	**100.0**

Reprinted by permission from Harris, Scutchfield: J Fam Pract, 4(4):749, 1977.

percent of family practice programs had their own fulltime OB/GYN specialist. Fifty-two percent of the programs had OB/GYN specialists available in the family practice center; in 48 percent of programs the specialists were present on a regularly scheduled basis.

Tables 1 and 2 display these results in terms of normal and complicated deliveries, respectively.

Crow HE, Roher MM, Carley WC, Radke KF, Holden DM, Smith GF: Non-rotational teaching of obstetrics in a family practice residency. J Fam Pract 10(5):831–834, 1980

The inclusion of obstetric care in a family practice setting rounds out the experience of providing total care for families, and provides a firm foundation for a practice to grow on. It is sometimes difficult, however, for community based family practice residencies to provide adequate patient volume for residents to be well trained in obstetrics, due to several factors: (1) decreasing numbers of "staff" patients available for resident management, (2) increasing numbers of both obstetrical and family practice residents, and (3) reluctance of private physicians to allow house staff significant participation in obstetrical care.

In response to these problems, the E.W. Sparrow Family Practice Residency has created its own obstetrical patient population composed of private family practice center patients and County Health Department Clinic prenatal patients. Educational autonomy has been achieved by this method, and appropriate liaison with obstetrics-gynecology is maintained through frequent use of consultative services. The obstetrical training of family practice residents is therefore relatively independent of the obstetrical staff and allows residents an opportunity to learn how to appropriately utilize consultants. Residents progress through varied levels of expertise with appropriate supervision and privileges at each level (Figure 1).

First year residents ("rotational" internship year) spend two months on the inpatient OB/GYN service, working with obstetrics residents and attending staff. They rotate through the regular and high risk OB prenatal clinics, take call every third night, and assist at or perform approximately 50 deliveries with the obstetrics attending physicians. They also rotate once a month throughout the first year to each of the two family practice community prenatal clinics.

During the second year, residents begin seeing their own private obstetrical patients, and spend one half day per week at one of the prenatal clinics as well. When on call (approximately every fifth night), they begin delivering their own private patients and the clinic patients. Due to the unique non-rotational aspects of the E.W. Sparrow Hospital Family Practice Residency Program, the second and third year family practice residents are taught primarily by the family practice faculty rather than by the obstetrics attending staff. Twenty-five percent of these family practice deliveries require obstetrical consultation; 75 percent are handled by the family practice residency alone with a family practice orientation.

This system allows several advantages over the traditional rotational format:

1. It facilitates role modeling by the family practice faculty to the family practice residents.
2. It increases the credibility of family practice as residents learn good obstetrical care from their own faculty.

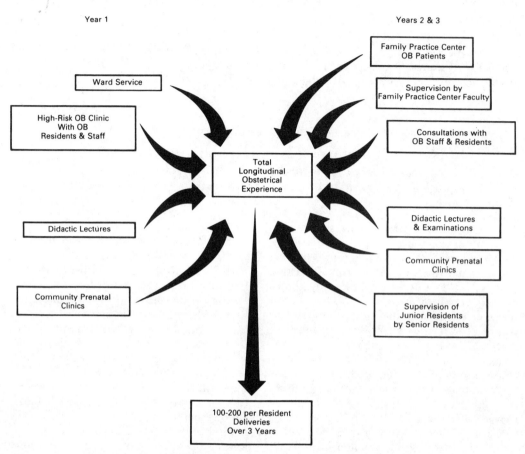

Fig. 1. Obstetrical experience. E.W. Sparrow Family Practice Residency. (Reprinted by permission from Crow, Roher et al: J Fam Pract, 10(5):831, 1980.)

3. It increases direct supervision of family practice residents by their own faculty, thus allowing for better evaluation.

4. It allows teaching of appropriate interaction with consultants, including learning how to deal with and resolve conflicts between consultants and family physicians.

5. It improves continuity of patient care by coordinating prenatal care and delivery rather than relying on an obstetrical service to provide patients for delivery only.

Steinert Y, Levitt R: The teaching of human sexuality in a family medicine training program. J Fam Pract 7(5):993–997, 1978

This article describes a teaching program on human sexuality in a Family Practice Center affiliated with the Department of Family Medicine at McGill University in Montreal. Its major goals are the transmission of information, the teaching of skills, and the desensitization of the health care professional in this area.

In the teaching of information and skills, an emphasis is placed on sexual development, sexual response, commonly believed sexual myths, and sexual dysfunctions. Skills which are taught involve sexual history taking and basic management principles. The major objective is not to make the physician a sex therapist, but rather to expose him to treatment possibilities.

The major aims of the program are carried out in a series of four seminars and in ongoing teaching. The seminars are held over a six-week period and each seminar is 90 minutes in length; the ongoing teaching takes place throughout the academic teaching year.

The first seminar—Learning the Usual—is focused on the development of human sexuality from infancy to old age. In discussing sexuality at each life period, the issue of sexuality vs. sex, internal and external influences affecting sexuality (e.g., culture, illness, and medication), and commonly held sexual myths are explored. The second seminar—Pinpointing the Significant—deals with sexual history taking. Its main objective is to emphasize the importance of taking a sexual history, to discuss common misgivings held by the health care professionals, and to illustrate the history taking process itself. The last two seminars deal with Sexual Dysfunction and Treatment. The description of various sexual dysfunctions and their treatment are aimed at providing the family physician with skills in the diagnosis of sexual problems and with knowledge of existing treatment modalities.

The first session on sexual dysfunction and treatment is focused on premature ejaculation, primary and secondary orgasmic dysfunction, and primary and secondary impotence. The second session continues with dyspareunia, vaginismus, retrograde ejaculation, and lack of interest. In these seminars, traits common to most couples with a sexual problem are outlined, each dysfunction is described, and the general principles and specific techniques of treatment are presented. Throughout the teaching, a problem solving, case-oriented approach is used.

Ongoing teaching consists of case discussions, consultation, supervision, and joint interviews. Case discussion is carried out on both an individual and a group basis.

On an observational level, a number of positive changes in the attitudes and behaviors of the residents, nurses, and staff physicians of the center have been noted. For example, many of the health care professionals have shown a heightened awareness of the importance of sexual health as part of the total health picture of the patient. This has been evidenced by an increase in the taking of sexual histories as part of the general history taking process and a more refined assessment once a sexual problem has been identified. The demand for supervision and consultation on cases where sexual problems have been identified has also increased.

Moore JT, Bobula JA: A conceptual framework for teaching geriatrics in a family medicine residency. J Med Educ 55:339–455, 1980

Nowhere is the need for training in geriatrics more apparent than in family medicine residencies. Primary care physicians now provide the bulk of health care delivery to the elderly and probably will continue to do so in the future.

The health needs of the elderly are sufficiently different from those of younger patients to require special skills on the part of physicians. Some of these differences and the requirements each makes on the physician are:

1. Many medical problems have different clinical presentations in the elderly; for example, myocardial infarction may be painless, and pneumonia may present with symptoms of organic brain syndrome.
2. Elderly patients are subject to problems in areas other than physical health status which influence the management of their health problems. Impairments in mental health, lack of social support systems, diminished economic resources, and decreased capacity for self-care require a multi-dimensional approach to data acquisition and patient assessment, and suggest the need for physicians to be able to work with other health professionals as a team.
3. Geriatric patients tend to have multiple and chronic problems that interact and complicate treatment.
4. Functional implications are especially important in the elderly. For example, the fact that a patient has a diagnosis of osteoarthritis, stroke, or marital maladjustment tells little that is helpful in

management; it is necessary to know the degree of impairment caused by specific problems.

The competency-based educational model is particularly useful for the development of geriatric training since it requires that fundamental questions be raised, such as: What should a resident be able to do in caring for the elderly? The first step in designing and implementing a competency-based curriculum is the selection of goals. After discussions with faculty and residents and a review of the literature, the faculty at the Duke-Watts Family Medicine Program chose to organize a curriculum around these four goals: understanding principles of geriatric medicine, acquiring and interpreting data, managing geriatric patients, and functioning as a member of a health care team.

A required one-month rotation based on the model described here was instituted in August 1978. The rotation has been well received by the 15 residents who have thus far participated in this rotation, at least in part because the expectations of the rotation have been clearly stated in the curriculum objectives and also because the objectives originated from faculty and residents in the residency itself. The authors believe that a required rotation based on well-defined objectives which is implemented after demonstration that the required competencies cannot be acquired efficiently otherwise will be more convincing to residents than a rotation developed without such planning.

Carson RA, Curry RW Jr: Ethics teaching on ward rounds. J Fam Pract 11(1):59–63, 1980

Ethics teaching in medical settings usually takes place in the classroom or at specially designated times and places, as in "ethics grand rounds." The authors have integrated ethics teaching into regular attending rounds.

For approximately two years the authors, an internist and an ethicist, have made ward rounds in a community hospital with family practice residents on a general medical inpatient service associated with the University of Florida College of Medicine. The hospital is a 450-bed, nonprofit general hospital with a medical staff of approximately 180 physicians, all in private practice. The family practice residency program is the only university based teaching service in the hospital. Three family practice residents staff the medical service to which they admit about 60 patients per month, with an average census of 20 patients. Faculty attending rounds are held six days a week, during which new patients are presented and the problems of all patients discussed. An ethicist accompanies the physicians on rounds once weekly. These Wednesday morning sessions are not what is coming to be known as "ethics rounds." Rather, they are regular ward rounds aimed at teaching family medicine by analyzing, criticizing, and reinforcing the care of sick patients as it is provided by residents under the close supervision of an attending physician.

Although the ethical problems confronted in the day-to-day practice or primary care medicine are many, a circumscribed number of questions came up again and again: Who should decide? Should this dying person's life be prolonged? How does one act on an uncertain prognosis? How does one conduct oneself with one's peers? The ends served by elucidating such questions on rounds are neither hortatory nor prescriptive but instructional. The ethicist functions in the clinical setting not primarily as an advisor or a consultant (although, on occasion, he advises and consults) and certainly not as a decision maker, but as a teacher of physicians-in-training. He does this by challenging assumptions, clarifying issues, making distinctions, pointing out deficiencies in reasoning, asking for reasons, and then probing them to see if they can withstand scrutiny.

Hopkins JR, Parker CE: Experience of family practice residents as athletic team physicians. J Fam Pract 7(3):519–525, 1978

This paper describes and discusses the educational aspect of a project designed to expose a group of family practice residents to sports medicine through work with college athletic teams. The Antelope Valley Hospital Medical Center Family Practice Program in Lancaster, California, has initiated an innovative project which involves residents serving as team physicians for local college athletic teams.

As part of a contract to provide health care for the college students, it was agreed that four resident physicians would, as a group, serve as the school's team physicians. The residents volunteered to participate in this project. Their responsibilities included preseason health assessment of all athletes, evaluation and treatment of illnesses and injuries, and attendance at all football games.

Prior to the beginning of the school year, instruction was given to the residents regarding the appropriate preseason history and physical examination, disqualifying conditions, skeletal and muscular development, psychological aspects of athletic competition, and interaction with coaches and trainers. A staff member of the Department of Athletics, a professional athletic trainer, met with the residents to acquaint them with his role. The roles of coach, trainer, and physician were defined, and lines of authority over injured players were established at the very outset. Resident backup and teaching was provided by the Family Practice Center (FPC) faculty, local Emergency Room physicians, an orthopedic surgeon, and the physical therapy department of the Antelope Valley Hospital. Athletes were required to complete a brief health history questionnaire and undergo a screening physical examination prior to beginning practice. Individuals particpating in more than one sport were evaluated only once during the year, prior to the earliest sport in which they took part.

Any positive finding encountered in the initial history and physical examination which required further consideration or investigation by the resident beyond the basic procedure was considered to be of educational value for the resident and is included in Tables 1 and 2. These include some conditions which, on further questioning or examination, were found to be insignificant or which, following appropriate therapy, were no longer of major importance to the athlete's health.

The pattern of demand for physician services revealed that 80 percent of the care delivered went to football players, with utilization paralleling the regular season (August 25 through November 20). Of the 136 encounters for illness and injury, 114 occurred during this period of time. Most injuries and illnesses were managed entirely by FPC personnel. Consultations were obtained from an orthopedic sur-

Table 1. *Summary of Positive Responses on Initial History*

Concussion	15
Asthma	8
Rheumatic fever	2
Fainting spells	2
Sprains	67
Spine fracture	2
Bee sting allergy	1
Currently on medication	2
Total	99

Reprinted by permission from Hopkins, Parker: J Fam Pract, 7(3):519, 1978.

geon for eight cases, a general surgeon for two cases, and a urologist for one case.

Many acute medical problems, particularly musculoskeletal injuries, are encountered during the year. It is possible for residents to follow injuries from the moment of trauma through rehabilitation and recovery in greater numbers than might be expected in other settings. Some exposure to preventive and psychological aspects of sports medicine is also provided.

Table 2. *Summary of Positive Findings on Initial Physical Examination*

Elevated blood pressure	34
Visual deficit (>20/200)	5
Dental caries	7
Dental appliance	4
Papilloma on tonsil	1
Heart murmur	10
Inguinal hernia	1
Varicocele	1
Hemorrhoids	2
Gonorrhea	1
Ligamentous laxity	15
Skin fungal infection	3
Warts	1
Total	85

Reprinted by permission from Hopkins, Parker: J Fam Pract, 7(3):519, 1978.

Snell GF: A method for teaching techniques of office surgery. J Fam Pract 7(5):987–990, 1978

Over the course of several years of involvement in family practice resident training, a method for instruction of the residents in basic concepts of skin suturing and office surgery has been developed by the faculty of the McKay-Dee Hospital Family Practice Residency in Ogden, Utah.

The equipment used for the teaching sessions is readily available in the primary care physician's office and in the Family Practice Center. It includes needle holder, skin hook, Adson tissue forceps, disposable scalpel with a #15 Bard-Parker blade, tissue scissors, and a skin marking pencil. A variety of suture material is utilized, including 4-0 Dexon, 4-0 Silk, 5-0 and 6-0 Nylon or Prolene. The "patients" to be worked on are pigs' feet prepared for surgical practice. The pigs' feet are scrubbed and shaved prior to their use. The prepared "patient" is then placed on a hand towel on a mayo stand tray which, in turn, can be set on a desk or table where the instruction session is to be held.

The instruction session is held shortly before the resident is to begin his Emergency Room rotation or, in some cases, at the beginning of his rotation on general surgery. Exercises for each instructional objective are listed in Table 1. The session is held on a one-to-one or one faculty member to two residents situation so that sufficient attention and observation can be rendered by the supervising faculty. A printed handout which describes certain aspects of wound care and has descriptions of both proper and improper suturing methods is given to each resident for his/her perusal and retention.

The pigs' feet teaching method is a popular and effective approach for learning basic suturing skills prior to actual rendering of patient care.

Table 1. *Educational Objectives and Learning Exercises*

Objective	Exercise Number	Wound Description
Simple suturing Wound apposition Suture placement Instrument knot tying	1	Y-shaped laceration
Apex suture	1	Y-shaped laceration
	4	Z-plasty
Wound trimming	2	Bevelled flap laceration
Layered closure	3	Elliptical incision
Undermining	4	Z-plasty
Excisional biopsy 'Dog ear' management	3	Elliptical incision
Wound revision	4	Z-plasty

Reprinted by permission from Snell: J Fam Pract, 7(5):987, 1978.

Scheingold L: A Balint seminar in the family practice residency setting. J Fam Pract 10(2):267–270, 1980

This paper attempts to show what a behavioral scientist with a psychoanalytic viewpoint can offer to young family physicians in a family practice residency. A beginning can be found in the work of Dr. Michael Balint, who made important theoretical and pragmatic contributions to family practice through the seminars for general practitioners which he led some years ago at the Tavistock Clinic.

Recognizing that physicians had neither the desire nor the training to become psychoanalysts, Balint raised the question of how psychoanalytic insights could be of assistance to the family physician. The answer is in the *understanding* of individuals and families that a family physician can develop over a long period of time. The length of this association, even if the contacts are episodic, puts the family physician in a unique position to be sensitive to the central psychological conflicts as acted out in many of his/her patients' lives.

In the Group Health Cooperative Family Practice Residency in Seattle, a Balint seminar series evolved according to the needs of the residents and the training of the faculty. Goals of the group within this residency were formulated at the beginning of the seminar: (1) encouraging residents' awareness of their own particular sensitivities with patients, (2) encouraging open sharing and trust among residents and faculty, (3) examining collegial relationships with other family physicians and with consultants, and (4) exposing attitudes or differing value systems that might be detrimental to patient care.

The first five sessions of the group focused on a wide variety of problems and tended at times to center more on the patient than on the physician. By the sixth session, group norms began to be established about the focus on the physician, so that more of the confronting was now initiated by group members than by the co-leaders, and relationships were now seen more in terms of, to use Balint's phrase, "clinical understanding." Themes now included the need to be liked by patients, feelings about patients who handle their own feelings in quite different ways, the interpersonal consequences and meanings of gift giving patients, the physician's response to sexual material brought up by the patient, painful dilemmas about quality care vs. clinic patient pressures, and a resident's feelings about the death of an infant. At the tenth session, the family practice co-leader presented a case. This session seems to have been a turning point, with the group able to sort out issues related to the reality of the patient's demands vs. the internal reality of the physician's expectation of himself. Within the next couple of sessions, the specific topics of discussion of the group changed a bit, partly as a result of a re-evaluation of the group's goals at the end of the twelfth session. The focus was still on the internal difficulties of the residents, but the topics broadened to include dealing with the stresses of a busy clinic practice, dealing with boredom, and the triggering of strong affect in the physician by the patient (in this case, anger). In addition, "follow-up" sessions were held in which cases previously discussed were brought up again and more recent developments examined.

The advantage of a Balint group in a residency setting is that the residents are already in a learning situation and are facing daily the important ethical and emotional dilemmas in family medicine. This has meant they seize readily on the opportunity to talk about their own and their patients' feelings, to learn that the presenting problem is not always as it seems, and to ask the questions: "What does this behavior mean?" "What does my feeling about this patient mean?" In other words, residents have developed a new way of thinking and introspecting, in some measure using psychodynamic concepts of relationships as discussed, modeled, and taught in the group.

Fitzgerald RD: Group process in teaching family dynamics to family practice residents.
J Fam Pract 9(4):631–635, 1979

Behavioral science training in family practice at Madigan Army Medical Center, Tacoma, Washington, has used small group seminars to teach family dynamics on an experiential level. The group process is similar enough to dynamics within families to facilitate understanding by introspection.

Small group dynamics and family dynamics both can be analyzed in systems theory concepts. Both have goals, characteristic roles, principles of homeostasis, boundaries, and resistance to change. While the group experience is not exactly the same as a family experience, the similarities are close enough to allow for the learning of concepts on a feeling level.

The objectives for the residents in the groups are: (1) self-awareness as physicians, (2) personal and professional growth, and (3) understanding of intra and interpersonal dynamics. This is accomplished by three primary methods: (1) case consultation, (2) discussion of personal and professional issues and development, and (3) introspection on the group process as it relates to interpersonal and family dynamics.

The group meets weekly for two hours. Some sessions are preplanned and some are open. The group is not restricted to use of group process and, in fact, spends the majority of the time in the case consultation format with each case usually generating some material for a more general discussion of personal and professional development. When group process is used, it is used in one of six ways:

1. The co-leaders may stop the group process in the here and now and comment on the relationships to either family dynamics or the helping process.
2. The leader(s) makes a group process comment after an interaction has taken place.
3. The leaders comment by making a summary kind of statement when group process occurs over a period of time rather than during a single event.
4. The leader comments on a future event.
5. The leaders create group process for the purpose of teaching and/or facilitating group development.
6. The group members comment spontaneously on the group process.

There are several similarities between the group and families not mentioned above which have occurred fairly consistently:

—The residents' relationship to the leaders leads to numerous examples of parent-child dynamics.

—Sibling rivalry takes a wide variety of forms.

—There always seems to be a "favored son" who is sort of a co-facilitator and the ways the leaders cope with that models counseling skills.

—There is usually a "rebellious child." ("All this behavioral science is just common sense and this group is a waste of time.") The rebellious child and the favored son frequently generate a lot of action.

—The "silent one" affords the opportunity to deal with projection by the other members at some point.

This "simulated family" provides the opportunity to experience the feelings of being a family member as well as some of the therapy experience. The leaders can model effective techniques in dealing with families. Considering the limited time behavioral science has to train physicians, this approach meets the need for a multidimensional format.

Anstett R: Patient discussion groups in the training of family practice residents. J Fam Pract 10(1):143–144, 1980

This paper suggests one approach which has demonstrated some success in establishing a patient oriented approach to illness in a family practice residency.

A variety of patient-resident discussion groups have been established by a number of the faculty at the University of Colorado Department of Family Medicine. A typical arrangement is to identify a number of patients or families with a specific medical problem or life situation, for example, having a new child in the house, having a particular chronic illness in a family member, or being a three-generation family. These discussions are moderated by a faculty member or members but quickly become open discussions including patients, residents, and faculty. Another successful approach has been to select an undifferentiated group of patients and to raise questions in and around the process of being ill. These discussions have generated conversation between patients and residents around such issues as patient compliance, the expectations patients have of their physicians, and the way patients respond to different kinds of physician styles. This format gives the chance for residents to hear directly from patients what it is they do that their patients like and do not like. Residents hear everything from what it is like to try to talk to somebody while you are in a flimsy patient's gown in a cold room, to what it feels like when the physician uses words that you do not understand.

Residents and patients seem to enjoy this group process immensely and what transpires seems to be not only informative but therapeutic as well. The patient-resident group discussion provides residents as well as patients with a forum to share their own perceptions of illness behavior.

Aluise JJ: Human relations training for family practice residents: A four-year retrospective review. J Fam Pract 4(5):881–888, 1977

The Family Practice Center of Akron, Ohio has developed and implemented a human relations training program as an integral part of the family practice residency curriculum. Following two years of planning and experimenting, a 12-month course of study was formalized in July 1975. Two full-time behavioral scientists are responsible for planning, coordinating, and teaching the curriculum. The curriculum includes a variety of learning experiences throughout the three years and represents approximately ten percent of educational programming and costs.

A logical progression for behavioral training would be *first* to prepare a family physician to become keenly aware of personal feelings and understand his/her reactions to people and their problems, and *second* to use this insight to focus upon the responsibility of the physician to perform in a nonjudgmental manner. There are five performance features of skill development which may cement learning experiences. These include *discrimination*— knowing when to do it, *problem solving*— how to make decisions, *recall*—knowing what to do, *manipulation*—how to do it, and *communication*—verbally expressing ideas and expectations. The primary methods of instruction at the Family Practice Center of Akron are weekly confer-

ences, audio/video reviews, and semiannual workshops.

A 28-hour introductory course is given during the first month of the residency for first-year residents. There are three regularly scheduled behavioral science conferences in each academic year. There is a weekly behavioral science/practice management seminar, a biweekly family health conference, and a weekly human relations seminar. Table 1 presents a list of topics for each of the three conference programs.

Table 2 presents an approximation of the hours residents spend in each educational method during the three-year residency program.

An evaluation consultant has concluded that several related factors have influenced the quality of the behavioral science curric-

Table 1. *Behavioral Science Conference Topics**

Family Health	Behavioral Science/ Practice Management	Human Relations Seminars
Pregnancy	Behavioral science objectives	Child rearing
Childbirth/postpartum	Theories of health and growth	Ethnic differences
Infant and the family	Applications of TA	Parental nurturance
Child neglect/abuse	Behavioral strategies	Sex-linked roles
Premarital visit	Depression	Freud's phases of psychosexual development
Working mothers	Anxiety reactions	
Enuresis	Crisis intervention	Sullivan and Erickson
Unwanted pregnancy	Reality therapy	Piaget's approach to cognitive development
Family interviewing	Leadership styles	
Human sexuality	Group process	Jung
Divorce and remarriage	Motivation and job enrichment	School phobia
Middle years and beyond	Office accounting practices	Child abuse
Death, a life experience	Medical/legal issues	Empty nest syndrome
	Insurance and estate planning	Family crisis
	Financial planning	Female alcoholic
	Family and children's services	Lonely elderly
	Child guidance center	Adolescent female
	Welfare and public assistance	Adolescent male
		Encopretic child
		Physically handicapped
		Adoption
		MD support systems
		Single parent

Reprinted by permission from Aluise: J Fam Pract, 4(5):881, 1977.
* Additional conference topics are selected and presented by family practice residents.

Table 2. *Behavioral Science Input per Resident for Three Years (2 full-time faculty, and part-time consultants)*

	First-Year Hours	Second-Year Hours	Third-Year Hours	Total Hours
Weekly conferences/seminars	60*	60	80	200
Workshops (semiannual)	30	30	30	90
Audio/video reviews	20	40	60	120
Resident projects and presentations	—	10	30	40
Practice management and leadership development	—	30	100	130
Total hours	110	170	300	580

Reprinted by permission from Aluise: J Fam Pract, 4(5):881, 1978.
* Includes 28-hour introductory course in July.

ulum: (1) existence of trust, rapport, and communication, so that all faculty and residents feel a part of the policy making; (2) sense of group identity and cohesiveness around common goals and results; and (3) selection process of residents which is based on individual qualities and capabilities and not similarity to faculty.

Shienvold A, Asken M, Cincotta J: Family practice residents' perceptions of behavioral science training, relevance, and needs. J Fam Pract 8(1):97–101, 1979

The present study was undertaken to determine the degree to which training in behavioral science-related areas has been obtained and how the residents have viewed the relevance of this training to their family practice experience. Fifty-six family practice residents representing programs in 23 different states were surveyed concerning their training experience in behavioral science. Questions covered three basic areas of concern: experiential content, subsequent relevance to family prac-

Table 1. *Rank Order of Areas Most Relevant to Family Medicine*

Rank Order	Area	Number of Residents
1	Counseling skills	38
2	Family dynamics and family therapy	18
3	Psychosomatics and understanding psychosomatic medicine in the relationships between psychosocial and physical aspects of disease	13
4	Behavioral techniques and interventions in patient problems	8
5	Physician-patient relationships	5
6	Intra- and interprofessional growth	5
7	The management of anxiety and depression	5
8	Drug abuse	1
9	Alcohol abuse	1
10	Adolescent psychology	1

Reprinted by permission from Shienvold et al: J Fam Pract, 8(1):97, 1979.

tice, and suggestions for curriculum improvement at the residency level.

The results point out definite deficits in predoctoral training, especially with regard to knowledge of medical psychology,

Table 2. *Rank Order of Suggestions for Improving Behavioral Science Training*

---

1. Integrate the behavioral science training into the total experience of the family practice residency.
2. Use videotapes as a feedback and supervisory mechanism.
3. Maintain staff psychologists rather than having consultants or psychiatrists.
4. Make the material more practical and applicable.
5. Provide for a consultation-liaison psychiatry rotation.
6. Provide for resident support and growth groups.
7. Provide preceptors who are better role models when behavioral science issues arise.
8. Emphasize the effect of physician reactions upon treatment of patients.
9. Provide residents with individual counseling and support during stress periods.
10. Increase the case conference model.
11. Minimize psychiatric techniques while maximizing behavioral techniques.
12. Expand the knowledge of psychopharmacology.
13. Make behavioral science more relevant in medical school so there is better understanding at that point.
14. Improve the resident selection procedures so that residents who have greater interests in behavioral science end up in family practice.

Reprinted by permission from Shienvold et al: J Fam Pract, 8(1):97, 1979.

psychiatric consultation to medical patients, and practical intervention skills. The residents' ratings of the relevance of their behavioral science training in medical school averaged 3.5 on a five-point scale. With respect to experience with videotaping, for example, 72 percent of the first year residents, 77 percent of the second year residents, and only 50 percent of the third year residents had had this experience.

The residents indicated that they felt the relevance of behavioral science to residency training was at an average of 4.6 on a five-point scale. Concerning the relevance of behavioral science to the practice of family medicine, the ratings were very similar with an overall rating of 4.5 on a five-point scale.

Table 1 presents the residents' view of areas of behavioral science which they have found most relevant to their family practice residency, whereas Table 2 outlines their suggestions for improving the teaching and formulation of behavioral science curricula.

It seems apparent from these results that the basic behavioral science curriculum needs a dual focus, with mental health aspects of psychology and medical psychology being integral parts in the development of the family physician. Although the specific nature of this curriculum may vary to meet the individual needs of a given family practice program, it seems that both areas need adequate treatment in order to prepare the family physician to meet the needs of his/her practice.

Werblun MN, Dankers H, Betton H, Tapp J:
A structured experiential curriculum in community medicine. J Fam Pract 8(4):771–774, 1979

In order for the family practice resident to become proficient in comprehensive care there must be an interwoven fabric of learning experiences in the three-year curriculum. Ability to utilize community medicine is an aspect of comprehensive care which is vital to the training of the family physician.

Competencies in community medicine most applicable in family practice include skills in:

public health and preventive medicine: disease prevention and early detection in individuals and groups
epidemiology in diagnosis and disease control
occupational health
utilization of community resources
organization and management of health care
assessing community health care needs
providing for community health education

Expertise in all areas of community medicine would reach far beyond the needs of the practicing family physician. The family practice resident needs to identify those skills to pursue which are most appropriate for his or her future practice, or personal interests.

Throughout the three-year training program, lectures and seminars are presented to provide the resident with the appropriate tools to understand various aspects of community medicine. During the first year of training, each resident is given the opportunity to visit and assess existing community medicine organizations. A written report on one of these agencies is required from each resident. Prior to the end of the first year of training, each resident will select from the following list of experiences the area of experiential learning he/she will pursue during the next two years:

1. Health care services research
2. Policy analysis and decision making
3. Community services
4. Community health education
5. Case study

This curriculum provides the residents with a base of knowledge in community medicine needed to apply the concepts of comprehensive care within his or her own practice and community. Additionally, the use of selective experiential learning resources enables each resident to tailor his/her experience to specific personal goals and needs.

Rosenblatt RA: On-call in a family medicine residency: Implications for patient care and residency training. J Fam Pract 6(2):327–331, 1978

This study was undertaken in order to scrutinize the type and quantity of interactions that occur after hours in a developing model unit of a family practice residency. The residency studied had just entered its second year of existence. Based at the University Hospital of the University of Washington, 18 residents in three years of the residency cared for 2,260 registered patients at the time of the study. Night call was shared by the 12 second- and third-year residents on a rotating basis, backed up by the faculty members. The purpose of the study was to record the volume and nature of the calls, the problems precipitating the calls, and the type of interventions used by the physicians to care for their patients. An attempt was made to see whether experience, i.e., third-year vs. second-year residents, or other variables affected the nature of the interaction.

All after-hours calls and visits during a two-month period in the model practice of the University of Washington's family medicine residency were analyzed. Data as to the nature and frequency of the telephone interactions were collected and analyzed, and the manner in which residents of varying experience handled these calls was compared.

The study showed that the volume of after-hours calls was about two calls per 1,000 registered patients per night, with about one half of all calls coming on the weekend. Seventy-five percent of the problems were handled by telephone contact alone; four percent of the calls ended in admission to the hospital. The vast majority of calls were handled by the residents themselves, without consultation. Third-year residents were less likely to attempt to modify patient behavior than their less experienced peers. Table 1 displays the major diagnostic categories encountered in this study.

Table 1. *Major Diagnostic Categories Generating After-Hours Calls*

Diagnostic Category	Percentage
Gastrointestinal (includes vomiting and diarrhea)	9
Infectious (includes upper respiratory infection)	9
Trauma (includes lacerations)	7
Genitourinary	7
Pregnancy	6
Neurological (includes headaches)	6
Problems of early infancy	5
Psychiatric	3
Otological (including otitis)	3
Respiratory	3
Dermatologic	3
Miscellaneous classifiable problems with frequency less than three percent	25
Not classifiable or no problem	14

Reprinted by permission from Rosenblatt: J Fam Pract, 6(2): 327, 1978.

The data presented here provide intriguing glimpses of random corners of the interaction between patients and physicians after-hours: patients are counseled, treated, reassured by telephone, and in most of the cases, the physician feels the call was legitimate and the patient better and happier for the encounter.

Curtis P, Talbot A, Liebeseller V: The after-hours call: A survey of United States family practice residency programs. J Fam Pract 8(1):117–122, 1979

This article reports the results of a 1977 survey of 245 family practice residency programs providing after-hours care. The objectives of the study were: (1) to clarify the involvement of family practice residents in this aspect of medical care, (2) to investigate the organization of after-hours care in the family practice centers as a possible training model for future family physicians, and (3) to establish whether or not specific educational activity was based on after-hours calls.

The data from this national survey of 245 operational family practice residency programs (as of June 9, 1977) show certain trends and similarities. Most of the programs tended to maintain clinic hours which approximated closely those of the physician's office in private practice; a minority also offered access to patients through evening and/or weekend clinics. Some form of after-hours coverage was provided by all the residency programs; the variability of coverage depended on the practice model selected by each particular training program. The longest period of after-hours coverage occurred on Sundays. The manpower used for providing care after hours was primarily family practice residents with backup from faculty physicians.

Methods of recording medical care after hours were considerably less effective and systematized than those provided during office hours. Program directors commented, in their responses, on the need for improved medical records, communication, and teaching of this part of medical care in the residencies.

The data also suggest that the educational commitment of residency programs to the teaching of after-hours medical care was only moderate (Table 1). Over a quarter of the programs provided no review of cases and another 25 to 50 percent dealt with cases only on an immediate and consultative basis with little evidence of systematized review.

Table 1. *Contexts Used To Review After-Hours Patient Encounters*

	Program	
Educational Method	**Number**	**Percent**
No method used	69	28
Group discussion and 1:1 teaching	61	24
Group discussion only	56	22
1:1 teaching only	51	20
Chart audit	8	3
Total	**245**	**97***
Educational Setting	**Number**	**Percent**
No setting reported	128	52
Morning report	74	30
Chart review	37	15
Other	6	2
Total	**245**	**99***

Reprinted by permission from Curtis et al: J Fam Pract, 8(1): 117, 1979.
* Rounding error; actually 100 percent.

If the various methods of education and service involved in the after-hours call are to be used effectively, it is evident that recording methods and information exchange between the medical providers need to be improved.

Warburton SW, Sadler GR: House call training in the family practice curriculum. J Med Educ 52:768–770, 1977

As part of its ongoing curriculum review of the four family practice residency programs in central New Jersey, the Department of Family Medicine of the College of Medicine and Dentistry of New Jersey-Rutgers Medical School raised the issue of whether specific training for the conduct of house calls should be added to the curriculum. A survey of the curricula of family practice residency programs throughout the state revealed that residents received little formal training in, or

evaluation of, their performance of house calls. Furthermore, the faculty did not have a consistent approach toward preparing residents to conduct house calls.

During the first year of the residency program, an understanding of the role home visits play in the comprehensive care of their patients is stressed to the residents. This is accomplished through a variety of lunch-time conferences dealing with various aspects of home care. For example, the residents are guided in reviewing their expectations of what should be accomplished on a house call and in recognizing not only the cost-efficiency of home care but also the advantages of maintaining a patient within the familiar surroundings of his home and family. They discuss the patient's "right to die" at home, give birth at home, and request home care for serious and/or chronic illness. In addition, residents are given a self-instruction package containing a selection of recent references related to home visits. As more pertinent references become available, they too are distributed to residents. The package also contains pretests and posttests to measure attitudes and knowledge about home care.

Concurrently, faculty members are being helped to strengthen their teaching skills in this area. They receive a self-instruction package which includes the same materials the first-year residents receive. In addition, they are given literature which discusses their position as a role model and as an active teacher when first-year residents accompany them on house calls.

In the residents' second year, when they begin to make house calls independently, the faculty's responsibilities change from role model to active supervisor. For example, prior to the residents' making a house call, the faculty members are encouraged to help the residents assess their expectations of what skills will be required as well as what information will be gathered. This discussion is resumed after the house call and focuses on the fulfillment of these expectations and the residents' attitudes toward the house call. This is done in addition to an ongoing chart audit, which focuses on the residents' intervention in the patients' medical and social problems.

Love DW, Hodge NA, Foley WA: The clinical pharmacist in a family practice residency program. J Fam Pract 10(1):67–72, 1980

A project of interdisciplinary family medicine education was conducted in which a clinical pharmacist served as a drug therapy consultant-educator in a family practice residency program. The project of clinical pharmacy consultative and educational services was established at the Family Medical Center (FMC) of the University of Kentucky.

A pharmacist established a clinical practice with the family physicians during the third year of her pharmacy residency program. The pharmacy resident practiced as a drug therapy consultant-educator for the physicians. She was available to provide drug information and advise about drug therapy, to teach in formal conferences, to prepare and disseminate a drug information bulletin, to make rounds with the physicians in the hospital, to provide a drug blood level consultation service, to interview and counsel patients, and to conduct a drug utilization review (DUR) project. The pharmacist did not dispense drugs or perform primary patient care.

It was hypothesized that changes in the attitudes of physicians about clinical pharmacists and about practicing with a clinical pharmacist would occur and, to enable documentation of this, assessments of their attitudes were made before and after the project by means of an interview. The physician attitudes assessed were in the subject areas of: (1) pharmacists and clinical pharmacy practice, (2) drug information and consultation service, (3) physician education, (4) drug utilization review, and (5) hospital rounds. Physicians were asked to describe their understanding of each subject, and their perception of the effect of the clinical pharmacist's activities on each subject area of their practice.

Table 1. *Physicians' Perceptions of the Effects of Clinical Pharmacy Services upon Their Practice as Elicited by the Questionnaire*

Service (number of respondents)*	Effect†		
	Beneficial	*Detrimental*	*None*
Giving drug information (24)	96	0	4
Being available for answering questions about drugs (24)	100	0	0
Providing drug information resources (24)	96	0	4
Conducting conferences (24)	96	0	4
Performing drug utilization review (24)	83	0	17
Making hospital rounds (19)	79	0	21
Counseling patients about drugs (16)	81	0	19
Monitoring drug blood levels (13)	54	0	46

Reprinted by permission from Love et al: J Fam Pract, 10(1):67, 1980.
* Number of physicians citing the service to be rendered to their practice.
† Measured as percentage of total number of respondents.

The physicians were asked to indicate whether the services of the clinical pharmacist were beneficial to, detrimental to, or had no effect upon their practice. Fifty-four percent or more of the physicians felt that the services that they perceived being rendered to their practice were beneficial (Table 1). No one perceived any service as being detrimental to his/her practice.

The interdisciplinary clinical training program described in this report was observed to have resulted in significant positive changes in the attitudes of the physicians about practicing with clinical pharmacists. Additionally, the pharmacist's perceptions of family physicians' training and practice were broadened. Mutual benefits resulted from this project of interdisciplinary family medicine education and similar models should be developed, documented, and reported in other family practice teaching programs.

Kantner TR, Vastyan EA: Coping with stress in family practice residency training. J Fam Pract 7(3):599–600, 1978

Training for a career in family medicine at a university teaching hospital offers residents some unique and rewarding educational opportunities. Such a program can also subject residents to certain stresses, one being a loss of identity with each other and with the family medicine department and faculty. Approximately three years ago at the Milton S. Hershey Medical Center of The Pennsylvania State University, an approach was developed to deal with this problem as well as to help residents cope with other stresses during their training, both of a personal and of a professional nature.

To deal with this problem of identity and also to provide mutual support for first year residents during this most stressful period of their training, a combined resident-faculty support group was created in July 1975. The specific objectives of the group were to: (1) foster a sense of *esprit-de-corps* among new residents, (2) provide opportunities for personal growth and development, and (3) provide opportunities to learn more about human interactions.

The group idea was introduced to residents during their orientation to the department the day before the start of their residency. Initially, all members of the group were expected to attend all meetings except for vacations, sickness, or emergency situations. Members wishing to leave the group were asked to share with the other participants their reasons for leaving. The groups were held for 1½ hours weekly, prior to the start of the residents' family medicine patient care time. The Chairman of the Department of Humanities at The Pennsylvania State University College of Medicine functioned as facilitator. Faculty and residents participated as equals with no attempt to structure the group "for the residents." A non-directive format was followed with initial sessions serving to introduce group members to each other. Subsequent sessions tended to focus on stresses experienced by residents on various specialty rotations, personal problems, interpersonal communication, and interpersonal interactions.

In addition to contributing to an increased sense of identity for residents in the program during their difficult first year of training, this program has helped residents and faculty develop better understanding of themselves as physicians and individuals. Group participation has enabled most persons to improve communication and interpersonal skills and to cope better with stresses of a professional and personal nature. The faculty and staff have found this process to be a most rewarding and worthwhile addition to the residency program.

Berg JK, Garrard J: The extent of psychosocial support of residents in family practice programs. J Fam Pract 11(6):915–920, 1980

There is increasing interest in addressing problems of residents and their families, as indicated by the existence of groups such as the Humanistic Medicine Task Force (American Medical Student Association) and the Committee on the Well-Being of Medical Students and House Officers (Stanford University School of Medicine). These groups advocate development of support systems for residents.

This paper has four purposes: (1) to document the availability of eleven kinds of psychosocial support in family medicine training programs, (2) to ascertain whether program characteristics (geographic region, type of program, size of residency) influence the availability of these kinds of support, (3) to explore the different patterns of support, and (4) to examine the range of variation in frequency of night call and length of vacation.

All approved family practice residency programs in the United States were surveyed to examine the frequency of eleven kinds of psychosocial support available to residents through their programs. A response rate of 96 percent was achieved ($N = 347$).

Family practice programs offer a considerable number of support elements to residents, with programs showing much homogeneity in the kinds of support offered. One program characteristic, size of program, does influence the kinds of support available, with small programs less likely than medium or large programs to offer the formal kinds of support examined in this study.

Of the eleven kinds of psychosocial support, three show statistically significant differences across type of program (see Table 1). Whereas both military (31 percent) and

Table 1. *Percentage, by Type of Program, of Residency Programs Providing Different Kinds of Psychosocial Support*

Kind of Psychosocial Support	Percent by Type of Program				
	Community Based (N = 49)	Univ.-Affil. Community Based (N = 173)	Univ.-Admin. Community Based (N = 52)	University Based (N = 57)	Military Program (N = 16)
Support groups	55	60	56	68	69
Family support groups	20	19	13	35	31
Part-time residencies	20	12	15	30	0
Professional counselors	88	82	79	88	81
Child care services	4	7	6	7	25
Formal gripe sessions	92	88	75	77	100
Seminars—medical issues	92	91	90	95	94
Seminars—personal and professional issues	74	69	67	77	94
Paid sick leave	92	89	90	93	94
Social activities	92	88	88	96	100
Financial advisors	47	51	48	46	25

Reprinted by permission from Berg, Garrard: J Fam Pract, 11(6):915, 1980.

university-based (35 percent) programs are more likely to offer family support groups than the other three types of programs (13 to 20 percent), it is university-based programs that lead in percentage of programs offering part-time residencies (30 percent) and military programs that lead in percentage of programs offering formal gripe sessions (100 percent).

Four patterns of support emerge from these data, each reflecting a specific orientation: (1) the psychological orientation, (2) the "bare bones" of support, (3) the support group orientation, and (4) the family orientation. In general, the kinds of support that address the residents' family needs are least likely to be available.

Wilson JL, Redman RW: Research policies and practices in family practice residencies. J Fam Pract 10(3):479–483, 1980

A questionnaire survey of all family practice residency programs in the United States was undertaken to gather information pertaining to the policies and practices of resident research projects. Questionnaires were returned by 281 program directors for a response rate of 80.7 percent.

The majority of the programs which responded require or encourage research by their residents. Cross-tabulations of the data relate several characteristics of residency programs to their positions on resident research. University based or affiliated/administered programs, programs with fewer residents and larger faculties, and programs in which the faculty are engaged in research tend to encourage or require research by residents although these findings are not consistent.

As displayed in Table 1, the majority of respondents (N = 181 or 64.4 percent) en-

Table 1. *Residency Program Position on Research as Component of Resident Education*

Position	Number	Percent
Not addressed—no plans to change	5	(1.8)
Not addressed at present—plan to consider in future	53	(18.9)
Resident research projects encouraged	181	(64.4)
Resident research projects required	42	(14.9)
Total	281	(100.0)

Reprinted by permission from Wilson, Redman: J Fam Pract, 10(3):479, 1980.

courage resident research projects; an additional 42 programs (14.9 percent) require a resident research project for completion of the residency requirements.

Residency programs that do not have a formal policy of encouraging or requiring resident research projects were requested to indicate the reasons for their position. The most frequently listed reasons were insufficient or inexperienced faculty or lack of adequate financial resources. Fifteen programs (25.8 percent) stated their residents were not interested in research; seven programs (12.0 percent) felt that research was not necessary in a residency program.

The relatively large number of programs (15 percent of the respondents) which require a resident research project was unexpected. This number, combined with the number of programs which encourage resident research, indicates that the emphasis in the literature on the importance of research experiences in family practice seems to have been absorbed by the majority of residencies. Many training programs appear to recognize the need for research and are responding to the challenge.

The creation of fellowship programs and other faculty development programs may alleviate the problem of lack of faculty experienced in research. Perhaps, also, this will furnish significant role models for residents and provide a further boost to research in family practice residency programs.

Geyman JP (Ed.): Profile of the residency trained family physician in the United States, 1970–1979. J Fam Pract 11(5):715–784, 1980

A full decade has passed since the formation of the American Board of Family Practice in 1969, which led to the development of formally structured three-year graduate training programs in this specialty. Over 5,000 family physicians have been graduated from U.S. practice residency programs, and it is now both possible and timely to assess the impact and products of these programs.

The overall goal of this monograph is to describe the practice patterns, perceptions, and geographic distribution of representative samples of residency trained family physicians in the United States. Four regional graduate follow-up studies are reported, representing different parts of the country and almost 600 graduates. Three of these studies involve well-established statewide networks of affiliated family practice residencies which agreed to collect similar and comparable information from their graduates. In addition, a separate but complimentary national study by the American Academy of Family Physicians is included which involves over 3,000 respondents.

Together these studies provide, for the first time, a profile of the residency trained family physician which has important implications for medical education and medical practice in this country. Among some of the highlights of these studies are the following:

1. The great majority of graduates (over 95 percent) are practicing as family physicians.
2. Single-specialty group and partnership practice attracts well over one half of graduates, with only about one fifth of graduates entering solo practice.
3. A broad spectrum of ambulatory and hospital practice is conducted by the graduates:
   —well over 90 percent of graduates hold hospital privileges in pediatrics, medicine, and family practice, including intensive care unit privileges in most instances
   —about two thirds of graduates nationally provide obstetric care, and over one third have some privileges for complicated obstetrics
   —almost two thirds of graduates serve as first assistants for major surgical procedures, while most include minor surgery in their practices
   —less than 4 percent of hospital privileges which have been requested have been denied in any category.
4. About three fifths of the graduates are involved in teaching, usually on a part-time basis.
5. The graduates of three statewide residency networks feel well prepared for practice as a result of their graduate training in the large majority of 60 content and process areas.
6. High levels of practice satisfaction are reflected by the responses of the graduates of these statewide networks.
7. Graduates are well represented in all sizes of communities, and gravitate to smaller and nonmetropolitan areas more than do other specialties.
8. Retention rates are consistently high in the states where graduates completed their residency training.

Concepts and Methods of Family Practice Research

COMMENTARY

MOST specialties in medicine have developed to encompass new areas of knowledge and/or technology, and have thereby begun with an active research base. Family practice arose on a different basis, in direct response to a broadly perceived lack of adequate primary care, and has therefore lacked an established research tradition.

As family practice has become established as a specialty with well-developed clinical and teaching programs, promising horizons for useful research have opened up which are now, for the first time, beginning to be addressed. Most research in the other clinical specialties has been carried out in secondary and tertiary care settings. Comparatively little work has been done in primary care settings to study the natural history of disease (especially common diseases), outcomes of care, effectiveness of screening and counseling, cost-benefit of medical interventions, and related areas. Careful research in these areas is obviously of great importance to the patient, to the whole of medicine, and to planning a more effective health care delivery system.

Two initial and fundamental tasks have been: (1) to conceptualize the major functional and content areas for needed research in family practice, and (2) to develop new research techniques de novo or adapt some existing research tools to the special needs of primary care settings. The papers and abstracts in this section address both of these issues, and represent substantial progress in both areas. Of particular interest is the diversity of research tools which are needed to study the process, content, and outcomes of patient care by family physicians in the community. Included in this section, for example, are papers which deal with the use of coding systems (adapted for ambulatory care problems), information management and data retrieval systems, models for collaborative research, specific outcome measures (e.g., morbidity and therapeutic index, health status index, impact-on-family scale), and other research techniques.

In spite of the differences which may exist from one country to another in patterns of family practice, there is much in common among family physicians around the world concerning the content, methods, and problems of family practice research. The directions and methods which emerge from the papers in this section are starting to form the necessary foundation for research in family practice, and are generally applicable beyond national boundaries.

Family Medicine as a Science*

Ian R. McWhinney

The remarkable progress made by academic family medicine in the past ten years has been made in spite of its limited scientific basis. As a body of knowledge, family medicine still has many of the marks of an immature discipline. Whether or not it grows to maturity in the next decade or two will depend very much on the wisdom with which we choose the direction of our research. It will be very important that we avoid the false trails which we could so easily take. Our research must be based on sound principles and a clear understanding of the nature of family medicine as a body of scientific knowledge.

In this paper I will suggest some guiding principles for the future development of family medicine research. I will begin by trying to answer some very basic questions which are important to my argument: what is a science? what is a technology? in what sense is clinical medicine a science and a branch of technology? I will then go on to develop the theme of family medicine as an immature discipline, using as my frame of reference the concept of mature and immature fields of science developed by Jerome Ravetz[1] in his book *Scientific Knowledge and Its Social Problems*. Finally, I will describe the course which I believe we should follow to bring our discipline to maturity.

It is important to emphasize that, in discussing the science of family medicine, we exclude a large and important part of our discipline. Family medicine is not only a science but an art. Although scientific research can make a contribution to the development of an art, knowledge of the art is not gained in this way. My purpose here, however, is to consider only those aspects

* Reprinted by permission from *The Journal of Family Practice,* 7(1):53–58, 1978.

of family medicine which come within the range of the scientific method.

What Is a Science?

One of the commonest fallacies about science—and one to which we have been prone in family medicine—is that by collecting information we are engaging in scientific research. It is true, of course, that the making of precise and reproducible observations on natural phenoma is an essential component of the scientific method. It is in its attitude to accurate observation —what Whitehead[2] called "brute fact"— that scientific thought differs from medieval thought. Medieval thinkers were intensely rational, but their arguments were based on *a priori* assumptions rather than the verified facts of experience. A devotion to facts, however, is not in itself sufficient to define the scientific method.

The other essential activity of science is the formulation of explanatory theories which can be tested against experience. It is theory which organizes and gives meaning to our data, helps us to formulate problems, and provides the basis for the interpretation of empirical findings. As a science matures, its body of factual information becomes embedded in an explanatory theory of increasing power and significance. "The factual burden of a science," wrote P.B. Medawar,[3] "varies inversely with its degree of maturity. As a science advances, particular facts are comprehended within, and therefore in a sense annihilated by, general statements of steadily increasing explanatory power and compass . . . In all sciences we are being progressively relieved of the burden of singular instances, the tyranny of the particular. We need no longer record the fall of every apple." Progress is made in science when a new and more powerful theory is born. The theory may be formulated to explain new facts, but not necessarily so. A new theory may be a new way of ordering facts which are already well known.

These two activities then—observation and theory building—are the essentials of the scientific method. They are also connected with each other in a way which is not always understood.

Although the scientist is devoted to "brute fact," the objects of science are not the raw data of our senses. One cannot observe without having some theory about the objects to be observed. The theory may not be an original one; it may not even be consciously held; it will nevertheless be a world view, derived from our culture and formal education, about how phenomena are to be classified and valued. "Observation is always selective," wrote Popper.[4] "It needs a chosen object, a defined task, an interest, a point of view, a problem. And its description presupposes a descriptive language, with property words: it presupposes similarity and classification, which in turn presupposes interests, points of view, and problems."

The objects of science, then, are intellectual constructs. In medicine, the "diseases" which we describe have no real existence: they are abstractions which we invent to bring order to a mass of data about illness. Abstraction is an essential part of the scientific method, but its danger is that we can so easily become the prisoners of our abstractions.

"The disadvantage of exclusive attention to a group of abstractions," wrote Whitehead,[2] "however well founded, is that, by the nature of the case, you have abstracted from the remainder of things. Insofar as the excluded things are important in your experience, your modes of thought are not fitted to deal with them. You cannot think without abstractions: accordingly, it is of the utmost importance to be vigilant in critically revising your modes of abstraction . . . A civilization which cannot burst

through its current abstractions is doomed to sterility after a very limited period of progress."

It is the "bursting through" of conventional abstractions to which Kuhn[5] ascribes the progress of science in his theory of paradigm change. Progress in science takes place, he argues, when an individual breaks out of the conventional abstractions and, as in a change of visual gestalt, sees the world in a different way. The fact that adherents of the conventional system of abstractions are often incapable of making this change of world view is the basis of many scientific controversies.

Before leaving the subject of the scientific method, one further point should be made about scientific theories. The sciences are not the only branches of knowledge that develop theories. In order to identify a scientific discipline, therefore, we need some criterion to discriminate between scientific and nonscientific theories. Popper has provided this in his criterion of demarcation.[4] A theory is scientific, says Popper, if it is capable of refutation. A theory can never be proved true, no matter how much supporting evidence is collected, for there will always exist the possibility of encountering falsifying evidence. To refute a hypothesis, however, we need only one falsifying instance.

As an example of a nonscientific theory Popper gives psychoanalysis, which, he maintains is impossible to refute because it is capable of explaining any observation, however conflicting. To say that a theory is not scientific, however, is not—or should not be—a pejorative statement. Theories often have great value in helping us to understand experience, even if they are not refutable. It is only that they should not be classified as scientific.

Medicine as a Science

Given this definition of science, can medicine be regarded as a scientific discipline in its own right? We have become accustomed in medicine to distinguishing between basic science and clinical medicine. These terms are not often defined but I often suspect that the term "basic" is used to imply that chemistry, physics, physiology, anatomy, and pharmacology are more scientific and fundamental than clinical medicine. This is really the opposite of the truth, for it would be impossible to apply advances in basic science without a body of scientific knowledge that is only obtainable from clinical observation. In the study of human illness, the ultimate test of any chemical or physical analysis must be: what are its implications for the survival and functioning of the whole organism? And this is a question which can only be answered by clinical observation. This is not only true of medicine, but of all studies of organisms and mechanisms. "Physics and chemistry can establish the conditions for their successful operation and account for possible failures," wrote Polanyi,[6] "but a complete specification of a machine in physico-chemical terms would dissolve altogether our knowledge of the machine . . . It is as meaningless to represent life in terms of physics and chemistry as it would be to interpret a grandfather clock or a Shakespeare sonnet in terms of physics and chemistry."

Clinical observation, then, is not only a scientific discipline, but is *the* science of medicine. It deals with precise, reproducible observations and it has its own body of theory. Our system for classifying illness is in itself a theoretical construct, and we also have theories of causation, decision making, and proof. Clinical medicine, like astronomy, ethology, anthropology, and a large part of biology, is an observational science. It is one of those sciences which, in Ryle's[7] words, tries to "establish the truth of things by observing and recording, by classification and analysis."

We must go on to acknowledge, however, that clinical observation has been a much neglected science in our own time. In his book, "Clinical Judgment," Feinstein[8] has commented: "Medical taxonomy has given him (the clinician) classifications for the host and for the disease, but not for the illness of the patient who is the diseased host. Lacking any formal means of classifying clinical observations, the clinician has no place to put the information when he communicates with himself or with his colleagues."

Medicine as Technology

Although medicine can be described as an observational science, most of medical knowledge would be more correctly classified as technological rather than scientific. As I hope to show later, the question is not entirely academic. It is true that science and technology have in modern times become so interwoven that it is difficult to tell them apart. It was not always so. Until the mid 19th century, science and technology pursued separate courses. Science was concerned with increasing our knowledge and understanding, largely for their own sakes. Technology progressed by the inventions of practical men, often based on craft skills of great antiquity. The analysis and specification of craft skills was, indeed, one of the chief ways in which technology developed. It is an indication of the gap which existed between science and technology that the industrial revolution was accomplished with hardly any help from science. "Except for the Morse telegraph," wrote Polanyi,[6] "the great London Exhibition of 1851 contained no important industrial devices or products based on the scientific progress of the previous fifty years."

Since that time, of course, science and technology have converged to such an extent that much of technology is now based on science, and technology contributes much new knowledge to science. One might be forgiven for thinking that there is no longer any useful distinction between them: scientists use tools, and scientific research itself is a technical and craft skill; technologists make precise observations and develop theories which can make an important contribution to our understanding. Moreover, the methods which technologists use for evaluating their tools are the same as those which scientists use for testing their hypotheses.

There are also, however, some important differences. Most of these need not concern us here but one, in particular, is important. A scientific discovery deepens our understanding of nature; a technological invention, in Polanyi's words, "establishes a new operational principle serving some acknowledged advantage." The test of a scientific discovery is the question, Is it true? The test of a technological invention is the question, Does it work? A scientific discovery can be superseded only by another discovery which brings us nearer to the truth. A technological invention can be superseded by another invention, or by a change in the way a process or its outcome are valued by society.

Where, then, does medicine stand? As I have already maintained, clinical medicine is an observational science, its subject matter being the phenomena of human illness. It is at the same time, however, a branch of technology devoted to the application of knowledge from many sources to the prevention, cure, and relief of illness. As in many modern technologies, progress takes place in different ways. Much technological innovation now comes directly from scientific discoveries, in medicine chiefly from those sciences which we have described as "basic." In medicine, however, as in other technologies, progress is still made by the specification and transmission of craft skills, and there exists, moreover, a significant residue of craft skill which has not been specified.

If we look at medical research in contrast with basic science research we find that much of it is indeed technological, that is, concerned with the development and testing of tools. I use the word "tools" here in its widest sense to include not only our material tools—instruments, drugs, etc—but also our intellectual and organizational tools: decision making processes,

psychotherapeutic methods, and systems of providing health care services.

Now let us turn to family medicine. Family medicine is, of course, one branch of clinical medicine. Like clinical medicine it has both scientific and technological components. Its scientific subject matter is the phenomena of illnesses as they present themselves to family physicians; its technological aspect is the development and evaluation of the conceptual, organizational, and material tools used by family physicians. The justification for its independent existence is that the tools are unique to the discipline, not derived from other branches of medicine, and that the phenomena can only be satisfactorily studied from within, rather than outside, the discipline. As an independent discipline, however, family medicine is of very recent origin, so we should not be surprised to find that it shows evidence of immaturity.

Family Medicine as an Immature Discipline

I have taken the idea of an immature field of inquiry from Ravetz,[1] who describes this as a field lacking in a body of stable factual knowledge. Students entering such a field, says Ravetz, "do not encounter a collection of standardized materials, presented in digestible form, and utterly reliable and incontrovertible in themselves." Instead, they are presented with "intuitive generalities dressed up as empirical laws, and insecure theoretical speculations masquerading as fundamental explanations." Can we say with honesty that this description does not apply to us? Perhaps we are not quite so bad as this. We may not pretend that our intuitive generalizations have the validity of empirical laws; our theory may be more securely based, our methods better tested. But do we have a body of factual knowledge about the phenomena encountered by family physicians? The answer to this must surely be no, unless it be second-hand knowledge which is entirely derived from other branches of medicine.

Workers in an immature field may respond either appropriately or inappropriately. The inappropriate response is to amass huge quantities of data, manipulate it with sophisticated statistical methods, and construct elaborate symbol systems which are then manipulated in formal arguments. These attempts usually fail because the results of research are vitiated by pitfalls which have not been identified in advance. In a mature field, these pitfalls are known and can be avoided. It is true, of course, that any innovative and growing discipline is bound to have signs of immaturity since, when new ground is explored, all the pitfalls cannot be known. A discipline which is soundly based, however, will be able to make forays into unexplored territory armed with well-matured criteria for the evaluation of results.

In exploring these new fields, however, family medicine has shown some signs of immaturity. We have done our share of accumulating masses of data with the idea that this is what science is all about. Although we have a distinguished tradition of clinical observation, much of our clinical research is based on records kept by untrained observers who were unaware that their records were going to be used for research. Mackenzie,[9] one of our most distinguished research workers, wrote: "One implement essential to the success of our enterprise is a trained observer. It is scarcely realized what a difference there is between a doctor who has systematically trained himself to observe and another who has perfunctorily examined his patients without attempting to improve his powers of observation." Nowadays we tend to assume that a training in research is a training in "methodology" rather than a training in observation.

In describing an appropriate response to immaturity, Ravetz has things to say which we would do well to ponder. First, we should not use physics as a model for what a scientific subject should be like. "It is not necessary," says Ravetz, "for a discipline to be fully "positive," in the sense of imitating physics, for it to make a contribution to the advancement of human knowledge." Technological subjects like medicine, agriculture, and engineering will inevitably—because of their subject matter—deal less with grand theories and abstract knowledge than with observation, classification, and description.

An immature discipline can make a useful contribution to knowledge if it concentrates on three things: technique, philosophy, and natural history.

Technique

A practical discipline can make much progress simply by describing, developing, and testing its tools. This is how much of modern technology developed from craft skills. The process is not as easy as it sounds, for many craft skills are extremely complex and defy specific description. Family medicine is no exception to this. General practitioners have developed diagnostic and therapeutic skills which we have only recently begun to recognize and describe. I think we have made as much progress in this aspect of our discipline as in any other. The way ahead can be seen quite clearly: we need to continue the process of describing and testing our techniques, both old and new: techniques of diagnosis, prevention, management, and organization.

In developing methods for the evaluation of our tools, we are fortunate in not having to start at the beginning. As a branch of medical science, we have in the discipline of epidemiology a well-developed method of evaluation. This is why, as Spitzer[10] has pointed out, epidemiology is an important basic subject for academic family medicine. Epidemiology provides a set of principles and methods: it is up to each discipline to apply these to its own problems, fully cognizant of the unique pitfalls which exist in every discipline. The research worker in family medicine, therefore, should be well versed both in the general principles of epidemiology, and in their application to his own discipline.

Philosophy

The purpose of philosophy in a scientific or technological discipline is to subject its basic assumptions to critical examination. It is surprising how often, in well-established disciplines, this process is neglected. I once asked a psychologist about his concept of mind. He had never given the matter a thought or been encouraged to do so in his training. We in medicine have no cause to feel smug, for we ourselves rarely examine some of our own basic assumptions. How many physicians have subjected to critical examination such everyday terms as health, disease, and illness?

A well-established discipline can often manage, at least for a time, without this critical examination of assumptions. A new and developing discipline must, if it is to survive, be based on a sound and well-constructed theory. If we are going to use terms like "continuity of care" and "the family as patient," we must say precisely what we mean by them and be aware of all their implications.

In the scientific aspects of family medicine the role of philosophy is to be, in Whitehead's[2] phrase, a "critic of abstractions." So far, family medicine seems to have accepted without question medicine's current system of abstractions, ie, its method of classifying diseases. We have done this even though it often fits poorly with the "brute facts" of general practice. We continue, for example, to perform morbidity surveys in which we accept without question concepts like "psychiatric illness." And we continue to find it very difficult to obtain results that are consistent from one physician to another.

I suggest that the next task for philosophy in family medicine is to re-examine our whole concept of illness and disease.

Perhaps we are on the brink of a change of paradigm in medicine. If we are, then I suggest that it is more likely to come from family medicine than any other field, because it is in family medicine that we see most clearly the incongruities of our current system of abstractions.

Natural History

It is in this field that our progress has been disappointing. The defects in our knowledge become apparent when we begin to teach. What can we teach our students? We can teach them our philosophy and we can describe some of our methods. But where is our body of knowledge about the phenomena of family medicine: the natural history of common complaints, the norms of individual behavior at all stages of life, the description and classification of families?

Of course, we are not alone. Modern medicine has neglected clinical research. It is particularly serious, however, that family medicine should do so, for there is no branch of medicine more suited to observational research. Family physicians see the whole range of diseases from the mildest to the most severe; they follow illness from its earliest symptoms to its latest stages; and they observe patients in their natural habitat—a habitat which they often share themselves. To indicate the rich harvest awaiting workers in this field I cannot do better than quote a passage from a recent article by Spitzer:[10] "The family physician has a distinctive perspective and the obligation to study intact human beings in free-living, non-institutionalized populations over long periods of time, observing transitions from health to disease and back to health, with a unique opportunity to observe, on a firsthand basis, many of the concurrent phenomena that affect health and disease, such as family, employment, housing, and exposure to risk factors.

"Some subject areas that deserve high

priority in family medicine research are calibrational studies focusing on clinical phenomena such as quantification of pain, quantification of the quality of survival, the development of explicit criteria for adequate clinical management of carefully defined conditions, demarcation of presenting complaints and their combinations as distinct from the demarcation of diagnoses, a taxonomy for behavior associated with disease or perceived disease, prognostic stratification of patients, and the calibration of the clinician himself as a reliable observer."

Anybody who peruses the family medicine literature will soon see that the task has hardly yet begun. Of all the papers published in *The Journal of Family Practice* since it started publication, how many are based on direct observation of clinical phenomena made by the authors themselves? We have studies based on the examination of records, we have review articles, we have papers on the description and evaluation of methods—all important and useful—but of research in the clinical science of family medicine, how little we have seen so far.

There is no doubt in my mind about the path to maturity: deep reflection on our modes of abstraction, continuing work on the development and evaluation of our tools, and the slow and steady accumulation of a body of data by meticulous clinical observation. Our immaturity is not a reason for despondency or shame; on the contrary it is a challenge which makes family medicine one of the most exciting of subjects. As Ravetz[1] concludes: "Immature fields with the hope of imminent maturation are, with all their attendant hazards, the place where the greatest challenge is to be found."

Acknowledgments

The quotation from WO Spitzer from The Intellectual Worthiness of Family Medicine, The Pharos of Alpha Omega Alpha, Vol 40:2, July 1977, is reprinted with the permission of the editor.

Quotations from JR Ravetz from Scientific Knowledge and Its Social Problems © Oxford University Press, 1971, are reprinted by permission of Oxford University Press.

REFERENCES

1. Ravetz JR: Scientific Knowledge and Its Social Problems. New York, Oxford University Press, 1971
2. Whitehead AN: Science and the Modern World. New York, Macmillan, 1925
3. Medawar PB: The Art of the Soluble. London, Methmen & Co Ltd, 1967
4. Popper KR: Conjectures and Refutations: The Growth of Scientific Knowledge. London, Routledge & Kegan Paul, 1963
5. Kuhn TS: The Structure of Scientific Revolutions, ed 2. Chicago, University of Chicago Press, 1970
6. Polanyi M: Personal Knowledge: Towards a Post-Critical Philosophy. London, Routledge & Kegan Paul, 1958
7. Ryle J: The Natural History of Disease, ed 2. London, Oxford University Press, 1948
8. Feinstein A: Clinical Judgment. Baltimore, Williams & Wilkins, 1967
9. Mackenzie J: Symptoms and Their Interpretation, ed 4. London, Shaw & Sons, 1920
10. Spitzer WO: The intellectual worthiness of family medicine. Pharos Alpha Omega Alpha 40:2, 1977

Research in the Family Practice Residency Program*

John P. Geyman

Research activity in family practice is becoming increasingly important as the specialty matures past its initial organizational and developmental phase. Family practice residency programs are directly involved in the definition and implementation of modern concepts in family medicine and frequently have available the necessary tools and resources for substantive research of various types. These programs therefore have both the opportunity and responsibility to become actively involved in research. Significant contributions have already been made in this area by faculty and residents in a number of family practice residency programs. This paper provides an overview of research areas in family practice, presents some examples of research to date, and suggests some practical approaches to facilitate further research efforts in family practice residency programs.

If one takes the Millis, Willard, and Folsom reports (1966) as the onset of active development of family practice as a specialty, the first decade—which, in many respects can be considered Phase One of the specialty's development—has now passed. The pressing tasks during this first stage have necessarily revolved around the organizational and logistic aspects of program development, and these have been well done. We are now entering Phase Two, and research in the discipline must become a vigorous element in this stage.[1] Since family practice residency programs are training family physicians for the future, they are inevitably involved in the definition and implementation of modern concepts in family medicine on the "cutting edge" of the developing academic discipline.

The word "research" has frequently had a "turn-off" effect on many who have been involved with family practice in the past. Many of us have seen research in other disciplines as overly focused on "esoteric" conditions and complex pathophysiologic mechanisms not directly applicable to the work of the family doctor. We have not yet developed and made visible valued and respected models of research and researchers in the settings of family practice teaching programs. This is quite natural since family practice as a specialty and family medicine as a developing, teachable academic discipline are relative newcomers in formal medical education.

Today's circumstances in family practice are quite different from those in the past, and a wide horizon for needed and important research in family medicine is now opening up at a time when the necessary tools and resources for research are becoming available. It is now not only possible, but *expected,* that the family practice residency program will use the problem-oriented medical record, maintain an active audit program, and utilize data retrieval methods involving accepted coding systems for ambulatory as well as hospital problems. Library search services are now available to most programs, thereby facilitating literature review. We are attracting young physicians of high caliber into family practice residencies, and the potential for original work in the field is great.

The purpose of this paper is to present an overview of research areas in family practice, give some illustrative examples of research to date, and suggest some practical approaches to encouraging research in a family practice residency program.

* Reprinted by permission from *The Journal of Family Practice,* 5(2):245–248, 1977.

320

Content Areas for Research in Family Practice

Webster defines "research" as the "diligent and systematic inquiry or investigation into a subject in order to discover or revise facts, theories, and applications," while Eimerl describes it as "organized curiosity."[2] Whatever definition for the word one accepts, it is clear that research in family medicine must be defined broadly, and that the patterns of traditional biomedical research are not directly applicable to the uncharted arena of the family practice approach to primary care.

Because they deal with the everyday problems of patients and families, family physicians have a number of inherent advantages related to research on a patient-care level. Some of these can be listed as follows:

1. The family physician sees all members of the family, of all ages and both sexes.
2. He/she has direct experience with primary or first contact care of unselected patients.
3. He/she has the opportunity to follow all of his/her patients.
4. He/she brings a multidisciplinary approach to health care.
5. He/she sees patients in any or all of the James Stages:
   Stage I. Foundations of disease.
   Stage II. Preclinical disease.
   Stage III. Treatment of symptomatic disease.
   Stage IV. Rehabilitation and management of medical conditions for which biologic cure is not possible.

Family physicians thus have a wider perspective of health and disease on the community level than anyone else in medicine.

The spectrum of avenues of needed research in family practice is wide. Although incomplete, Table 1 presents a simple taxonomy with four major categories of research in family practice, together with sample subject areas in each category.

By way of example, the following list reflects the diversity of important original work which has already been completed and published during the past several years in this country by faculty and residents in family practice residency programs:

"A Data Bank for Patient Care, Curriculum and Research in Family Practice"[3]
"A Critical Review of Periodic Health Screening Criteria"[4]
"A Study of Thyroid Disease in Family Practice"[5]
"Low Back Pain in the Primary Care Setting"[6]
"Six Years' Experience with Pelvic Inflammatory Disease"[7]
"Behavioral Perspectives in Coronary Care"[8]
"An Audit of Obstetric Care in a University Family Medicine Department and an Obstetrics-Gynecology Department"[9]
"Classification and Coding of Psychosocial Problems in Family Medicine"[10]
"Why Home Visits? 'Analysis of 142 Planned Home Visits"[11]
"The Consultation Process and Its Effects on Therapeutic Outcome"[12]
"Primary Care Research in a Model Family Practice Unit"[13]
"Comparative Profiles of Residency Training and Family Practice"[14]
"Types of Family Practice Teachers and Residents: A Comparative Study"[15]
"Practice Objectives and Goals: A Survey of Family Practice Residents"[16]
"The Impact on Patient Satisfaction of the Introduction of Family Medicine Residents"[17]

Some Practical Approaches to Facilitating Research

For a program director to be persuaded of the importance of research, and then simply to establish a research rotation for residents is not only insufficient but headed for failure. The planning, design, conduct,

Table 1. *A Taxonomy for Research Areas in Family Practice*

Epidemiological and Clinical Research	Health Services Research	Behavioral Research	Educational Research
Single illness studies Morbidity Natural history Prevention Early diagnosis Management Case reports	Consumers Health and illness behavior Needs and demands Consumer participation Patient compliance Effects of health education	Doctor-patient relationships Health team and changing roles Impact of societal changes on primary care	Medical student interest in family practice Teaching aids for family practice Family practice residency programs Educational objectives Role of problem-oriented record and medical audit Program costs Model family practice clinic costs and revenue
Practice studies Content Common diseases Common problems Variation with geographic setting Consultation rates Changing patterns	Providers Numbers and distribution Efficiency (utilization) Physician performance Referral patterns Costs of primary care Solo practice Family practice group Multi-specialty group Allied health manpower studies	Family dynamics Normal Abnormal Changing patterns Developmental aspects of family life cycles	Self-assessment methods Family practice residents Practicing family physicians
Family studies Morbidity Prevention Role of genetic counseling Crisis intervention	Task definition Health team studies Cost and efficiency studies Drug and laboratory procedure studies Experimental models for delivery of primary care (including comparison of family practice and multi-specialty approaches)	Counseling Methods Results	Continuing medical education Needs of family physicians Physician performance
	Interface Patient outcome studies Costs and incentives Cost-benefit ratios Facilities and utilization Role of health hazard appraisal		

analysis, and publication of a research project is often based on the curiosity and personal interest of one individual or a small group of individuals. Research is therefore a delicate, creative process, which can be facilitated by building a supportive environment but cannot be legislated by fiat.

In view of these considerations, however, a number of positive steps can be taken to promote creative efforts and original work by residents in family practice, the future leaders of the specialty. The following principles are suggested as practical ways to facilitate research in family practice residency programs:

1. *An attitude of critical inquiry must be developed and maintained among all residents and faculty in the program.*[18] The origin of any research project is the asking of a question. We should encourage residents to raise questions about the effectiveness of diagnostic and therapeutic approaches in patient care as well as any related aspects of health care in family medicine.

2. *The residency program should implement and make available for everyday use the basic tools for research in the family practice setting.* These include the problem-oriented medical record, active audit programs, a coding system, data retrieval methods, and library search resources. A number of helpful papers have already been published on various research methods in family medicine.[19-35] The program can easily subscribe to *Abridged Index Medicus* for its library, and the nearest medical library is usually prepared to conduct MEDLINE searches on request.

3. *The faculty should demonstrate interest in research as a valued and necessary element in the program.* The real priorities in a program are often unwritten and implicit in the environment. Research cannot be effectively encouraged in a family practice residency unless faculty members take a special interest in new ideas, en-

courage critical thinking, and reinforce each resident's efforts in pursuing studies of particular interest. Even more effective than these approaches is the active involvement of faculty members in some area of original work, for it is in this kind of role modeling that the residents will perceive genuine commitment to research activity.

4. *A research project, not a rotation, should be strongly encouraged for all residents.* If a program is to establish a meaningful emphasis on original work and creative activity, it is reasonable to expect that each resident, by the completion of his/her residency training, will have completed a research project in an area of special interest. Quite beyond the individual gains in learning derived by the resident in pursuing a selected subject in some depth, each resident will necessarily add to his/her ability to obtain and organize new information and to think critically. This experience will add to the future family physician's interest in his or her practice and will increase the capacity to pursue significant continuing medical education. A research project invariably requires time for germination of ideas, development of a plan of study, conduct of the study, analysis, and presentation of results. This process is not readily adaptable to a block rotation, but is best carried out over a period of one or two years.

5. *Back-up resources in research methods should be identified and made available to residents.* Just as the program director identifies resources and arranges for teaching in the various clinical curricular areas, similar efforts should be taken to identify individuals in the community and/or in affiliated institutions with expertise in such areas as research design, statistical analysis, and other related aspects involved in the conduct of a research project. Residents should have help available in the planning, conduct, and analysis of their research projects. Most communities with suffi-

cient clinical teaching resources to maintain a family practice residency program also have these kinds of resources available. Programs which are affiliated with medical schools can frequently obtain help from visiting faculty in these areas, and in some instances collaborative studies may be carried out with the medical school itself.

6. *Residents should be provided with an opportunity to present and share the results of their research studies.* An essential part of the program's activities in research is a periodic conference involving all of the residents and faculty for the reporting of research studies. Some programs are finding that an annual two-day conference provides an effective opportunity for the sharing of original work, serves as a stimulus for residents to finish their projects, and provides them with the additional learning experience of presenting their work to their colleagues. An atmosphere should be sought which permits dialogue and critique of the research methods and of the validity and implications of results. Active resident involvement should be encouraged in the planning and conduct of these conferences.

7. *The range of research and original work must be defined broadly.* There is a potential hazard in taking too circumscribed an approach to research in this specialty, for family medicine is an integrated and functional clinical discipline. We need clinical and epidemiological research just as much as behavioral research, and health services research just as much as educational research. Priorities for kinds of research should be based on local and individual interests and capabilities. Research projects by residents may involve case reports, audits of care, prospective or retrospective studies of clinical problems, or may address a wide variety of practical problems arising from an inquiry of personal interest to the resident. Whatever

the project, each resident should be expected to conduct an appropriate literature review as part of the completed study.

Discussion

In 1966 McWhinney noted the absolute importance for the survival of any specialty of the development of the academic discipline and of an active area of research.[36] This must become a central task of Phase Two in family practice development, now that the initial organizational and logistic efforts of Phase One are largely completed. It is, therefore, not just a desirable option, but *essential*, that graduate students in family medicine (ie. family practice residents) be involved in this process. They have much to contribute and much to gain.

As "model" practices with both the opportunity and responsibility to develop, test, and implement improved approaches to health care of families, family practice residency programs are ideal settings for research in family medicine. If the teaching practices and Family Practice Centers in these programs are considered "laboratories," and if the basic research tools which have been described earlier are implemented in each program, then family practice residencies can contribute immeasurably to research in family medicine.

Research in family practice is at an embryonic but promising stage. The horizons for useful research are wide and basic research tools are now available. The quality and energy of our research efforts are vital to the more precise definition of family medicine as an academic discipline and to the continued development of the specialty of family practice. We must now raise the priority for research and integrate active research efforts into our teaching and patient care programs throughout the country. The payoffs of this direction are considerable—increased quality of teaching programs, expansion of the body of knowledge which family physicians will teach, an ongoing stimulus for continuing medical education, increased practice satisfaction, and, most importantly, better health care for our patients and their families.

REFERENCES

1. Geyman JP: On entry into phase two in family practice development. J Fam Pract 4:15, 1977
2. Eimerl TS, Laidlaw AJ: A Handbook for Research in General Practice. Edinburgh, E & S Livingstone Ltd, 1969
3. Marsland DW, Wood M, Mayo F: A data bank for patient care, curriculum, and research in family practice: 526, 196 patient problems. J Fam Pract 3:25, 38, 1976
4. Frame PS, Carlson SJ: A critical review of periodic health screening using specific screening criteria. (a four-part series) J Fam Pract 2:29, 123, 189, 283, 1975
5. Shank JC: A study of thyroid disease in family practice. J Fam Pract 3:247, 1976
6. Haight RO, Marsland DW, Temple TE: Low back pain in the primary care setting. J Fam Pract 3:363, 1976
7. Hess GS, Burr BD, Lawrence R, et al: Six years' experience with pelvic inflammatory disease. J Fam Pract 1(2):13, 1974
8. Geiger WJ: Behavioral perspectives in coronary care. J Fam Pract 2:245, 1975
9. Ely JW, Ueland K, Gordon MJ: An audit of obstetric care in a university family medicine department and an obstetrics-gynecology department. J Fam Pract 3:397, 1976
10. Cole WM, Baker RM, Twersky RK: Classification and coding of psychosocial problems in family medicine. J Fam Pract 4:85, 1977
11. Guy LJ, Haskell EG, Hutson AC, et al: Why home visits? Analysis of 142 planned home visits. J Fam Pract 4:337, 1977
12. Rudy DR, Williams T: The consultation process and its effects on therapeutic outcome. J Fam Pract 4:361, 1977
13. Wentz HS, Tindall HT, Zervanos NJ: Primary care research in a model family practice unit. J Fam Pract 1(1):52, 1974
14. Johnson AH, Wimberly CW: Comparative profiles of residency training and family practice. J Fam Pract 1(3):28, 1974
15. Onenk N, Heffron WA: Types of family practice teachers and residents: A comparative study. J Fam Pract 2:195, 1975
16. Longenecker DP: Practice objectives and goals: A survey of family practice residents. J Fam Pract 2:347, 1975
17. Blanchard CG, Treadwell TW, Blanchard EB: The impact on patient satisfaction of the introduction of family medicine residents into a model practice facility. J Fam Pract 4:133, 1977
18. Geyman JP: On the need for critical inquiry in family medicine. J Fam Pract 4:195, 1977
19. Farley ES, Froom J: The age-sex register. J Fam Pract 1(1):44, 1974
20. Froom J: The diagnostic index E-book. J Fam Pract 1(2):45, 1974
21. Froom J: Family folders. J Fam Pract 1(2):49, 1974
22. Smith SR: Application of the tracer technique in studying quality of care. J Fam Pract 1(3):38, 1974
23. Farley ES: Implications of filing charts by area of residence. J Fam Pract 1(3):43, 1974
24. Froom J: The problem-oriented medical record. J Fam Pract 1(3):48, 1974
25. Kane RL, Leigh EH, Feigal DW, et al: A method for evaluating patient care and auditing skills of family practice residents. J Fam Pract 2:205, 1975
26. Keller K, Podell RN: The survey in family practice research. J Fam Pract 2:449, 1975
27. Baker C, Schilder M: The "E-box": An inexpensive modification of diagnostic indexing. J Fam Pract 3:189, 1976
28. Bass M: Approaches to the denominator problem in primary care research. J Fam Pract 3:193, 1976
29. Froom J: Assessment of quality of care by profiles of physicians' morbidity data. J Fam Pract 3:301, 1976
30. Newell JP, Bass MJ, Dickie GL: Defining the practice population. J Fam Pract 3:517, 1976
31. Bass MJ, Newell JP, Dickie GL: The value of defining a practice population. J Fam Pract 3:525, 1976
32. Newell JP, Dickie GL, Bass MJ: Gathering encounter data. J Fam Pract 3:633, 1976
33. Dickie GL, Newell JP, Bass MJ: Encounter data and their uses. J Fam Pract 3:639, 1976
34. Westbury RC: The analysis of family practice workloads by seriousness. J Fam Pract 4:125, 1977
35. Given CW, Simoni L, Gallen R: The design and use of a health status index for family physicians. J Fam Pract 4:287, 1977
36. McWhinney IR: General practice as an academic discipline. Lancet 1:419, 1966

The Use of Epidemiologic Methods in Family Practice*

Joseph E. Scherger

Epidemiologic methods of research can be readily used in family practice. Since the 19th century, family physicians have used epidemiologic methods in making important contributions to the understanding of disease. Using these methods requires an organized practice including patient registers, encounter data, and detailed records. Descriptive studies can define certain characteristics that are related to disease. Case-control and cohort studies can provide evidence for the association of risk factors and disease. A stepwise outline for carrying out a study is presented.

Epidemiology is the study of disease in groups of people. It is a discipline of methods rather than a body of knowledge. The family physician, being the first contact for medical care in the general population, is in an ideal position to use the methods of epidemiology in the study of disease.

This paper is focused toward how the practicing family physician might use epidemiologic methods. Basic methods are described for studying disease in population groups applicable to family practice and references are provided for more detailed descriptions of research design. Emphasis is placed on studies that can be performed by family physicians themselves or with a little help, not on more sophisticated studies that an epidemiologist might do on family practice populations.

Some epidemiologists make a distinction between epidemiologic research and clinical research.[1] The distinction is that epidemiologists study populations for the development of disease, while clinical researchers study patients with diseases for their progress and outcome. With respect to the family physician who relates to the general population both before and after the development of recognized diseases, this distinction is blurred. Many epidemiologists are crossing over and becoming involved with clinical research. The methods are the same provided that groups of people are studied. This paper describes basic epidemiologic methods for studies by family physicians on groups of people. The term "disease" is used in its broadest definition, ie, a state of "dis-ease," or any definable problem that a patient brings to a physician.

Historical Precedents

Since prior to specialization virtually all physicians were generalists, much of the early descriptions of disease came from general practitioners. Because methods for studying diseases in population groups were not known, these early descriptions came from anecdotal experiences with individuals or small groups of patients.

Epidemiologic concepts and methods were developed during the late 18th and early 19th centuries. Epidemiologic methods were popularized by John Snow in 1854 in his study of cholera in London.[2] Since then there has been a string of general practitioners/family physicians in England who have made major contributions to the knowledge of disease using epidemiologic methods. William Budd (1811–1880), a rural general practitioner, kept careful notes and first described the mode of spread of typhoid fever.[3,4] James Mackenzie (1853–1925) made observations on

* Reprinted by permission from *The Journal of Family Practice*, 6(4):849–854, 1978.

the irregularities of the pulse and greatly improved the accuracy of diagnosis and prognosis in heart disease.[4,5] Mackenzie wrote in 1916 what is true today:[5]

> The life of a general practitioner is not considered one that can help much in the advance of medicine; . . . You know well that if a man aspires to research work it is to the laboratories or to the hospital wards he is sent. As a result of my experience, I take a very different view, and assert with confidence that medicine will make but halting progress, while whole fields essential to the progress of medicine will remain unexplored, until the general practitioner takes his place as an investigator. The reason for this is that he has opportunities which no other worker possesses—opportunities which are necessary to the solution of problems essential to the advance of medicine. . . .

Will Pickles (1885–1969), a general practitioner in rural England, began at the age of 40 to carefully record data on the infectious diseases in his practice.[4,5] From his observations he was one of the first to describe Bornholm disease (epidemic pleurodynia); he contributed to the understanding of the incubation period of infectious hepatitis (catarrhal jaundice); and he was the first to describe "farmer's lung." Pickles became the first president of the Royal College of General Practitioners and delivered the Cutter lecture at the Harvard School of Public Health in 1948 on epidemiology in country practice.[6]

More contemporary work has been done by John Fry in England on the epidemiology of common diseases seen by the family physician.[7] His recent text provides descriptions of common illnesses based on carefully collected data from his practice along with recommendations for management. His descriptions vary significantly from standard textbooks in which the observations were made largely on hospitalized patients.

With the development of the discipline of family practice in Canada and the United States, epidemiologic studies are beginning to be done by North American family physicians. Some of these will be cited in the discussion of methods.

Practice Prerequisites

Family physicians have unique opportunities for making observations on disease, but must have their practices organized to collect information. The methods of data collection must be simple and inexpensive to be practical for the practicing physician.

Most of the historical studies cited above were the result of the physician carrying a notebook to record observations. This simplest method has some merit but many limitations. The information will be limited to what the physician decides beforehand to record and will probably change over time.

Other methods of organizing patient information which can be used for epidemiologic study are becoming widely used in family practice. A uniform registration of all patients in a practice will provide a denominator (population at risk) to which a group of patients can be related. This registration form must contain at a minimum the age, sex, race, and date of entry of each patient. Other useful information would be marital status, education, and socioeconomic level.

The use of an encounter form for each patient visit is a very valuable source of information. It should contain at a minimum the date of visit, identification of patient and provider, and a listing of the problems dealt with during the encounter. This information can be manually collected or filed in a computer. From such encounter data, a physician can index or profile the diseases seen in practice and select certain diseases for audit or study. The most common problem with interpreting encounter data and comparing it with other practices is the variation in number of return visits a patient may make for the same problem.

The patient register or the encounter data will provide access to another valuable source of information, the patient record. The use of problem-oriented records allows for an organized source of information that is necessary for studies. A more detailed description of the need for and use of patient registers, encounter data, and patient records is provided by Newell[8] and Eimerl.[9]

The use of the patient register as the denominator or population at risk can be criticized as not being reflective of the general population, or the true population at risk. Also, encounter data from one practice can be criticized as not being a representative group of all persons with a disease. These limitations must be considered for each practice when reporting observations. A discussion of the problem of appropriate denominators in family practice research is provided by Bass[10] and White.[11]

With these prerequisities, various epidemiologic methods of study can be performed by family physicians. A more detailed description of the methods described below can be found in epidemiologic texts such as Freidman[1] (highly readable and simplified), and MacMahon[12] (more detailed standard text).

Descriptive Studies

Studies which describe the nature of disease in groups of people have been the most commonly used epidemiologic method in family practice. Descriptive studies are concerned with describing relationships between a disease and certain characteristics of a population. These characteristics should be divided into the categories of: *Person* (To whom does a disease occur?), *Place* (Where does it occur?), and *Time* (When does it occur?). Personal characteristics are usually the most detailed and should include age, sex, race, and others, such as marital status, education, and socioeconomic level where appropriate.

Because family physicians have the opportunity to observe disease at its earliest stages, they may contribute greatly to the understanding of the natural history of disease. Family physicians often comment that many diseases, for example rheumatoid arthritis, look different in their offices than as described in textbooks of medicine. Reference was made previously to the work of John Fry in describing the natural history of common diseases.[7] Other similar work by family physicians is that of Hodgkin[13] and McWhinney.[14] These are sparse examples of the vast amount of knowledge that could be obtained about the early nature of disease.

The simplest method of descriptive epidemiology is that of collecting a series of cases of a certain disease in practice and describing them as a group in relation to the characteristics mentioned above. This series should be representative of all the cases of this disease in the practice, or all the cases over a period of time, to avoid describing a biased group. These cases can be obtained through encounter data, and their description will depend on appropriately detailed patient registers and records. Recent studies of this type in family practice have been done on patients with asthma[15] and low back pain.[16] Both of these studies reveal disease characteristics which are different from those usually described for specialty clinic populations.

These studies are limited, however, in not describing the frequency or *rate* of the disease in the population studied. Calculating a rate requires knowledge of the population from which the patients were taken (denominator group). The rates most commonly used in descriptive epidemiology are *prevalence* and *incidence*. The prevalence of a disease is the number of cases in the defined population at a certain point in time:

$$\text{Prevalence} = \frac{\text{Number of Cases}}{\text{Study Population}} \text{ (usually per 1,000)}$$

The incidence of a disease is the number of new cases that occur in a defined population over a period of time:

$$\text{Incidence} = \frac{\text{No. of New Cases}}{\text{Study Population}} \text{ (usually per 1,000/yr)}$$

Recent descriptive studies in family practice have been done on chest pain[17] and thyroid disease[18] containing information on prevalence or incidence. These studies have also shown striking differences from the usual emphasis of subspecialists and have implications for the education of family physicians. They also provide a better understanding of the symptom or disease in the general population.

If a family physician fulfills the practice prerequisites, he/she could use descriptive epidemiology to look at his/her entire practice. One study described for a single family physician: the most frequent reasons for visits, the incidence of illness in major categories for different age groups, the types of illness under a category such as infectious disease, the distribution of patients by age, number of illnesses and visits, and the distribution of referrals.[19]

In a major study which helped define the content of family practice, encounter data from 118 family physicians in Virginia with 88,000 patients were tabulated to describe the rank order of diagnoses by frequency, disease category, and age/sex distribution in family practice.[20–22]

Though descriptive studies can provide very important information, they fail to provide the excitement of analyzing the causation of disease or the efficacy of treatment. Two methods of analytic epidemiology readily applicable to family practice are case-control studies and cohort studies.

Case-Control Studies

When a family physician observes an apparent association between an exposure and the development of a problem, he will generate an hypothesis regarding this association. Unfortunately, he may make clinical decisions on the basis of this hypothesis without confirming it in the literature or testing it. If he does check the literature and is unable to find a satisfactory description of this association, it behooves him to test his hypothesis before making clinical decisions on it. This test may provide the first medical evidence for this association. Usually the simplest and cheapest way to test for a hypothesized association in clinical practice is with a case-control study.

In a case-control study, a representative group of patients with the problem under study is compared to a control group without the problem for differences in the frequency or rate of the hypothesized exposure. The most important part of a case-control study is the careful selection of cases and controls. This is done through the use of encounter data for the cases and the patient register for the controls. The cases should be representative of the population of patients with the problem. The number of cases selected should be great enough to be likely to provide significant differences in the data. The size that is necessary depends on the strength of the association, and usually the minimum size group is 25. This may require a collaborative effort using the practices of more than one physician.

The control group should be as much like the group of cases as possible with respect to the characteristics of person, place, and time, differing most significantly in an absence of the problem under study. For example the controls should have the same distribution of age, sex, and race as the cases. This will avoid having confounding factors affect the results of the study, ie, factors other than the hypothesized exposure which are related to the disease and differ in the two groups. If feasible, each member of the control group can be matched to a member of the cases, giving a paired arrangement.

The results of a case-control study, if they confirm the hypothesis, are usually described as a ratio or *relative risk:*

$$\text{Relative Risk} = \frac{\text{Rate of the exposure in cases}}{\text{Rate of the exposure in controls}}$$

Though case-control studies may appear rigid and difficult, they can be done readily in family practice. The family physician performs a crude case-control study when he observes that ten patients come into his office in one day with diarrhea and a history of being at a community picnic the night before. The association is confirmed upon observing that a few or none of his patients with other problems were at the picnic. A more sophisticated example might follow an observation that many young women with elevated blood pressures are taking oral contraceptives. To test this association, now well known in the literature,[23,24] a family physician might use encounter data to select cases of women in a certain age group with elevated blood pressure and use the patient register and patient records to select a control group with normal blood pressures. He would then compare the two groups for the rate of taking oral contraceptives.

There are numerous possibilities of case-control studies that could be done by family physicians. Many factors that are related to the development of disease are unknown, yet exist closest to the physician who sees the earliest manifestation of disease. The psychosocial factors related to disease development are largely untested.

Though the more definitive case-control studies are performed through university centers using large groups, smaller studies, which are usually imperfect, done by single or small groups of physicians, often give the first clues of an association. Family physicians can join with local university centers and participate in collaborative studies, a model for this having been described by Hesbacher et al.[25]

Cohort Studies

Cohort studies are generally the most valuable method in epidemiology when they can be applied. They provide the most direct measurement of the risk of disease development. A cohort is a group of people with a common characteristic, usually an exposure, that is followed over a period of time for the development of disease. The method is simply observing for certain events in the cohort chosen for study.

Because family physicians by nature follow their patients over long periods of time, cohort studies can be performed readily in family practice. These studies are usually done prospectively, and their main disadvantage is that they require waiting a period of time for results. A cohort study can be done retrospectively by selecting a study population in the past and then observing what happened over a period of time, but often the records lack the necessary consistent information.

As with a case-control study, the decision to do a cohort study is made after generating an hypothesis about an association or course of events. The decision regarding which method to use depends upon the nature of the problem and how quickly the physician wants to have results. If both are feasible, the cohort study is usually preferred since it allows a direct observation of the hypothesized association under a study protocol. In the example of the association between oral contraceptives and elevated blood pressure, a cohort study would be the selection of a group starting on oral contraceptives and following them over a period of time for the development of elevated blood pressures.[23] Epidemiologic methods are complimentary and cohort studies are often done after descriptive or case-control studies.

Several cohort studies could be done at the same time by one or a group of family physicians, providing an "organized curiosity" to the practice. Some examples of cohorts for study are: diabetic or hypertensive patients for the development of complications, a group with an industrial exposure for the development of lung disease, separated couples for changes in sickness behavior, all patients over 70 years for certain problems, breast-fed and bottle-fed infants for early infection, postmyocardial infarction patients for future employment in a community. The list is endless. It is important in beginning a study to have a protocol for what patients will enter the study, what is to be observed, and how the observation is to be done. In most instances, the protocol will not be different from good medical practice and will not be an added expense.

A specialized type of cohort study is the experimental trial. Here a certain intervention, such as a drug or other treatment, is given to the cohort group and results are observed. Experience has shown that in order for the results of an experimental trial to be meaningful, a carefully selected control group should also be observed. The control group is usually given a placebo intervention. If possible, both the patients and the investigators should be blinded (unaware) as to the treatment or control groups during the intervention and observation, hence the term double-blind, controlled clinical trial. A family physician can perform small-scale experimental studies, for example, studying the efficacy of a patient education technique or a new treatment modality such as diathermy. Usually experimental studies require elaborate protocols to prevent bias and are expensive, requiring a collaborative effort with a university center. In all experimental studies, the ethical considerations and informed consent must be addressed.

Carrying Out a Study

If a family physician decides to use one of these epidemiologic methods to study a problem, he must be organized to be suc-

cessful. The following steps for carrying out a study have been synthesized from Friedman,[1] Newell,[8] and Eimerl:[9]

1. Define the problem and the question(s) to be answered in the study. Write them down. Generate a hypothesis if appropriate.
2. Look at what is known about the problem. The regional university library or local medical society may have an information service which can be very helpful in searching the literature.
3. Write out a rough draft of a protocol or study plan. This will be modified after steps 4 and 5.
4. Obtain advice regarding the study plan. Local physicians who have done similar research can be helpful. Someone knowledgeable in epidemiology and/or biostatistics should review the study plan with respect to the necessary group sizes and data analysis.
5. Present the plan to important local persons that should know about the study, for example, hospital administrators, local health officers, and the medical society.
6. Collect the data. Be sure to have standardized forms that are used for every case. It is often helpful to pretest these forms on a few cases for unanticipated problems.
7. Analyze the data. Look at examples of similar studies for the use of tables and diagrams. Samples from this paper are: descriptive,[1,7,11,15–22] case-control,[1,11] and cohort.[1,11,24] Perform or have performed for you the appropriate statistical tests.[26,27]
8. Report the data. This is usually separated into an introduction, a statement of the methods, the results, and a discussion. Again, a look at examples of similar studies is helpful.

If the hypothesis is confirmed by the study, it should be critically evaluated. What other factors might explain the observed difference or association? Could the results be due to some bias in the sampling? Virtually every study, no matter how conclusive, needs to be repeated using the same or different epidemiologic methods.

Conclusions

Most family physicians have an awareness that the body of medical knowledge in standard texts does not quite fit what they observe in practice. An understanding of basic epidemiologic methods of research that can be readily applied to family practice can make one eager to investigate this hiatus. The possibilities are vast. Applying research to patient care in order to better understand patient problems should lead to increased physician satisfaction and improved patient care.

Acknowledgment

The author wishes to thank James L. Gale, MD, of the Department of Epidemiology for reviewing the manuscript and providing helpful suggestions.

REFERENCES

1. Friedman GD: Primer of Epidemiology. New York, McGraw-Hill, 1974
2. Snow J: Snow on Cholera. New York, Commonwealth Fund, 1936
3. Pickles WN: Epidemiology in Country Practice. Bristol, John Wright, 1939, reissued, 1949
4. Pemberton J: Will Pickles of Wensleydale. London, Geoffrey Bles, 1970
5. Mackenzie J: The Principles of Diagnosis and Treatment in Heart Affections. London, H Frowde, 1916
6. Pickles WN: Epidemiology in country practice. N Engl J Med 239:419, 1948
7. Fry J: Common Diseases: Their Nature, Incidence, and Care. Philadelphia, JB Lippincott, 1974
8. Newell JP: Information from family practice: Why and how? Can Fam Physician 21(4):47, 1975
9. Eimerl TS, Laidlaw AJ: A Handbook for Research in General Practice. Edinburgh, E & S Livingstone, 1969
10. Bass M: Approaches to the denominator problem in primary care research. J Fam Pract 3:193, 1976
11. White KL: Primary care research and the new epidemiology. J Fam Pract 3:579, 1976
12. MacMahon B, Pugh TF: Epidemiology: Principles and Methods. Boston, Little, Brown, 1970
13. Hodgkin K: Towards Earlier Diagnosis: A Guide to General Practice. New York, Longman, 1973
14. McWhinney IR: The Early Signs of Illness. Springfield, Illinois, Charles C Thomas, 1964
15. Haight RO, Marsland DW, Mitchell GS: Clinical and educational implications of a longitudinal audit for asthma. J Fam Pract 3:481, 1976
16. Barton JE, Haight RO, Marsland DW: Low back pain in the primary care setting. J Fam Pract 3:363, 1976
17. Blacklock SN: The symptom of chest pain in family practice. J Fam Pract 4:429, 1977
18. Shank JC: A study of thyroid disease in family practice. J Fam Pract 3:247, 1976
19. Research in family practice: What's small-town solo practice really like? Patient Care 9(12):97, 1975
20. Marsland DW, Wood M, Mayo F: A data bank for patient care, curriculum, and research in family practice: 526, 196 patient problems. J Fam Pract 3:25, 1976
21. Marsland DW, Wood M, Mayo F: Content of family practice: Part 1: Rank order of diagnoses by frequency. J Fam Pract 3:38, 1976
22. Marsland DW, Wood M, Mayo F: Content of family practice: Part 2: Diagnoses by disease category and age/sex distribution. J Fam Pract 3:48, 1976
23. Weir RJ: Blood pressure in women taking oral contraceptives. Br Med J 1:533, 1974
24. Laragh JH: Oral contraceptives—induced hypertension: Nine years later. Am J Obstet Gynecol 126:141, 1976
25. Hesbacher P, Rickels K, Zamostein B: A collaborative research model in family practice. J Fam Pract 4:923, 1977
26. Armitage P: Statistical Methods in Medical Research. New York, Wiley, 1971
27. Colton TC: Statistics in Medicine. Boston, Little, Brown, 1974

Some Non-Random Views of Statistical Significance*

Alfred O. Berg

Although research in family medicine is growing rapidly, few family physicians have had experience or training in statistical methods. Statistical significance and P values are often misunderstood and frequently misapplied. "Significance" is arbitrary; the actual P value is of greater interest than a significant/not significant statement; P values do not measure the strength of an association; statistical significance is not equivalent to "actual" significance; P values are largely dependent on sample size; and data "dredging" is guaranteed to yield spurious results. Competent statistical consultation, careful study planning, and recognition of statistical pitfalls are important to anyone who does research, and knowledge of these areas is useful as well to anyone reading the medical literature.

Research in family medicine is a growing field, yet few family physicians have had formal training in research methods. Discussions of P values dimly recall medical school lectures to the effect that "the smaller the better," but few have had occasion to calculate them or become familiar with their more subtle applications. This paper will point out some of the frequent errors and misapplications of tests of statistical significance, emphasizing use and interpretation of P values. After a definition, examples will be given drawn from the medical literature, illustrating some of the common problems, and concluding with recommendations and suggestions for those involved in research and for those reading the results.

Definition

No one knows who published the first P value, but it cannot have been before the 1930s, since it was only during that decade that Fisher developed the whole idea of statistical inference.[1] Quite simply, any event has a probability of occurrence somewhere between zero and one. A P value is the probability that, if the experi-

ment or study were exactly repeated, the size of the differences or changes demonstrated in the study could have been due to chance (random error) alone.

Examples

> "... the difference was not significant at $P = 0.10$."

> "... the difference was significant at $P = 0.10$."

These two examples illustrate that statistical significance is entirely arbitrary. In both cases, the probability that the observed difference could have been due to chance is one in ten, yet interpretations vary. There is no single level at which significance is guaranteed. Even a P value of less than 0.0001 does not assure that the event could not have been due to chance, only that it would be very unlikely.

A researcher was recently introduced to a game which had a 1 in 10,395 chance of being solved on the first try. It happened that he *did* solve it on the first try. The point is that rare things do happen.

The larger the number of comparisons in a research study, the more likely it becomes that some proportion of the findings will lead to spurious conclusions. If one sets a significance level of $P = 0.05$, it

* Reprinted by permission from *The Journal of Family Practice*, 8(5):1011–1014, 1979.

is sobering to realize that five percent of all research findings published "significant" at that level are due to chance alone.

". . . but the difference was not significant."

This is even worse—no P value at all. If the author set an arbitrary significance level at P = 0.001, and rejected the finding because P was only 0.002, one might argue with the conclusions. It is always better to calculate the P values exactly and to report them. This allows the readers some freedom to make up their own minds about "significance."

". . . Group I was older than Group II (P = 0.005)."

In this particular case the readers were never told *how much* older Group I was than Group II. This illustrates that P values do not measure the strength of an association. One should always give a measure of the effect being tested—a difference, a percent change, or whatever.

A reviewer was recently given the preliminary findings of a large, well-designed study comparing patients in a family practice setting with those in an internist's practice, but the "findings" consisted only of pages and pages of P values, with no measures of how large the differences were. A P value without some measure of effect is of no value whatever.

". . . the mean hematocrit in the first group was 38.6, in the second 37.5, and the difference was highly significant (P = 0.003)."

This example illustrates the difference between statistical significance and actual significance. Statistical significance is largely a function of sample size, or how many subjects were studied. The larger the sample, the more likely it is that a difference observed will be statistically significant. In the above example, one could argue whether the authors proved anything, since a difference of less than three percent in hematocrit is unlikely to have clinical consequences, and certainly does not help one predict a given outcome.

A recent mail survey of physicians was designed to elicit attitudes on preventive medicine. On a five-point scale, five being most positive, internists average 4.1 and family physicians, 4.3 The difference was statistically significant (P = 0.02) because there were large numbers of physicians in each group, but the finding is of very little value in predicting the attitude of a given internist or family physician, or in making a strong statement about true differences in attitudes, because the observed difference was so small.

"If you required treatment with an experimental drug, and drug A had just been shown effective over placebo on a sample of 500 patients (P = 0.05), and drug B had just been shown effective over placebo on a sample of 20 patients (P = 0.05), which drug would you choose?"

This is an example of the interaction between sample size and the "power" of a statistical test on the sample. The correct answer is to choose drug B, since it is very difficult to achieve statistical significance with such a small sample (hence the difference in *effect* must have been quite large), whereas it is fairly simple to achieve significance on a sample of 500, even if the difference in effect was very small. Calculating the power of a test is outside the scope of this paper, but, in general, the larger the study, the more likely one will be able to detect small differences between the study groups.

"The average numbers of clinic visits made by the experimental and control families were 6.4 and 7.8 per year, respectively, and the difference was not statistically significant (P = 0.32) . . . One can conclude that the educational program had no effect on the number of visits."

In this example, careful reading of the paper itself showed that only ten families were in each of the two groups, experimental and control. Using other data provided in the article, the chances of this study discovering a true difference of as much as 80 percent between the two groups was only fifty-fifty. This illustrates another aspect of the "power" problem mentioned in the previous example.

Frequently, a small study will fail to demonstrate statistically significant differences between the study groups, and the conclusion is made that no differences exist. When one calculates the power of the test, however, one finds that the results may be consistent with large differences in the overall population, but that the differences were missed because too few subjects were studied. In other words, watch out for "no significant difference" findings in small studies.

> ". . . patients were compared on 78 characteristics, and only income and marital status differed between the two groups."

This sort of analysis is called "dredging" by some, a "fishing expedition" by others. The point is that the more tests one does, the more likely it is that significant differences will be found. In the above example, if the significance level was 0.05 (note that it is not given!), on the basis of chance alone one would have expected the authors to come up with three or four significant differences, not just two. There are some statistical ways around this problem, but very few researchers use them.

> "The average decrease in serum cholesterol after changing diets was 22 mg percent, but the difference was not statistically significant ($P = 0.09$)."

This example is more subtle than the preceding ones. Here the only problem is that the statistical test used is not identified. (Alert readers will note that the test names have not been stated in *any* of the previous examples). In this case, working backwards from the author's data, it is apparent that the unpaired t test was employed. Had the more appropriate paired t test been used, the observed difference would have been statistically significant at $P = 0.02$. This illustrates the desirability of naming the statistical test used, in addition to giving the measure of effect and the exact P value. It is uncommon that only one statistical test might be appropriate in

a given situation, and choosing between the several tests available is often a difficult decision. The reader should have the opportunity to judge the appropriateness of that decision, without having to laboriously retrace the author's calculations in order to guess at the statistical test employed.

Conclusions and Recommendations

No single discipline has a monopoly on confusion with P values. The examples chosen for this analysis were from journals in several medical specialties. A few summary comments are appropriate for those contemplating a study using statistical methods and for those who must read the results:

1. Obtain statistical consultation early, before the study begins. Few family physicians have the background or the interest for much statistical work, and many are uncomfortable with anything more complicated than a chi-square test. Find a consultant who is interested in your study and who is personally approachable. This is easier said than done. Even individuals with significant statistical training occasionally have difficulty obtaining the kind of statistical help they need.

2. Plan the analysis before the study begins. Know what kind of differences you would like to find, and how much money is available to spend on the study. It is possible to calculate the size of the study needed to answer your research question, and, in any event, you need to figure the power of the study to determine a specified difference once the size is established. You may find that the proposed study would be too expensive, but sometimes you may actually be able to trim costs by reducing the study size.

   Plan the comparisons to be made in advance, and limit yourself to those. Avoid dredging the data—you are certain to "discover" meaningless relationships.

3. Always give some measure of the effect observed—a percent change, an absolute difference, a relative risk, a difference in means, or whatever. Only then should the statistical test be performed. It is occasionally a good idea to state the effect and calculate a confidence interval without *ever* giving a P value. For example, a difference of 15 percent, with a 95 percent confidence interval of 0 percent to 30 percent means that one is 95 percent certain that the "true" difference in the population is somewhere between zero percent and 30 percent (in this case not a very impressive finding).

4. If you do choose to do significance tests, name the test used, and present the actual P values along with the effect measures. Allow the readers flexibility to make up their own minds about the appropriateness of the test, and whether or not the result is significant.

5. Distinguish between statistical significance and "actual" significance in the discussion. Very small P values do not mean that you have discovered something important.

6. Recognize that even with the best techniques and intentions, chance catches up with you. The whole idea of P values is based on the fact that random errors *do* exist. You may well discover some relationship which does not hold up under further testing. It is impossible to do an absolutely definitive study, as countless examples from medical history attest. Be comfortable with that.

7. If you wish to become heavily involved in research, or if competent statistical consultation is not available, further reading or special courses in the area may be necessary. Several excellent resource books are available.[2-5]

REFERENCES

1. Fisher RA: The Design of Experiments. Edinburgh, Oliver and Boyd, 1935
2. Armitage P: Statistical Methods in Medical Research. New York, John Wiley, 1971
3. Remington RD, Schork MA: Statistics with Applications to the Biological and Health Sciences. Englewood Cliffs, NJ, Prentice-Hall, 1970
4. Snedecor GW, Cochran WG: Statistical Methods, ed 6. Ames, Iowa, Iowa State University Press, 1967
5. Afifi AA, Azen SP: Statistical Analysis: A Computer-Oriented Approach. New York, Academic Press, 1972

A Method for Assessing the Outcome of Acute Primary Care*

Robert L. Kane, Jerry Gardner, Diana Dryer Wright, David Sundwall, George Snell, F. Ross Woolley, C. Hilmon Castle

Some 1,700 acute care episodes were studied to assess the outcomes in terms of the extent to which patients regained their usual functional status. Involving active follow-up of each patient, the study serves as a prototype for measuring several components of quality of care including actual outcomes, patient expectation of outcome, physician expectation of outcome, and patient satisfaction with outcome and care. Because this study was conducted in a family practice residency training setting, we hope that it will serve as a model of how such information may be used to increase residents' sensitivity to the course of illness commonly seen in primary care, and to encourage the residents to set expectations for the care they give.

It can safely be said that medicine has entered the Age of Accountability. Concern about the quality of care—what it is and how to measure it—is very evident in the professional literature and in federal regulations. Although many have tried to resist this pressure as an infringement on professional sovereignty, this movement should provide great opportunity for family practice.

As Lewis noted, evaluation of quality of care has come full circle—from the most basic outcome measurements, such as mortality, through an emphasis on structure and process review, and back to outcomes again, now with a more sophisticated point of view.[1] This evolution has been associated with a shift in emphasis from hospital care for the acutely ill to the more diffuse management problems of ambulatory care. Although hospitals were the natural targets for the first efforts to obtain data on patients with similar, definable problems, relatively complete documentation, and substantial per unit costs, there is increasing recognition of an equal or even greater need to understand the factors that affect quality in the broader area of primary care.

The efforts made to correlate the outcomes of care with certain professional standards for what ought to be done in a given instance have been frustrating.[2] In the ambulatory setting, where patient record keeping may be less complete, the emphasis on outcome rather than process is particularly appropriate. The development of quality-of-care studies in the primary care setting offers an opportunity to understand more about this type of care—how it works and what makes a difference; these goals reflect the desire of some family practitioners to become more actively involved in applied research.

This article describes a method of looking at the outcomes of one aspect of primary care. A prospective study was implemented to obtain data on approximately 1,700 patients who sought treatment for acute illnesses at two model clinics run by the Family Practice Residency Training Project at the University of Utah Medical Center. The article presents a model showing how similar studied might be made in a family practice setting. It illustrates what types of useful information might be obtainable by a family practitioner as he seeks to improve the quality of his care.

* Reprinted by permission from *The Journal of Family Practice*, 4(6):1119–1124, 1977.

Methods

One clinic was housed in the University Hospital and the other in an affiliated, community hospital. The physician staff consisted of first-, second-, and third-year family practice residents, attending physicians on the family practice faculty, and physician assistants.

In order to focus on the episodes of care that would offer some possibility of producing a functional change as a result of the physician's intervention, all patients who presented with an acute complaint during the nine-month period of the study were asked by interviewers we had trained, to participate as they entered the clinic for their appointments. (In the case of children, the parent was interviewed.) Patients who were seen for treatment of chronic problems without exacerbation, for general health maintenance such as pre-natal care, and patients who required hospitalization in the course of treatment were excluded. The study was explained to patients in terms of the doctors' desires to obtain better follow-up information about their patients; a bilingual, written statement was given to each participant stating that the interviewer would call before coming to his home for additional information.

There were very few refusals to participate. Approximately eight percent of the patients could not be reached for follow-up, and another six percent experienced a second, separate episode of illness before follow-up. These were omitted from the final analysis. Repeated clinic visits for the same problem were included in the same episode. Occasionally a patient returned after follow-up with a new illness and was enrolled for a second episode. The overall study design is diagrammed in Figure 1.

Clinic Visit

Each patient was interviewed before he was seen by a physician; his age, sex, usual functional status (defined as that approxi-

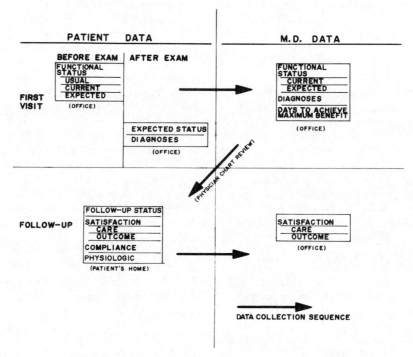

Fig. 1. A schematic representation of the study design.

mately six months prior to the clinic visit), his presenting functional status (as reflected by the degree of impairment imposed by the current illness), and the status the patient hoped to achieve or return to after treatment were recorded. The interviewer determined from the patient's responses to questions about his usual and recent activities what the functional status was; the interviewer used a previously tested six-level index that was adapted from Williamson.[3] The levels chosen were (1) full activity without symptoms, (2) full activity but with presence of an underlying physical or laboratory abnormality without symptoms, (3) symptomatic but with full activity, (4) symptomatic with restricted activity, (5) limitation of mobility, and (6) confinement to bed. Approximately seven percent of the patients were unable or unwilling to estimate their follow-up status. This group was handled as a separate category in the analysis when necessary.

After the patient had been seen by a physician, he was again asked by the interviewer to describe briefly his impression of the nature of his illness according to the information conveyed to him by the physician and to note any change in the follow-up status expected for him. Only four percent of the patients were still unable to estimate their follow-up status at this time. As many as three diagnoses were recorded per patient, using the H-ICDA code; thus, either symptoms or specific diagnoses—whichever accurately represented the level of resolution of the diagnostic process—could be specified.

Sometime on the same day, each physician was asked to give his estimation of the patient's current functional status, the diagnoses, the length of time necessary for the patient to receive the maximum benefit from treatment, and when and what level of function the patient should achieve. If treatment for several problems was involved, the time estimate was made for the major acute diagnosis; the maximum time allowed for treatment to achieve results before a follow-up visit was set at six months. The physician could

delay making his estimate of expected status until laboratory data were returned if he desired.

Independent Case Review

In the interim before follow-up, an independent physician reviewed the chart of each patient to determine what data were needed at the follow-up visit. A minimum data base for each study patient, consisting of weight, hematocrit, blood pressure, and urinalysis, had been established. These data were gathered at the time of follow-up if they had not been recorded in the chart or if they had been abnormal and no subsequent normal values were recorded. Similarly, laboratory tests ordered for the specific problem were repeated for the same reasons. The reviewing physician had also noted for the interviewer any specific instructions regarding medication, diet, activity, etc, that the physician had given the patient. At this time the reviewing physician also compared the care provider's estimation of presenting functional status to the interviewer's determination so that gross discrepancies might be detected or to account for the existence of an underlying disease which would place the patient in functional-status classification 2 (see Table 4). In general, unless there was contravening evidence in the chart, when discrepancies in reported symptoms were discovered, the interviewer's impression was used because it fit the criteria established.

Follow-up Visit

At the time specified by the physician, an interviewer saw each patient in his home to determine his follow-up functional status. The interviewer also performed any of the tests needed to complete the minimum data base or to evaluate the effectiveness of treatment, such as blood pressure checks, throat cultures, urine cultures, and so on. Some test was required for approximately ten percent of the patients. If unexpected abnormalities were found, the interviewer immediately called the clinic to obtain instructions or to make an appointment for the patient to see his own physician for further follow-up.

A compliance score, derived from the average of reported behavior in any of four possible areas (medication, diet, activity, and other), was computed for each patient and then dichotomized. Finally, the interviewer questioned the patient about his satisfaction with the care he had received and his satisfaction with the outcome he had achieved. A single specific question was asked about whether or not the patient was satisfied with his care and a second separate question focused on his satisfaction with the outcome.

The interviewer later conveyed the information on follow-up status and patient satisfaction, along with any other comments the patient made about the episode, to his physician and asked that the physician state his satisfaction with the care and the outcome also. This, unfortunately, allowed the physician to be influenced by the patient's opinions, but it was necessary so that the physician could know the actual outcome.

For the purpose of this analysis, a good functional or physiological outcome was defined as one in which the patient's follow-up status was equal to or better than his usual status prior to illness. The patient's expected status was also compared to the follow-up status to assess whether the expectation was met. The two measures of satisfaction represented a third type of outcome score.

The physicians were expected to treat their patients in the usual manner during the study: no attempt was made by the investigators to influence their behavior. The possibility that some physicians might change their practice behavior during the study because of information gained from the follow-up interviews was considered, however. The physicians were informed about the study in advance, and a vigorous attempt was made to encourage their cooperation and to minimize the time and paperwork required of them, particularly so that follow-up visits would not be delayed by a backlog.

Cost Factors

The costs for each episode of care were recorded by specific components (physician, laboratory and x-ray, medication, and other) and totaled. Data on physician office-visit costs, laboratory and x-ray expenses, and other fees were obtained from the clinic and hospital billing records. All billings charged between the clinic visit and the estimated time of maximum benefit were included. Fees discounted for employees or welfare patients were recorded at the full usual charge. The physician fee schedule used was competitive with local private providers, although the clinics were partially supported by federal grant funds and the residents were paid by salary. Medication costs were determined from the price charged in the hospital pharmacy for all medications prescribed by the physician, whether or not the prescriptions were filled. "Other" costs were minimal and were not analyzed separately. Cost subcategories were analyzed in terms of both relative (percent of total) costs and actual dollars.

Process Evaluation

In addition, two process measures of quality of care were employed. First, after all data had been collected, we performed process review on the charts of all patients with diagnoses for which explicit criteria for ambulatory care had been developed by the local Professional Standards Review Organization. The criteria for this review varied in length from 5 to 37 items and were designed to be a standard for minimum acceptable performance. Because this provided no absolute standard for relative levels of good or poor care, the normative standard of care against which each case was compared was the average number of items missed for each diagnosis by this population of physicians. Diagnoses for which there were very few cases were not included in the process review.

Second, as part of the teaching program, a sample of each resident's charts was reviewed periodically by other residents and the faculty, according to standards based on the correct use of the problem-oriented record.[4] For this study, the individual items on which the resident was reviewed were abstracted into five general categories and an overall summary statement regarding quality of care. The questions were as follows:

1. Was the problem list properly prepared?
2. Was the problem list used?
3. Was the data base complete?
4. Was treatment appropriate for the problems listed?
5. Was follow-up adequate?
6. General rating of care.

Results

With so many individual pieces of information available, the spectrum of possible analyses is quite broad. First, the relationship between the chosen outcome measure and a variety of patient, provider, and disease characteristics can be learned. Second, functional outcome can be compared to other outcome and process measures to evaluate their relative strengths and usefulness as approaches to assessing quality in ambulatory care. Both types of analyses can assist the private physician in determining how his own patient population may be unique, and what aspects of his professional behavior are especially strong or merit extra attention.

Among the total 1,761 patients who made up the final sample of this study, 76.5 percent experienced good outcomes;

but 23.5 percent of these patients with supposedly acute complaints had not returned to their usual status by the time of follow-up. There were a small number, less than three percent of the total sample, who had been thought to be entirely normal prior to their acute illness, but, through either the discovery of underlying chronic disease or the failure of treatment, they had a persistent laboratory abnormality on follow-up which left them with a bad outcome despite resolution of the acute symptoms. However, for the other 21 percent, the poor outcome represented a major decrease in daily functional activity.

It is important to keep in mind that the illnesses chosen for assessment consisted in large measure of presumably self-limited conditions. Several explanations of the failure of this group of patients to regain their usual status can be entertained: they may have developed new problems, although those with clearly identifiable new episodes of illness were eliminated. More likely, the original problem may have been misdiagnosed. A more serious complaint may have been mistaken for a self-limited condition. In addition, some of the poor outcomes may be the result of complications of treatment, a particular concern in otherwise self-limited conditions.

Patient factors that could be related to outcome include age, sex, compliance, and patient understanding of the illness. Although the proportion of older patients in this population was small (six percent were over the age of 50), the percentage of bad outcomes did not increase substantially with age (Table 1), indicating that this factor alone did not greatly influence the overall results. Sixty percent of the patients were female, but the difference between males and females in outcome was slight (78 percent vs 75 percent good outcomes). A total of 1,518, or 86 percent of all patients, were requested to comply with one or more instructions; 1,328, or 87 percent, did comply. Compliers had 78 percent good outcomes, while noncompliers had 70 percent good outcomes, not a great

Table 1. *Outcomes by Age of Patients*

Age	Percent with Good Outcome	N
<1	73	91
1–5	78	255
6–15	78	339
16–30	80	662
31–50	69	313
51+	62	101

Table 3. *Relationship between Length of Time until Follow-up Visit and Outcome*

Days to Achieve Maximum Benefit	Percent with Good Outcome	N
<1 week	80	566
1–2 weeks	79	769
3–4 weeks	72	158
>4 weeks	66	268

difference; 75 percent of the patients without instructions achieved good outcomes.

To determine if outcome could be related to the degree to which patients understood the nature of their illness as communicated to them by their physician, we matched the diagnoses reported by each patient against those reported by the physician. As shown in Table 2, patients with poor knowledge scores (or, alternatively, instances of poor physician communication) had at least as high a percentage of good outcomes as did those who knew exactly what was wrong with them.

Another possibility that might have affected the outcomes was that the physicians might have underestimated the length of time necessary for patients to achieve benefit from treatment. (It has already been pointed out that if they overestimated to the extent that the patient contracted a separate illness before follow-up, the case was removed from the study.) However, as seen in Table 3, there was only a slight decrease in the percentage of good outcomes as the length of time until follow-up increased; this tends to refute the likelihood that this was an important contributing factor.

Because some patients are more severely affected by illness than others and because some types of disease have inherently different recovery rates, the relative percentage of good outcomes was compared according to the different levels of presenting functional status and for each of the diagnoses with more than 50 cases. There were nine such diagnoses and 988 patients in this category; other problems were very widely distributed, with the largest categories being forms of respiratory disease (mentioned 581 times), and injuries (187 times); 650 complaints were non-specific signs or symptoms. The percentage of good outcomes did not vary with the different levels of impairment at the time of the first visit for that episode (Table 4), but among the common diagnoses examined individually, abdominal pain and headache stand out with remarkably poor outcomes (Table 5).

Looking at other outcome measures, 95 percent of all patients achieved the follow-up status that they anticipated after being seen by the physician. Approximately four percent of the patients changed their estimation after having been seen by the physician; three fourths of those who changed

Table 2. *Relationship between Patient's Knowledge of Diagnosis and Outcome*

Knowledge/ Communication*	Percent with Good Outcome	N
Perfect (4-digit match)	77	1475
Correct disease type (3-digit match)	73	138
Correct organ system (2-digit match)	79	132
None (no match)	81	16

* Because the 4-digit positions of the H-ICDA code categorize diagnoses by organ system and type of disease, a 4-digit match between two diagnoses was considered perfect agreement, a 3-digit match represented patient knowledge of correct type of disease, and 2-digit matches were matched by hand by an independent physician to make sure that signs or symptoms appropriate to a specific etiologic diagnosis were not missed.

Table 4. *Outcome by Presenting Functional Status*

Presenting Functional Status (Severity)		Percent with Good Outcome	N
2	Asymptomatic with lab abnormality	76	45
3	Symptomatic	75	997
4	Restricted activity	79	646
5 and 6	Limited mobility	74	73

their estimate actually were less accurate. Six percent of patients were initially unable to estimate their follow-up status but made an accurate estimate after their visit.

Satisfaction

Ninety-six percent of the patients were satisfied with the care they received, and 90 percent were satisfied with their outcomes. As might have been expected from the structure of the study, the figures for physician satisfaction were virtually identical. However, in those instances where patients were not satisfied with their care, 71 percent of physicians were satisfied with the care; and where patients were not satisfied with the outcome, only 44 percent of the physicians were satisfied with the outcome. Among the patients who actually experienced bad outcomes, 92 percent were still satisfied with the care they received, and 65 percent were satisfied with the outcome

Table 5. *Outcomes for Selected Diagnoses*

Frequent Diagnoses	Percent with Good Outcome	N
Otitis	80	134
Pharyngitis	83	192
URI	81	261
Flu	80	49
Abdominal pain	64	88
Rash and dermatitis	73	52
Back and neck pain	70	53
Cough and bronchitis	71	96
Headache	63	52

itself. Among the patients who failed to achieve their expected outcome, more (97 percent) were actually satisfied with their outcomes than among patients who did achieve their expectations (89 percent).

Satisfaction with care and outcome were not found to be related to cost. It is thus difficult to postulate a rational basis for patient satisfaction or to argue for it as a useful, overall outcome measure.

The cost data were valuable in showing how funds were allocated to different medical services and how outcome was related to cost. The average total cost per episode was $20.71. Physician and office fees were $12.75 (71 percent); laboratory and x-ray fees, $4.35 (nine percent); and medication, $3.22 (18 percent); other costs made up less than two percent of the total. For patients with good outcomes, the average total cost was less than for patients with bad outcomes ($20.04 vs $22.89).

Better process scores were also found to be related to good outcomes, but the implications to be drawn from process data must be limited by the small number of cases on a small spectrum of mainly infectious diseases rather than the broader range of ambulatory care problems.

Discussion

Additional relevant data that could be gathered in a similar primary care setting would include whether the physician had previously seen the patient or if the visit was an initial encounter; the number of appointments scheduled and kept; and the patient's impression of the nature of his illness before he saw the physician. These data could be used to test the rationale for continuity of care—that a knowledge of a patient's usual state of health and previous response to treatment regimens would enable the physician to achieve a good outcome with fewer intermediate steps. This would permit the physician to omit safely steps in the care process that might lower their performance scores when compared with process criteria but, if it were safe and effective, the proportion of good outcomes should remain high.

Also, because incidental office charges could distort the amount of the physician fee when used as an indicator of physician time, it would be helpful to know what actual utilization of other resources was associated with each unit of treatment, follow-up, or complication. Finally, because a substantial portion of the patients either changed their expectation or developed a new one after talking with the physician, it would be interesting to see how this related to the type of disease and various other communication factors.

A study like the one described can be particularly useful as a part of an educational program; a central argument for all forms of evaluation has been the educational benefit to be derived. The private practitioner, accustomed to treating the individual patient, may lack a sufficiently critical perspective of his overall performance or his performance relative to his peers. The experience of examining outcomes offers an opportunity that other techniques do not—it establishes an internal system of quality assessment in which the ultimate validator is *whether or not the patient achieved the results that the physician intended.*

As this study suggests, neither the patient nor his physician at the present time has a clear concept of what should be expected of their interaction in the health-care delivery system. Many experts have recommended that the patient be taught what to expect, and many practicing physicians would concur that more realistic goals would benefit many patients. We have not yet reached the stage where each physician sets the individual patient's goals and communicates these in turn to the patient. Each physician is the product of training, which has traditionally insisted upon the possibility of maximum improvement for each patient, if only all our knowledge and skills are properly applied. Recent data have, however, shown that this

is not always the case. The physician is, therefore, called upon to see for himself what will make a difference in his own practice; and the emphasis on outcomes offers him a way to do this.

One important goal for this type of outcome assessment might reasonably be that the family practice resident would change both his attitudes and his behavior to reflect his concern for outcomes and his recognition of the need to think prognostically. This might take a tangible form through a modification of the way in which he keeps his records. We would hope to see the now familiar SOAP-format of the problem-oriented record expanded to include two new concepts: prognostication and concern for patient outcome.

The assessment of a patient should include not only the highest level of diagnoses justified by the data but also a prognostic statement indicating the degree of improvement (or deterioration) expected and the anticipated time course. Similarly, the plan would include a specific method for follow-up, so that the actual outcome could be ascertained. While this might necessitate a return visit, other means to assure contact should also be considered lest we continue to misinterpret no news as always meaning good news.

This would require a mechanism for obtaining direct feedback on the patient's ability to function after treatment and the degree to which he cooperated with instructions so that treatment corrections could be undertaken at appropriate times. This system of follow-up need not, however, be dependent on a physician's time, since it has already been shown that a clerk with some initiative can gather much useful data by telephone.[5] In fact, most patients recognize and appreciate this effort to improve their care and report greater satisfaction with their care when they know that the physician is interested in what happened to them after seeing them.

Documentation of prognosis and outcome measures in the records of family practitioners would mark a major step forward for the specialty. The regular amassing of such data could provide a rich resource for useful research. The continuous process of prognosis-with-feedback would also sharpen the skills of the practitioners and perhaps alert them to important additional factors to consider when dealing with primary care problems.

Family practice is a discipline in transition. We have been shown the need for new ways of thinking in regard to the way problems are presented[6] and the diagnostic taxonomies most appropriate.[7] It is now time to reinforce this need for increased attention to prognosis and evaluation. This type of progress provides the kind of information from which new knowledge derives. It is the kind of research appropriate to family practice.

Acknowledgment

Work for this study was supported by Public Health Service Award No. 1 R01 HSO 1596, "Quality Assessment Methods in Primary Care."

REFERENCES

1. Lewis CE: The state of the art of quality assessment. Med Care 12:799–806, 1974
2. Brook RH: Quality of Care Assessment: A Comparison of Five Methods of Peer Review. DHEW Publication No. HRA-74 3100. Washington DC 1973
3. Williamson JW. In Hopkins CE(ed): Outcomes of health care: Key to health improvement, in methodology of identifying, measuring and evaluating outcomes of health service programs, systems and subsystems. DHEW Health Services and Mental Health Administration. Washington, DC, 1970, pp 75–102
4. Kane RL, Leigh EH, Feigal DW, et al: A method for evaluating patient care and auditing skills of family practice residents. J Fam Pract 2:205–210, 1975
5. Kane RL, Woolley FR, Gardner HF, et al: Measuring outcomes of care in an ambulatory primary care population: A pilot study. J Community Health 1:233–240, 1976
6. Hodgkin K: Towards Earlier Diagnosis: A Family Doctor's Approach. London, ES Livingston, 1966
7. McWhinney I: Beyond diagnosis. N Engl J Med 287:384–387, 1972

A Morbidity and Therapeutic Index in General Practice*

C. Bridges-Webb

The use of a morbidity and therapeutic index in general practice is described. The system can monitor practice activities, morbidity, prescribing and patient characteristics for individual practices or surveys. A triplicate prescription form is used for data collection, with minimum inconvenience to the doctor. Complete patient confidentiality is maintained. Some problems of classification and coding are discussed.

The importance of the study of morbidity in general practice has been recognized in the past twenty years, both as an indicator of community health problems and as a means of describing the nature and scope of general practice.[1] Many individual general practitioners have undertaken surveys of morbidity in their own practices, often rising the E-book or diagnostic index developed by the British Royal College of General Practitioners.[2] This has the added advantage that it provides each individual practitioner with an index of diseases in his own practice. Major morbidity surveys were undertaken in Australia in 1962–63[3] and in 1969–74,[1] though for various reasons in neither instance was the diagnostic index method used.

Interest in the extent and nature of prescribing in medical practice has developed even more recently with recognition of the importance of problems of cost, side effects of drugs, habituation, suicide and over-prescribing—the latter controversial and often poorly justified, since statistical information about benefits as well as disadvantages is conspicuous by its scarcity. In relating prescribing to morbidity, the 1969–74 Australian morbidity survey broke new ground, though there were some major disadvantages in the failure to identify patients and link contacts, and the short sampling period for each doctor.

The development of a morbidity and therapeutic index in general practice, using the experience gained in the Australian Morbidity and Prescribing Survey is described. The system can routinely monitor patient characteristics, morbidity and prescribing for individual practices, or provide such information for a wider survey.

The Practice Situation

The morbidity and therapeutic index has been developed in the general practice unit of the Department of Community Medicine, University of Sydney. This is conducted in Croydon as a private fee for service practice with a receptionist, one full-time general practitioner and two members of the department part-time, and provides a full range of general practitioner services including family planning, obstetrics, office procedures, home visits and care of patients in nursing homes and hospitals when appropriate.

The practice uses the RACGP medical record system, modified to allow one folder per family instead of one per individual, with a family profile form specially designed to collect and record information relevant to the whole family. Each family and individual is allotted a serial number, and colour coding and terminal digit filing are used.

* Reprinted by permission from *Australian Family Physician*, 9:365–368, May, 1980.

Aims and Objectives

The morbidity and therapeutic index has been designed to provide information about:

Practice activities—services, referrals
Problems and diagnoses (morbidity)
Drugs and medications prescribed (therapeutics)
Patients and families

The aim has been to do this on an ongoing basis, at minimum inconvenience to the doctors, at minimum expense, collecting the minimum of information to meet specified objectives but with capacity for flexible alteration or expansion to meet future requirements. Its scope has therefore quite deliberately been restricted, but in its development the possibility of extending its use to other practices and of using it as the basis for a more comprehensive project, has been kept in mind.

At present, the specific objectives are:

To monitor the practice activities on a month-to-month basis in respect of:
–the number and kind of services rendered,
–the number of problems or diagnoses dealt with,
–the number of drugs prescribed, and the number and nature of referrals.
To relate practice activities to the age and sex of patients and to morbidity.
To determine morbidity seen in the practice and relate it to the age and sex of patients.
To determine the number and nature of drugs and medications prescribed and relate this to the age and sex of patients and to morbidity.
To provide an annual summary list of families and patients showing sex, month and year of birth for each person, the diagnoses for which each patient has been treated, with the number of medical encounters and the names of all drugs prescribed for each diagnosis.

To provide, when required for any given diagnosis or group of diagnoses, a list of patients with that diagnosis and the drugs prescribed for that diagnosis.
To provide, when required for any given drug or group of drugs, a list of patients for whom that drug was prescribed and the diagnoses for which the drug was prescribed.

Method

Data are collected using a triplicate copy of any prescription written (or a triplicate form alone when a prescription is not written) at all patient encounters, including indirect ones such as when a prescription or certificate is provided without the patient being seen on that occasion (Figure 1). Telephone consultations are included only if this results in a note being made in the medical record, or a prescription or other document is written.

The triplicate form provides for the collection of the following data:

Doctor or other professional providing the service.
Date.
Patient identification by family number, sex, month and year of birth.
The service rendered—usually in terms of the medical benefit number, but some other items are also included. Only the main service is recorded.
Diagnoses or problems actually dealt with at this encounter. A second form is used and linked if there are more than three. The encounter status (first encounter for new illness, follow-up, the first encounter for recurrent episode of a chronic disease, or altered diagnosis at follow-up compared with the diagnosis previously made at the first encounter) is recorded for each diagnosis or problem. The problem number recorded is used only to link the diagnosis and any drug prescribed.
Drugs prescribed are automatically re-

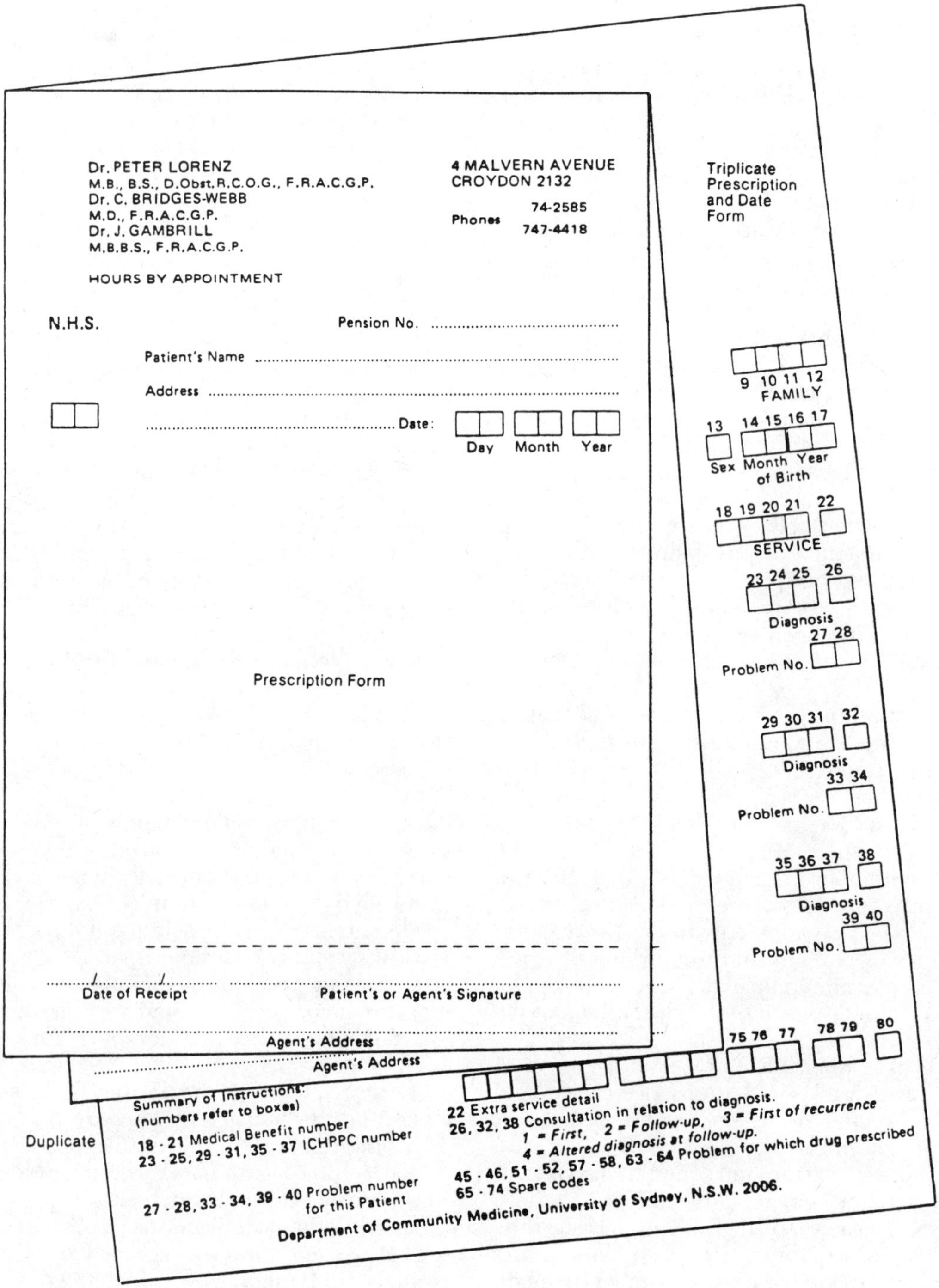

Fig. 1. Morbidity and therapeutic index: Triplicate prescription recording system.

corded on the triplicate form when the prescription is written, and are later coded.

Referrals to specialists and hospitals and for diagnostic tests are recorded and coded on the bottom of the form.

The doctor must record a certain minimum of information in writing or by coding—date, identification of the patient, service rendered, diagnosis(es) and encounter status, referrals (if any). This adds on average about two minutes to the encounter time.

Completion of the coding is done by a part-time research assistant, who also batches the data on a monthly basis and submits it to the University Sample Survey Centre for computer processing and analysis. Before this is done the upper portion of the triplicate form is detached so that confidentiality is preserved, since the only patient identification is by family number, age and sex, the key to which remains in the practice. The data are processed on to four files relating to encounters, diagnoses, drugs and patients, so that output tables may be obtained in terms of any of these units. Processing is in monthly batches, but output on any occasion may use data accumulated for up to twelve months.

Classification of Problems and Diagnoses

The International Classification of Health Problems in Primary Care, developed by the World Organization of National Colleges, Academies and Academic Associations of General Practitioners/Family Physicians (WONCA) is used to code and classify problems and diagnoses. This is internationally recognized, and is compatible with the World Health Organization (WHO), International Classification of Diseases (ICD). It is available as a conveniently sized reference book with an alphabetical index.[4]

The 378 rubrics include not only conventional medical diagnoses, but also social and emotional problems and the undifferentiated symptoms and problems which are frequently presented in primary care. It is important that participating doctors have available and are familiar with the classification used, as a guide to the nature and specificity of diagnosis required. Even so, problems of consistent recording arise, particularly in relation to a problem-oriented approach, since it is often a matter of arbitrary decision as to which manifestations of disease are recorded separately. For example, a patient with ischaemic heart disease may have associated arrythmia, congestive failure and angina. It would be possible to record this as only one diagnosis if the other conditions are regarded only as manifestations of the one basic disease; on the other hand, it is equally reasonable to regard each or any of these conditions as a problem in its own right and to record all four. The principle of multiple coding is recommended by WHO in the ICD, and in our practice we tend to record all the problems. However, we have not yet resolved the question entirely to the satisfaction of even the three doctors involved.

Apart from the question of the number of problems to be recorded during any given encounter, there is also the problem of how specific such recording should be, and how consistency of definition of rubrics can be achieved. A useful general principle is to be as specific as possible so that, for example, duodenal ulcer is diagnosed rather than peptic ulcer or indigestion. However, on what criteria should such a diagnosis be based? Is X-ray or endoscopy required to justify such specificity, or is clinical judgement enough? In an endeavour to resolve such difficulties for the purpose of classification and morbidity studies, the International Classification Committee of WONCA is at present preparing a companion volume of definitions of rubics included in the classification.

Classification and Coding of Drugs

At present there is no widely recognized general system for classifying and coding drugs. The system used by the Commonwealth Health Department in Australia relates only to drugs which are pharmaceutical benefits. The widely used MIMS (Monthly Index of Medical Specialties) provides a useful classification but not a coding (numbering) system, and another commercial organization, Intercontinental Medical Statistics, uses a similar but different classification; both code all preparations individually by brand names.

The WHO classification of drugs, medicaments and biological substances which is included in Volume 2 of the International Classification of Procedures in Medicine was not available when the Morbidity and Therapeutic Index commenced, and it was therefore necessary to develop an ad hoc classification and numbering system based on the MIMS classification, with small modifications in order to produce a system compatible with that used by the Commonwealth Health Department and with the draft of the WHO classification. This provides for a four digit hierarchical numbering system allowing for identification of 19 major groups of drugs, 64 subgroups, and individual identification of drugs and major preparations (for example, oral, injectable) but not distinguishing different brands or minor differences in preparations (such as tablets, capsules).

Results

The index has been in use since October 1977, and much information is available for all or part of this period, although there is some variability due to the deliber-

ate development and evaluation aspects of the project to this stage.

The computer produces tables which are based on the statistical package for social sciences, in some cases with minor modifications to meet the project objectives. There is obviously scope for a very large number of tables to be produced, but the principle of producing the minimum that will meet the present objectives is followed. From these, a number of regular consolidated tables are produced by the research assistant:

Monthly totals of encounters, diagnoses and drugs.
Number and type of encounters (services) by provider (doctor).
Number of diagnoses by provider.
Encounter status of diagnoses by provider.
Number of encounters, diagnoses and drugs by age and sex.
Number and nature of referrals.

These meet the aims of monitoring practice activities, prescribing and patient characteristics. Morbidity and prescribing information has so far been tabulated more to determine that the system works, rather than to produce specific information.

An annual summary list of all families and patients with their diagnoses and drugs prescribed has been produced which assists in patient care, and is useful for referral purposes or to provide the patient with a personal record summary when appropriate.

So far, the diagnosis list has been used only to obtain a list of all patients who have had an adverse reaction to a drug (which is one of the diagnostic rubrics) in order to investigate this topic by extracting details from the relevant medical records.

Later the drug list will be used to enable us to investigate the characteristics of all patients for whom certain drugs were prescribed.

Acknowledgments

This project has been supported by a Health Programme Grant for Evaluative Research and Development from the Commonwealth Department of Health; a University Research Grant; and a Medical Research Grant from the University of Sydney.

Mrs. Helena Britt and Mrs. Leonie Gibbons have arranged coding and analysis of data. Drs. J. Dowsett, J. Gambrill and P. Lorenz have recorded information. Mrs. Tania Rtshiladze has provided secretarial assistance and typed the manuscript. To them all I owe thanks for a job well done.

Author's Update

The Morbidity and Therapeutic Index provides useful research information but contributes relatively little to patient care. A mini-computer is now being installed in the practice to enable development of an indexed computer medical record summary system. This will be comprehensive enough, with fast enough turnaround, to be of real value in patient care while allowing even more extensive epidemiological, operational and evaluation research information to be generated without increasing the staff workload.

REFERENCES

1. Bridges-Webb, C (Ed.) The Australian Morbidity and Prescribing Survey 1969–1974. Med J Aust 1976; 2:Suppl. No. 1
2. Eimerl, TA and Laidlaw, AJ. A Handbook for Research in General Practice 1969; pp. 39–62, E & S Livingstone Ltd, London
3. National Health and Medical Research Council. Report on a National Morbidity Survey 1969; NH & MRC, Canberra
4. WONCA. International Classification of Health Problems in Primary Care 1979; Oxford University Press

The Design and Use of a Health Status Index for Family Physicians*

Charles W. Given, Lewis Simoni, Rita Gallin

This paper describes a Health Status Index (HSI) which is part of a patient encounter form in a family practice center. The Index, which is used to profile a patient's health status longitudinally, combines physical and psychosocial measures of health. Based on its use in the center and through the presentation of data on patient health status, the authors illustrate how the Index can facilitate the evaluation of care and the management of practice. More specifically, they suggest that such data assist physicians in: (1) evaluating the effect of different modes of treatment on the duration and severity of ill-defined symptoms and complaints; (2) identifying high-risk patients for special attention; (3) indicating treatment modalities which produce more desirable outcomes; (4) determining the efficiency of different modes of treatment and of continued care; and (5) addressing chronological, as well as interpersonal and interprofessional, questions of providing continuous care for the chronically ill.

The family physician has responsibility for first contact, continuous care, and the management of available health resources on behalf of his patients.[1-3] In this paper we describe a Health Status Index (HSI) and discuss how it can assist family physicians in discharging these responsibilities. First, we define the component measures of the HSI and report the way in which it is completed in a family practice center. Then, using data collected via the Health Status Index, we discuss how it can assist physicians in the evaluation of care and the management of their practices.

Description of the HSI

The Health Status Index is one element of a patient encounter form which provides data for a health information system in a family practice residency training center. This center has a staff of 21 residents and two board-certified family physicians who manage over 1,000 patient visits per month. The HSI, which is used to profile a patient's health status longitudinally, com-bines physical and psychosocial measures of health (Table 1). Symptoms are a physical measure of illness based upon the physician's observations and examination of the patient. Discomfort and inability to perform major activities are psychosocial measures of the existence of morbidity based upon the patient's reports. The definitions and classification of the psychosocial measures were adapted from those used by the National Center for Health Statistics in the United States National Health Survey.[4]

The categories of health included in the HSI are used to evaluate patient health status at three points in time: prior to the onset of the illness for which care is sought, at the time of the visit to the center, and three months after the visit. The first patient visit for an illness is considered to mark the onset of that condition. The patient's usual status prior to this onset is used as his baseline measure of health.

The severity of the patient's illness is defined by the degree of change in his status over two or more points in time. Comparing status prior to the onset of an illness with status at the time of each visit summarizes the impact of the illness on the patient.

The duration of an illness is defined by

* Reprinted by permission from *The Journal of Family Practice*, 4(2):287–291, 1977.

Table 1. *Definition of Health Status by Major Activity for Pre-School and School Age Children, Housewives, Workers, and Retired Persons*

Health Status	Definition	Specification of Major Activity				
		Preschool	*School*	*Housewives*	*Workers*	*Retired Persons*
Not symptomatic: performs usual major activity	People who are asymptomatic	Takes part in ordinary play with other children	Goes to school	Does house-work	Works at any job or business	Performs usual retired activities
Symptomatic: experiences discomfort, performs usual major activity	People in whom symptoms are pronounced (i.e., affect comfort) so that person recognizes change in usual health status	Symptomatic, experiences discomfort (same for all categories of persons)				
Activity restricted	People who are unable to engage in major activity, confined to house, almost completely inactive, not bed disabled	Does not take part in play activities other than sedentary, e.g., watch TV, look at books	Does not attend school	Does not keep house	Does not at-tend work or business	Is confined to house
Bed disabled	People who stay in bed all or most of the day—more than 1/2 of hours person is usually awake	Stays in bed (same for all categories of persons)				
At risk	People with terminal illness	At risk (same for all categories of persons)				

the length of time between onset and recovery or, in the case of long-term, continuing conditions, from onset to death. For an acute illness, recovery may be defined as the time when a patient resumes that status prior to the onset of illness. For chronic conditions, the HSI may be used to define the progression of the illness over some period of time. It is up to the judgment of the physician to determine if the observed changes in status for an individual patient represent an acceptable progression for that illness.

Completion of the Health Status Index

The HSI is completed by the attending physician for all patients at the time of each visit to the center (Figure 1). The patient is asked his usual health status prior to the onset of the present illness and his status at the time of the visit. These are recorded by the physician, along with his estimate of the patient's expected status in three months. This estimate is based on information available to the physician, including data from the patient's history, physical examination, laboratory and/or x-ray procedures, and diagnosis.

For the purposes of the HSI, the physician's estimate of the patient's status in three months is used to differentiate acute, short-term illness from chronic, long-term problems. The use of a three-month time period to separate acute from chronic conditions is based on a convention established by the National Center for Health Statistics in their surveys of the health status of the United States population. In these studies, illnesses or conditions first noticed more than three months before an interview are considered chronic. Thus, a chronic, long-term problem is not subject to clinical definitions of resolution within three months and an acute, short-term problem is. Though acute conditions may be exacerbated by co-existing chronic con-

ditions, they are considered to be etiologically separate from chronic conditions in the HSI. Therefore, a urinary tract infection in a diabetic patient would be considered a short-term problem, while an acute episode of the diabetic condition, such as ketoacidotic shock, would be considered to be related to the chronic condition.

When the physician decides a problem is short-term, he checks "short-term problem," notes whether a prescription drug was ordered, and estimates the number of days required for the patient to return to his functional status prior to the onset of the present illness. When the physician decides that an illness is not subject to resolution within three months, he checks the box labeled "long-term problem," indicates whether or not a prescription medication is being used to manage this problem, and estimates the patient's expected status in three months.

Table 2 describes the completion rate of the time components of the HSI for patients diagnosed as having one of ten common diseases at the time of their first visit to the center in 1975. The Table also includes the rates for patients with all other diseases and for those with no disease at the time of their first visit in 1975. These completion rates are based on a total of 2,674 patient visits. Exclusive of patients with no disease at first visit, status prior to visit had an average completion rate of 89 percent. Status at time of visit had a slightly lower rate of completion, but the average percent completed, exclusive of patients with no disease, was 87 percent. The third component of the HSI, expected status in three months, was completed on an average of 87 percent of the time for all groups of patients except those without disease at the time of their first 1975 visit. This high rate of completion suggests that even where residents were asked to estimate or predict future outcomes, they generally were willing to provide an assessment. Thus, we have received reasonably good compliance among the residents in completing the HSI.

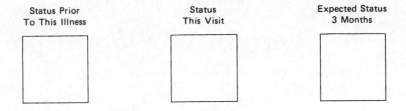

Status Prior
To This Illness

Status
This Visit

Expected Status
3 Months

1) Not symptomatic. Performs usual major activity.

2) Symptomatic. Experiences Discomfort. Performs usual major activity.

3) Activity Restricted.

4) Bed Disabled.

5) At Risk.

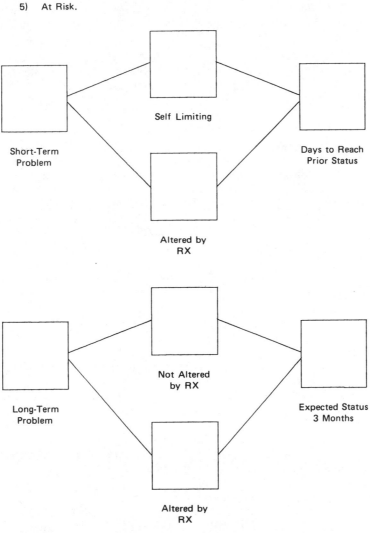

Fig. 1. Health status index.

Table 2. *Completion Rates of HSI January through December 1975, for First Visit in 1975 by Patients Having One or More of Ten Frequently Occurring Diseases, Other Diseases, and No Diseases*

Disease	Number of Patients	Status Prior to Illness Complete		Status This Visit Complete		Expected Status Three Months Complete	
		Number	Percent	Number	Percent	Number	Percent
Hypertension	139	125	90	128	92	117	84
Upper respiratory infection	140	127	91	120	86	112	80
Diabetes mellitus	65	56	86	58	89	52	80
Depression	28	25	89	24	86	22	79
Urinary tract infection	49	47	96	45	92	44	90
Arteriosclerotic heart disease	18	14	78	13	72	12	66
Vaginitis vulvitis	48	45	94	43	90	43	90
Bronchitis	48	45	94	43	90	43	90
Arteriosclerosis	12	11	92	10	83	9	75
Osteoarthritis	11	9	82	11	100	9	82
Other	1557	1422	91	1393	89	1311	84
No disease	569	370	65	376	66	312	54
Total	2674						

Uses of the Health Status Index

Studies of general and family practice indicate that a significant proportion of patients seeking care present with ill-defined symptoms and complaints which do not fit standard classifications of disease.[5,6] The Health Status Index can assist family physicians in assessing and treating these problems by providing a collection of integrated observations on the course of patients' illnesses. Katz and colleagues,[7] and Akpom, Katz, and Densen,[8] for example, have shown how measures of function can be combined with symptoms, clinical indicators of disease (laboratory tests and x-rays) and risk factors to create meaningful classifications of patient illnesses. The family physician can use such classification schemes to categorize ill-defined problems into homogeneous groupings in order to describe changes in the course of these illnesses and to evaluate the effect of different modes of treatment on the duration and severity of these problems. These schemes need not exclude standard disease classifications, but can provide additional information to assist the family physician in defining the course of and in treating ill-defined problems.

The HSI can also assist the physician in defining the course of long-term continuing conditions. For example, during a five-month period of observation, the health status of nine of 20 patients with essential hypertension improved, the status of one patient deteriorated, and the status of ten patients remained unchanged. Of the ten patients whose status remained unchanged, five had no coexisting chronic condition, two had osteoarthritis, two were obese, and one had diabetes mellitus. Three of the nine patients whose status improved had no other chronic condition, one had osteoarthritis, three were obese, one had ischemic heart disease, and one had mitral stenosis. The one patient whose status deteriorated had ischemic heart disease and osteoarthritis. None of the 20 patients, however, sought care for acute conditions which might have distorted observed changes in health status. The presence of coexisting chronic conditions, therefore, did not appear to have any systematic effect on changes in health status. The one exception, perhaps, was the case of the patient who deteriorated over the observation period. This patient was the only one with a coexisting condition (osteoarthritis), as well as evidence of target organ involvement (ischemic heart disease) associated with the hypertension.*

Data such as these can assist family physicians in managing their practices. As they are accumulated they describe a distribution of outcome status over time that establishes outcome norms or standards for different illnesses. These norms can be used to compare patients' courses of illnesses and to identify those who deviate from the norm. They can also be used to examine the appropriateness of patient care, and to identify treatment modalities which produce more desirable outcomes. For example, physicians may wish to question whether or not it is acceptable for patients with hypertension to be symptomatic at the beginning and end of an observation period. If such an outcome is suspect, the physician might review in more detail the care given those patients whose status remained unchanged. Based on an audit of the patients' medical records, he may conclude that care is adequate and that the patients' status could not be improved, or he may decide to alter some aspect of care for these patients to achieve more desirable outcomes. Equally important, when desired outcomes are compared with information describing the resources employed to produce them (eg, the cost of personnel and services), they enable the physician to determine the efficiency of different modes of treatment and of continued care. The Health Status Index, thus, helps the

physician to successfully manage his practice not only by identifying those treatment modes that shorten the duration or reduce the severity of illness, but also by delineating those costs to himself and to the patient that are associated with producing desired outcomes (Table 3).

Finally, the Health Status Index can assist family physicians in providing continuous care, especially for the chronically ill, by describing the impact of the disease process on the patient and by indicating when additional health resources are needed to manage the patient. For example, as patients become restricted in their major activities and confined to bed for longer periods of time, physicians can plan with family members for the care of these patients. Can such patients continue to be cared for at home, or should plans be initiated to secure an appropriate level of institutional care? The measures included in the HSI not only alert physicians to these questions, but they also provide a common language which doctors, nurses, social workers, and representatives of community agencies can use to discuss the options available to the patient. Thus, the HSI assists the physician in addressing chronological, as well as interpersonal and interprofessional, questions of providing continuous care for patients.

In summary, we believe a Health Status Index such as that described can assist family physicians in providing first contact and continuous care for their patients. Further, the HSI can assist physicians in managing their practices and in allocating the resources available in the larger health system for the benefit of their patients. The HSI is extremely valuable for describing the course of most acute and chronic diseases seen within a family practice center and is a good measure of patient outcome. It provides a summary measure of patient health and a mode of communication of patient needs among different health-care providers. The HSI, thus, can be an important instrument in the delivery of family-oriented health care.

* The validity of this HSI was examined in a recent study of hypertensive patients.[9] In this study measures were recorded on 99 hypertensive patients at the beginning and end of a five-month period using the Health Status Index and an Index of Severity which included systolic and diastolic blood pressure and involvement of target organs. Of the 99 patients studied, 40 improved on both measures. Twenty-one patients deteriorated and 38 remained unchanged on the Severity Index. Nineteen patients deteriorated and the status of 40 remained unchanged on the HSI.

Table 3. *Average Number of Visits April through August 1975 and Average Charge per Visit by Change in Health Status of 20 Hypertensive Patients*

	Improved	Deteriorated	No Change
Average number of visits	4	6	5
Average charge per visit	$12	$25*	$10
Total number of patients	9	1	10

* The high average charge per visit for the one patient whose status deteriorated appears reasonable in view of the number of coexisting diseases which were identified.

Acknowledgment

Work on the Health Status Index, and the Health Information System of which it is a part, was conducted by the Office of Health Services Education and Research of the College of Human Medicine, Michigan State University, under a subcontract with the Michigan Cooperative Health Information System of the Michigan Department of Public Health, pursuant to a contract No. HRA 106-74-35 between the National Center for Health Statistics and the Michigan Department of Public Health.

REFERENCES

1. Baker C: What's different about family medicine? J Med Educ 49:229–235, 1974
2. Draper P, Smits HL: The primary-care practitioner—specialist or jack-of-all trades. N Engl J Med 292:903–907, 1975
3. Hennen BK: The dimension of continuity in family practice. J Fam Pract 2:371–374, 1975
4. US Department of Health, Education and Welfare, National Center for Health Statistics: Health survey procedure. PHS Publication 1000, Series 1, No. 2. Washington DC, US Government Printing Office, 1965, p 45
5. Murnagham JH: Review of the conference proceedings. In Murnagham JH (ed): Ambulatory Care Data: Report of the Conference on Ambulatory Medical Care Records. Philadelphia, JB Lippincott, 1973, p 30
6. McFarlane AH, Norman GR: Methods of classifying symptoms, complaints, and conditions. In Murnagham JH (ed): Ambulatory Care Data: Report of the Conference on Ambulatory Medical Care Records. Philadelphia, JB Lippincott, 1973, pp 101–108
7. Katz S, Ford AB, Downs TD, et al: Chronic disease classification in evaluation of medical care programs. Med Care 7:139–143, 1969
8. Akpom CA, Katz S, Densen P: Methods of classifying disability and severity of illness in ambulatory care patients. Med Care 11(suppl):125–131, 1973
9. Given B: Relationship between Process and Outcome Components of Patient Care: An Evaluation Model, dissertation. Michigan State University, East Lansing, 1976

Approaches to the Denominator Problem in Primary Care Research*

Martin Bass

As increasing numbers of morbidity studies from family practice are published, the need for comparability is essential. This can only be accomplished through the use of age-sex specific incidence and prevalence rates. While patient visits or discrete patients visiting are often used as denominators for rate calculations, only the at-risk population reduces the variability due to practice patterns and includes those persons who do not visit during that interval. Three methods of determining the at-risk population are presented: registration, percent utilization, and episodes of illness distribution. The episode of illness approach was tested in five teaching practices and found to give results similar to the registered population only when the total population was included. No method is ideal, and the further search for testing of new approaches is important.

The family physician has a very worthwhile contribution to make in mapping out large areas of disease and dysfunction. He is the first and, in many cases, the only professional to see many problems and illnesses. Thus, he is in an excellent position to describe ambulatory illness, the factors which influence it, and its course over time. Once agreement has been reached on how to record and code our experience, it is not a difficult matter to count the number of cases of influenza, or arthritis, or complications from oral contraceptives. The problem arises when we want to express our experience in a manner that allows us to compare it with the experience of other physicians, or other countries— or even with our own previous experience —so that we can increase our knowledge of the natural history of illness. To say that 50 cases of infectious mononucleosis were seen this year tells about my experience, but little about the illness itself. The significance of this number depends on the number of patients seen this year, their age distribution and the illness experience of the community cared for. The solution

to the problem of comparing data is to express findings in terms of rates which are or can be used by all concerned.

The Denominator Problem

Comparable rates require similarly defined denominators. Easily obtainable denominator values are: the number of patient visits in one year and the number of discrete patients seen in one year. These two values can be obtained from a count of the daily register or the E-book, or they can easily be produced by a computer. Because they are so readily available, they are often used. While these two values, patient visits and patients utilizing, are useful in describing the workload of the practice, they contain too many sources of variability to allow adequate comparisons of incidence and prevalence rates among practices. The primary drawback is that the composition of a physician's yearly visits depends largely on his method of practice —that is, how often he recalls patients for follow-up and the frequency of preventive examinations. To count only those patients who were seen tells us nothing about those patients who did not visit the doctor dur-

* Reprinted by permission from *The Journal of Family Practice*, 3(2):193–195, 1976.

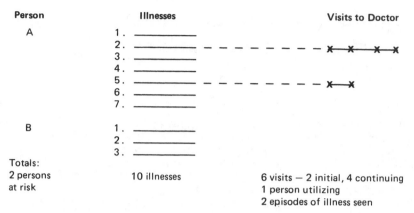

Fig. 1. Illustrative illness behavior of two patients during one year.

ing that interval, even though they were at risk.

I would like to offer a simple example to illustrate the confusion that might arise out of the use of these several possible denominators. Figure 1 illustrates the illness pattern of two patients in one year. Two individuals, A and B, in a single practice, experience seven and three episodes of illness, respectively, in one year. Patient A visits the doctor for two of these episodes. For one episode he is asked to return three times, and for the other he is asked to return once. Patient B does not visit the doctor for any of his episodes of illness. In the office, we have seen and recorded A's two illnesses and six visits. What is our denominator for the expression of our experience in this year? Is it the six visits (two initial and four continuing), the one person utilizing, the two episodes of illness, or the two persons at risk? I would suggest that persons at risk is the most acceptable denominator for office morbidity studies. Ratio equations expressing office morbidity over persons at risk contain only two major sources of variation: the illness pattern of the community, which is the variable of particular interest; and the illness behavior of the individuals, which though it varies considerably from person to person tends to average out within the practice as a whole. An additional source of variation, that of differing practice composition, can be avoided through the use of age-sex specific rates.

How to Determine the At-Risk Population

To express morbidity using proper incidence and prevalence rates, the at-risk population must be known. The established method is to register the population.

1. Registration

Registration entails noting at least the age, sex, and commitment to the practice of all individuals who are under the physician's care. This is the system used in Britain where patients are registered with one physician. This is the practice age-sex register kept as a companion to the E-book.[1] The major problem with this type of age-sex register is difficulty in keeping the register current.[2] This results because of:

1. losses (those not at risk, but registered)
   –patients who move without notification
   –patients admitted to institutions for long-stay care
   –deaths
   –individuals who are away from the

household (students, separations)
– use of other medical facilities
2. gains (those at risk, but not registered)
– late registration of newborns
– individuals who postpone registration until they need medical service

Registration is best for practices with little change, because updating the register is time-consuming and less accurate for practices with a high turnover. For the calculation of rates, the midyear population at risk is usually a good approximation. A reasonably accurate register at each New Year is sufficient to arrive at this figure:

$$\frac{\text{Population at beginning of year} + \text{Population at end of year}}{2}$$

Medical facilities that provide a total service under prepayment schedules may produce good age-sex registers from their accounting procedures. But for many physicians interested in research, registration is time-consuming, expensive, and of questionable accuracy. Other less expensive, more convenient approaches have been sought to determine the at-risk population.

2. Percent Utilization

This method entails multiplying the number of patients utilizing by a correction factor to determine the population at risk. The correction factor is determined for an area by a separate study or through analysis of health insurance statistics. In Saskatchewan, Dr. John Garson has used this approach to produce an at-risk denominator for a morbidity study involving 23 physicians from all parts of the province.[3] The provincial insuring agency records can be analyzed to determine what percent of the population sees their general practitioner. In Britain, 67 percent of the population are seen annually, with variation according to the different age and sex groups.[4] In the

teaching practices of the University of Western Ontario, this figure varies between 70 and 75 percent. By noting the number of patients of each age and sex group seen during the study and multiplying by the appropriate correction factor, the number of people at risk can be calculated. This approach is being considered for multicentered studies, where utilization statistics are available from government-operated, prepaid medical care insurance plans.

3. Episodes of Illness Rate

Dr. James Kilpatrick of Virginia Commonwealth University, while analyzing the data from the Second National British Morbidity Survey, uncovered an intriguing relationship.[5] He noted that the numbers of patients seen with one, two, three, etc, episodes of illness bear a constant relationship to each other. The ratio of successive episode frequencies is constant. This is a unique property of the geometric distribution. For those interested in the mathematics:

> If $f(e)$ represents the frequency of individuals with e episodes, the geometric distribution specifies that $f(e) = (1 - q)\, q^e$ ($e = 0, 1, 2, \ldots$) where q is the constant ratio between successive frequencies; ie, $q = f(e + 1)/f(e)$. Note that $(1 - q)$ is the frequency of individuals with zero episodes.[5]

For the purposes of the Second National Morbidity Survey, any face-to-face contact between doctor and patient is counted as a consultation. An episode of illness, on the other hand, is defined as a period of illness for which there were one or more consultations. Episodes tend to reflect the number of problems seen by the general practitioner.

Dr. Donald Crombie of the Birmingham Research Unit of the Royal College of General Practitioners, has applied this principle to the reported episode rates to 50 general practices with verified regis-

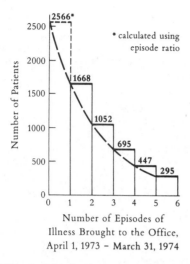

Fig. 2. Distribution of episodes of illness—for one year—St. Joseph's Family Medical Centre, London, Ontario (excluding prophylactic procedures & prenatal care).

tered populations.[6] The calculated populations came to within five percent of the registered populations in 49 cases. In the 50th, the physician was known to be a poor recorder and the result was markedly deviant. Since there is no known theoretical reason that the episode rate should take the form of a geometric distribution, we wondered if this finding was specific to practice in Great Britain. Perhaps in North America, with our different methods of practice and different population, the relationship would not be found.

To explore the validity of the episode rate, we used this approach on our registered population at one family medical

center of the University of Western Ontario, London, Ontario. It necessitated calculating episodes of illness. This was possible because each presentation of a problem is categorized as being either the initiation of a new episode or as one visit in a continuing episode.[7] Figure 2 shows our results for all visits between April 1, 1973, and March 31, 1974. The average ratio between episode frequencies is .65. By using the relationship:

$$\frac{\text{Persons with one episode}}{\text{Persons with zero episodes}} = .65$$

the number of people that presented zero episodes of illness was calculated and, by adding this value to the previously known number of persons utilizing the center, a total number of persons at risk was obtained (7,182). The calculated result for the total population was one percent higher than our registered 1973 year-end population (7,102). From Table 1, it is seen that the ratios for the total population are consistent. With the smaller numbers involved in the male and female categories, variability is more pronounced. Our initial results are encouraging for this approach.

Conclusions

The following points can be made concerning the state of the art on this subject:

1. Attention to the denominator, its type and composition is important for com-

Table 1. *Episode Ratios and Estimated At-Risk Population of the Family Medical Center for Period April 1, 1973 to March 31, 1974*

	Ratio of Successive Episode Frequencies				Episode Rate Estimate of At-Risk Population	Registered Population December 1973
	2/1	3/2	4/3	5/4		
Total population	.63	.66	.64	.66	7182	7102
Males only	.58	.66	.55	.70	3119	3242
Females only	.68	.66	.71	.64	4073	3856

parability of results in morbidity studies.

2. The population at risk is the most satisfactory denominator.

3. Registration is the best present method of determining the at-risk population, but problems may exist in its accuracy and it is time-consuming.

4. New methods of denominator determination are needed before family practice research can involve the majority of practicing physicians in morbidity studies.

5. The Episode Rate and Utilization Correction Factor are two untested methods that offer promise.

Acknowledgments

The author is grateful for the assistance of Dr. JP Newell, Dr. G Dickie, and Dr. IR McWhinney. Dr. DL Crombie, Dr. JZ Garson and Dr. SJ Kilpatrick provided thoughtful insights.

Dr. Bass has been supported by a National Health Scholar Award.

REFERENCES

1. Eimerl TS, Laidlaw AJ: A Handbook for Research in General Practice. Edinburgh, E & S Livingstone, 1969

2. Morrell DC, Gage HC, Robinson NA: Patterns of demand in general practice. J R Coll Gen Pract 19:331–342, 1970

3. Garson JZ, Garson C: Report of a pilot recording project in family practice. Presented at the University of Western Ontario Workshop on the Denominator Problem, London, Ontario, October 11, 1974

4. Crombie DL: Changes in patterns of recorded morbidity. In Taylor D (ed): Benefits and Risks in Medical Care. London, Great Britain, Office of Health Economics, 1974

5. Kilpatrick SJ: The distribution of episodes of illness—a research tool in general practice? J R Coll Gen Pract 25:686–90, 1975

6. Crombie DL: The denominator problem. Presented at the University of Western Ontario Workshop on the Denominator Problem, London, Ontario, October 11, 1974

7. Newell JP: Information from family practice—why and how? Can Fam Physician 21(4):47–53, 1975

A Family Medicine Information System: The Beginning of a Network for Practicing and Resident Family Physicians*

*Larry A. Green, Roger L. Simmons, Frank M. Reed,
Perry S. Warren, John D. Morrison*

This Family Medicine Information System is presented as a problem-oriented, family-oriented, selectively automated medical information system useful in family medicine residencies, as well as in the office practice of family medicine. Still developmental, the system is already used in five residencies and five practices by 97 providers caring for 13,205 families with 34,989 members. The automated function is integrated by a family registration document and an encounter form, and is organized into three modules: patient accounts, practice analysis, and patient management.

Several examples of how this system is being used are offered to illustrate its breadth of application. Calculations are presented which indicate that the system is economically competitive with commercially available billing systems while offering increments of: (1) access to information on the part of the practice 23 hours per day; (2) family orientation; (3) flexibility in cross relating patients, services, providers, diseases, and costs; and (4) ready comparisons across teaching, nonteaching, urban, and rural settings.

Future directions for this system are toward: (1) implementation in additional practices; (2) more intelligent automated analysis; (3) application directly into the physician/patient encounter; (4) the exercise of its research potential; and (5) the maintenance of the data bank.

This Family Medicine Information System (FMIS) is a selectively automated medical record and information system for family medicine residencies and private practices. It is designed to serve the practicing family physician who has developed "the mind set of critical inquiry."[1] Using the information required to register patients and bill for services and little or no additional provider work, the FMIS relates families, providers, services, diseases, and costs across urban, rural, teaching, and nonteaching settings. It consists of: (1) a paper record developed in the University of Colorado family medicine residencies, similar to the record described by the University of Rochester,[2] and (2) automated aspects developed by the Mountain Plains Outreach Program and Community Electrocardiographic Interpretative Service.

The Mountain Plains Outreach Program is a consortium composed of Rose Medical Center, the University of Colorado Medical Center Departments of Family Medicine and of Preventive Medicine, the School of Nursing, the Dental School, Colorado State University, and the US Department of Health, Education, and Welfare's Health for Underserved Rural Areas Program (HURA). The goal of the Mountain Plains Outreach Program is to address the reasons why physicians do not enter practice in rural areas and to provide the necessary support systems to attract well-trained primary care physicians who intend to remain in rural communities. The FMIS was developed to support practice operations, patient care, physician and patient education, and research.

The Community Electrocardiographic Interpretative Service is a non-profit, physician-operated company that performs research and development in computer-

* Reprinted by permission from *The Journal of Family Practice*, 7(3): 567–576, 1978.

assisted clinical systems. Prior to its involvement in the FMIS development, the Community Electrocardiographic Interpretative Service had developed and operated similar systems for ECG interpretation, medical history, physician consultation and education, and clinical data storage and retrieval. The group became involved in the FMIS because of its interest in demonstrating that computer-assisted ambulatory care data management can be a powerful tool to the practicing and training physician in urban and rural areas.

The basic premises of the FMIS include: (1) systems describing family medical care are needed; (2) the information required to bill for services and operate a private practice includes much of the information required to analyze the practice from the viewpoints of patient care, education, and research; (3) data systems must assist, not disrupt, the day-to-day practice of family medicine; (4) the family physician's system should be family-oriented; (5) flexibility to relate multiple factors across multiple settings should be assured; and (6) the system must be affordable.

The system is now operational in ten practices representing urban, rural, teaching, and nonteaching practices, including residents and fully trained family physicians. This paper presents the basic anatomy and physiology of the data system and, by examples, the way this system is beginning to be used. As of March 1978, 13,205 families representing 34,989 patients have generated 44,114 encounters involving 16,189 active patients. Ninety-seven providers have made 56,743 diagnoses. Participating practices are located in communities as small as 1,000 persons and as large as Denver.

General Description

The FMIS is bionic, ie, it integrates manual and automated parts. The manual part consists of an effective chart system and is very important. However, the automated part is the focus of what follows.

The automated sections of the FMIS include a complete patient accounts module, a practice analysis module, and a patient management module. The information required for these three modules is collected onto two documents. The Family Information Sheet (Figure 1) is the registration document that describes families in the practice. It records basic demographic and fiscal responsibility information about the entire family. It is completed when the first member of the family becomes a patient in the practice. Data for all members of the family are recorded even though they may not be patients in the practice. The Encounter Form (Figure 2) records the patient's identification, problems, and all services performed or ordered for each patient visit.

The patient accounts module accepts charges for all services, prepares insurance forms, writes family statements, and produces fiscal reports such as the family ledger, aged accounts receivable, detailed charge and receipt listings, and monthly summaries of all the charges, receipts, and adjustments to patient accounts.

The practice analysis module prepares each quarter an age/sex registry, age/sex distribution of patients seen, morbidity reports, and service (procedures, patient visits, laboratory) reports for each provider and practice, and for the entire system. These reports allow each provider to compare his/her experience with other providers in the same practice or residency and with all other practices in the system.

The patient management module enables the users to extract any cohort of patients. The cohort can be presented as a list or as mailing labels for use in outreach, audit, and research.

Anatomy

The anatomy or structure of the automated FMIS includes a nervous system, some muscles, and a skeleton.

The nervous system is the brain power of the system's users (who control its de-

FAMILY INFORMATION

Family Name _____

No. _____

Prov. _____ Prov. No. _____

Referred by: _____

Date: _____

Day _____ Mo. _____ Yr. _____

Confirmed ☐

Entered ☐

HEAD OF HOUSEHOLD INFORMATION

NAME	CODE	SEX	RACE	DATE OF BIRTH DAY MO. YR.	RELATIONSHIP TO HEAD OF HOUSEHOLD	F.M. PATIENT	LIVING AT HOME	SHARED CARE	RECEIVES BILL
						Y N	Y N	Y N	
Occupation						Y N	Y N	Y N	
Business Phone						Y N	Y N	Y N	
No. in Family						Y N	Y N	Y N	
BC/BS Group No.						Y N	Y N	Y N	
BC/BS Individual No.						Y N	Y N	Y N	
BS Subscriber's Name						Y N	Y N	Y N	

FAMILY ADDRESS (INCLUDE STREET NAME, NO., APT NO., CITY, STATE, ZIP)

RESIDENCE PHONE

Medicare Health Insurance Claim No. (Health Insurance Benefit No.) _____

Medical Assistance Care No. (Medicaid No.) _____

Any Other Insurance: _____ Company _____

Subscriber or Policy No. _____

PLEASE COMPLETE ONLY FOR FAMILY MEMBERS OTHER THAN HEAD OF HOUSEHOLD WHO CARRY PERSONAL HEALTH INSURANCE

Name _____

Business Phone _____

Address (If different from above) _____

Occupation _____

Medicare Health Insurance Claim No. (Health Insurance Benefit No.) _____

BC/BS Group No. _____

Medical Assistance Care No. (Medicaid No.) _____

BC/BS Individual No. _____

Other Insurance: Company _____

BS Subscriber Name _____

Subscriber or Policy No. _____

Name _____

Business Phone _____

Address (If different from above) _____

Occupation _____

Medicare Health Insurance Claim No. (Health Insurance Benefit No.) _____

BC/BS Group No. _____

Medical Assistance Care No. (Medicaid No.) _____

BC/BS Individual No. _____

Other Insurance: Company _____

BS Subscriber Name _____

Subscriber or Policy No. _____

HEAD OF HOUSEHOLD WILL RECEIVE BILL FOR ENTIRE FAMILY UNLESS OTHERWISE DESIGNATED

Fig. 1. Family information sheet.

Encounter Form

PATIENTS NAME

LAST   FIRST   MI

ATTENDING PHYSICIAN   PROVIDER

DATE OF ACCIDENT

OFFICE   PATIENT NUMBER   DAY   MO.   YR.   PR   DAY   MO.   YR.

RETURN TO WORK   Y   N   DATE

DATE OF BIRTH   DATE OF SERVICE

HOSPITALS:
ROSE   58   AURORA 61   B.S.
CO. GEN   97   SWEDISH 60   M/CARE
CHILDREN'S 2   PORTER   4   M/CAID

PVT.   NONE

PLACE: OFFICE   HOME   NURSING HOME

OUT PAT HOSP (OP)   IN PAT. HOSP (IP)

WORKMAN'S COMP.   3RD PARTY   LIABILITY   ACCIDENT

NO SHOW ☐   CANCELLED ☐   WALK IN ☐   LEFT ☐   RESCHEDULE ☐

REASON FOR VISIT (PATIENT'S OWN WORDS)

SERVICES		CHARGES
OFFICE VISITS		
NEW PT. BRIEF	90000	
NEW PT. LTD.	90010	
NEW PT. COMP.	90020	
EST. PT. BRIEF	90040	
EST. PT. LTD.	90050	
EST. PT. INTERM	90060	
EST. PT. COMP.	90080	
ANNUAL PHYSICAL	90088	
COLLEGE PE (17-21)	90082	
CHILD PE (6-16)	90085	
CHILD PE (0-5)	90091	
WELL CHILD PKG.	90090	
OB PKG.	59400	
OB DELIVERY	59410	
PRENATAL VISIT	59420	
POST PARTUM VISIT	59430	
EMG. OFFICE VISIT		
HOME VISIT	99500	
NURSING HOME VISIT	90350	
COUNSEL. 25 MIN. I/G		
COUNSEL. 50 MIN. I/G		
HOSPITAL VISITS		
ADMIT DATE DISCHG. DATE		
INIT. LTD.	90200	
INIT. COMP.	90220	
HOSP. CARE—ROUTINE	90250	
INTERM	90260	
CRIT. CARE		
FROM: TO:		
INIT. CRIT. CARE	90293	
VST. CRIT. CARE	90270	
OTHER		
NURSE VISIT	90030	
NEWBORN CARE	90285	
FRACTURE CARE		
ASSIST. SURG.		
EMG. ROOM VISIT		
MISC.		
SPECIMEN DRAW.	99000	
DRAW. & CENTR. SVC.	99005	
COMPLETION OF FORMS	99080	

LABORATORY		LOC	CHARGES
ALK. PHOS.	84075		
ANTI BODY SCR.	86260		
BILIRUBIN	82250		
BUN	84520		
CBC	85010		
CHOLESTEROL	82465		
CREAT. CLEARANCE	82575		
CREATININE	82540		
CULT( )	87080		
DIFFERENTIAL	85040		
ELECTROLYTES	80004		
ESTRIOL	83235		
GC CULT	87063		
GLUCOSE—F	84330		
GLUCOSE—2°	84330		
GLUCOSE—R	84330		
GLUCOSE—TT			
GRAM STAIN	87000		
HB	83032		
HCT	85055		
HEMA CULT	82270		
LIPID PROFILE	83710		
LIVER PROFILE	80006		
MCV	85011		
MONOSPOT	86300		
PLATELETS	85580		
PKU	84040		
POTASSIUM	84140		
PREG. TEST	83160		
PRO-TIME	85610		
PTT	85730		
SGOT	82465		
SED RATE	85650		
SMA 6-12	80012		
SMA 18-22	80013		
STOOL OVA-PARA	87010		
STREP SCREEN	87061		
T3	83440		
T4	83450		
THYROID PROFILE	80003		
TRIGYCER	84475		
UA COMP.	81000		
UA DIPSTICK	81816		
UA MICRO	81015		
URIC ACID	84550		
URINARY PROTEIN 24°			
VDRL	86411		
WBC	85030		
WET PREP	87010		
OB PROFILE	08991		
OTHERS			

PROCEDURES		CHARGES
ANOSCOPY	46600	
AUDIOMETRY	92505	
ASPIRATION JOINT	20610	
CAST Apply/Change/Repair	20610	
CATH. BLADDER		
CIRCUMCISION	54150	
CRYOSURGERY		
CERVIX	57505	
SKIN	17100	
OTHER		
DEBRIDEMENT	11030	
DRESSING CHANGE	06114	
EAR IRRIGATION	92900	
EKG 12 LEAD	93000	
EKG RHYTHM	93040	
ELECTROCAUTERY	17110	
EXCISION, BIOPSY	11100	
I & D	10060	
IUD INSERTION	58300	
LACERATION		
LOCATION		
LENGTH		
SURGERY		
PAP SMEAR	88101	
SIGMOIDOSCOPY	45300	
SIGMOIDOSCOPY W/BX	45305	
SPLINT		
TONOMETRY	92100	
VASECTOMY	55250	
VISION SCREENING	05401	
VITAL CAPACITY	94150	
RADIOLOGY		
CHEST X-RAY		
OTHER		
IMMUNIZATIONS/INJECTIONS		
DPT 06768 ☐ DT 06769 ☐ TT 06861 ☐		
OPV 06827 ☐ RUBELLA 06807 ☐		
MUMPS 06813 ☐ MEASLES 06806 ☐		
TINE 06864 ☐ PPD 06837 ☐		
INFLUENZA 06793 ☐ MMR 90700 ☐		
THER. INJ. 90705 ☐		
DRUG:		
DOSAGE:		
OTHER (SPECIFY) ☐		

MEDICATION

PROB NO. ☐☐☐ / ☐☐☐ / ☐☐☐ / ☐☐☐

	SERVICES	
	SUPPLIES/LAB	
CASH/CHECK	PROCEDURES & INJECTIONS	
	TOTAL CHARGES	

POSTED ☐

SUPPLIES

WRITTEN DIAGNOSIS FOR INSURANCE

ADDITIONAL INSTRUCTIONS

DISPOSITION

NEXT APPOINTMENT

WITH (PROVIDER)

AMT. OF TIME   5   15   30   45

CONSULTANT/HOSPITAL

SIGNATURE

PATIENT COPY
RETAIN FOR YOUR RECORDS

Fig. 2. Encounter form.

sign and function), coupled with a time-sharing computer system. This computer is a Digital Equipment Company PDP 11/40 with 96,000 characters of main memory and 80 million characters of disc storage. It uses a Meditch Interpretative Information System (MIIS) operating system and programming language. The MIIS system, a dialect of Massachusetts General Utility and Multiprograming System (MUMPS), is supplied by Medical Information Technology of Cambridge, Massachusetts. This system allows multiple practices to use the computer simultaneously, each with its own partition in the memory. It appears to the user that he/she has a personal computer in his/her office.

The muscle of the system is supplied by users at the practice site combined with complex applications programs at the computer center. These programs were derived from the Business Office System of the Cardiovascular Clinic in Oklahoma City. Through this practice-computer center interaction, the data entry, some report generation, and the interrogation of the data base are usually done at the practice, while the computer center assists with complex tasks.

The skeleton of the automated FMIS is formed by a communication network leading to each practice from the computer center. In eight of the ten practices using the system, the skeleton is built with leased telephone lines connecting the computer with one or two computer terminals at the practice site. At two sites, communication between the practice and the regional computer center is done by mail and/or messenger.

Physiology

In general, the functions of the automated FMIS are to ingest family, medical, and fiscal data about the patient populations of the practices, and analyze the data to produce useful patient accounts, practice management, and patient management reports.

The *patient accounts* functions are similar to other well-designed, automated billing systems. Briefly, the purpose of this module is twofold: first, it is intended to provide a practice with assistance in maintaining an adequate cash flow; secondly, the data used in performing the first function are also used to generate files used for practice analysis and patient management reports.

The *practice analysis module* provides quarterly reports describing the patient population of the practice, problems and diagnoses of this population, and services performed or ordered by the provider. The first of these takes the form of two reports: the age/sex registry and the age/sex patient distribution report.

The age/sex registry is a graphic representation of those family members registered in the practice. It displays the percentage of males and females in each of 16 age groups who have been registered and who claim to be patients of the practice. These percentages are displayed for each provider, each practice, and for the entire system. The display of these data allows easy comparison of one provider's patient population with that of other providers in the same practice and of the population of one practice with all the practices using the system. Since the users of the FMIS currently include training practices as well as private practices in urban and rural areas of Colorado, the graph for all patients represents a cross-section of the family medicine patient population in the state. This characteristic allows meaningful comparison among geographic regions, teaching and nonteaching settings, and urban and rural settings.

The age/sex patient distribution report takes the same form as the registry and displays the number and percentages of patients seen during the time period covered by the report. It is important to note that this is not an encounter or patient visit report, since a patient visiting multiple times during the period will only be counted once. In addition to its usefulness for studying and comparing the distribution of patients seen by a provider, a practice, and all practices, this report, compared to the age/sex registry, determines what portion of the registered population is actually visiting the provider, the practice, or all practices.

The practice analysis reports include a *morbidity report*. This quarterly report describes the problems seen by each provider, each practice, and all practices. The problems are listed in a ranked frequency distribution with the most frequent problem first, the next most frequent second, and so on. The rank of each problem in the provider's practice and in all practices is displayed along with the provider's rank. Also listed is the number of times the problem has been recorded, the number of patients with the problem, their percentage of the visiting patient population, and the maximum and mean number of visits for the problem.

Again, as with all reports in the practice analysis module, the morbidity report allows study of the experience of any single provider in comparison with the experience of other providers in the system. It also provides a basis for monitoring the incidence and prevalence of primary care problems in an entire state.

The *service analysis* generates three reports. This series first describes for each practice the number and percentage of all services, patient visits, and charges provided by each physician. The second section lists for each physician the number and percentages of services in each of several categories: office visits, hospital visits, laboratory services, surgical procedures, consultations, radiology services, and other medical services. The third section provides a detailed list of each service in the category shown in the previous section. The services are ranked by frequency of occurrence for the provider, his/her practice, and for all practices.

There is a special part of the practice analysis module that allows documentation and analysis of a resident's experience during his training. The basic FMIS collects information for services performed for which the practice charges, but not all residents' services are charged. Residents carry a 3×5 card for recording services performed that are not charged. These data are added to charged services in the FMIS files to produce a residency experience file. Thus, the entire experience of the resident can be reported during and at the completion of training. These reports allow curriculum modification to optimize training experience and documentation of the residents' skills, useful in requesting hospital privileges.

Applications

Much of the literature referring to automated medical record systems has been presented from an academic view. Sometimes, reference is made to use by practicing family physicians, but this applicability is mainly in fiscal management. In addition to this important function, the FMIS gives the family physician the ability: (1) to escape the false stereotype of the nonresearch-oriented keeper of the URI turnstyle, and (2) to participate in the invigorating exercise of studying his own work. This section presents specific examples of how the FMIS was used this past year in a Colorado family medicine residency and in a practice begun in September 1977, served by a residency-trained family physician working in a community of 3,000 people. The examples were selected not to be exhaustive, but to indicate the flexibility of the FMIS in the hands of its users. Six categories helped organize the examples:

1. Teaching/Learning

1. The physician in the practice has selected continuing education courses to further understanding of the problems he most frequently encounters. Since his nurse has a provider number, her morbidity index and service reports also indicate her continuing education needs.

2. The weekly conferences in the resi-

dency were designed to include management of most frequent diagnoses; for example, during one report period, 379 prenatal visits were performed involving 95 patients producing the second most common diagnosis. Therefore, at the beginning of the academic year, the first series of conferences offered were in prenatal care and the management of third trimester complications.

3. The morbidity report from the last quarter of 1977 indicated lacerations were the tenth most common diagnosis in the entire system, but were 31st in the residency. Bruises and contusions were 20th in the system, but 61st in the residency. The conclusion was that residents received an inadequate exposure to trauma and one that differed from that of practicing physicians in Colorado. Therefore, there has been a revision of the Emergency Room curriculum and the addition of a rural practice experience which, the information system has indicated, will include more exposure to trauma.

4. Especially important is the feedback to individual physicians concerning their performances. When one physician recognized that his most frequent laboratory procedure was a protime while the remainder of the system ranked that tenth, he immediately inquired about the age of his patient population and some specific diagnostic categories. This prompted the use of the age/sex registry and the morbidity index. Thus, the inquisitive posture was promoted.

2. Evaluation

1. The residency wants individual residents to experience an appropriate sample of family practice. No corrective actions were judged necessary for Dr. A when her experience was reviewed as follows. Doctor A, during the last quarter of 1977, conducted 156 encounters involving 82 patients and made 200 diagnoses. Her top ten diagnoses were prenatal care, general health maintenance, diarrhea, postnatal care, pain in a limb, upper respiratory tract infection, depressive neurosis, menometrorrhagia, perinatal problems, and abdominal pain. Of Dr. A's services, 32 percent were rendered as office visits, 28 percent involved the laboratory, 16 percent were surgical, three percent were provided in the Emergency Room, and seven percent involved hospital visits. Doctor A's average charge for an office visit was $15.80. Her most common laboratory procedure was a urinalysis, which was the second most common laboratory procedure in the entire system as well as in the practice. Doctor A sees many more boys under the age of five, men between the ages of 25 and 30, and women between the ages of 20 and 25 than does the rest of the practice or the entire system. Doctor A inserted two IUDs during the report period, did one sigmoidoscopy, and had nine patients admitted to the hospital. On similar review, another physician, however, was discovered to have seen no patients with otitis media. Therefore, a physician who had otitis media as his second most common diagnosis was notified and was able to demonstrate the disease readily to the physician not having otitis in his practice.

2. A pediatric (age 12 to 24 months) immunization status audit of the practice was conducted in January 1978, and showed only 33 percent compliance. Names and telephone numbers of inadequately immunized patients were produced, and these patients were contacted and immunized. Re-audit six weeks later found over 95 percent of these children receiving appropriate immunization.

3. The standard morbidity reports indicated, in the last quarter of 1977, that the average pregnant woman in the residency had 12 prenatal visits. This was interpreted as an acceptable performance. On the other hand, the average number of visits for a person who had acute otitis media was 1.6, which implied inadequate follow-up.

3. Administration

1. One of the first needs of the practice was determination of malpractice insurance rates. In addition to filling out the usual questionnaire, it was possible to provide the insurance carrier with data on diagnoses and procedures done in the practice. This resulted in a 50 percent reduction in malpractice insurance rates over what was previously projected. Annual review is available at insurance renewal time.

2. A local prepaid insurance group is attracting a large number of patients, many of whom are residency patients. It became increasingly important for the Family Medicine Center to be a participant in the prepaid program. The program, however, was concerned about laboratory utilization by physicians in training. Information generated by standard reports documented that the amount of the patient's dollar spent on laboratory services averaged 19 cents for the physicians in the residency. This assured the administration of the prepaid group that these resident physicians do not overspend on laboratory services.

3. Since the system automatically prepares claims for Medicare, Medicaid, Blue Shield, prepaid groups, and commercial insurance, physician and staff involvement in the insurance claim process is minimized. The FMIS also assists in the collection of fees by providing a modified aged accounts receivable report which includes the address and telephone number of families with delinquent accounts. Furthermore, it offers the ability to assign a collection message to the monthly statement, either automatically or manually.

4. Service

1. The FMIS facilitated on-site evaluation of a group of patients by a specialist. All female patients between 35 and 50 years of age with irregular menses were identified and evaluated by a gynecologist at the practice site. Not only was this more convenient for the patients, but it promoted the continuity of their care and furthered the education of their physician.

2. In the fall of 1977, the faculty and residents determined the population which they wished to have receive an immunization against influenza. The patients meeting the criteria were readily identified. Simultaneously, mailing labels were produced and those patients were notified of the office schedule designed to facilitate their receiving the immunization.

5. Patient Education

1. An item of intense public health concern in the community was streptococcal infection. At the conclusion of the last quarter of 1977, it was possible to demonstrate that the incidence of streptococcal pharyngitis was lower in the practice than the average in the rest of the FMIS system. Newspaper articles aimed at public education on streptococcal infection were published using data generated by the system.

2. The residency's head nurse teaches classes on breastfeeding. The FMIS assists her by identifying all of the pregnant women in the practice and notifying these expectant families of the availability of these classes.

6. Practice Planning

1. The FMIS assisted the practice in the determination of the appropriate time to bring on a new partner. The growth projections suggest that a new partner might be necessary 15 to 18 months after the practice opened.

2. When the opportunity to hire a full-time pediatrician for the residency arose, the FMIS indicated that 45 percent of the visiting patients were under the age of 20 and over one third of the hospital admis-

sions were newborn babies, suggesting that a pediatrician would be a timely addition to the residency faculty.

Cost

One of the stated goals of the development of the Family Medicine Information System was to create a cost effective, automated billing and data system applicable to both training centers and actual family medicine practice sites. The system must take the place of staff time and/or improve the quality of the tasks performed. While the FMIS may not replace an insurance clerk, it allows more effective utilization of staff time and an expanded and improved level of working knowledge about the practice, the providers, the patients, and the management systems. The ten practices using the FMIS are in various stages of development and growth and utilization of components of the Family Medicine Information System. As a result of this development and growth, it was necessary to examine utilization and cost of the system by each individual practice. The compilation of the information provided enough data and cost information to develop two illustrative models.

The first is a one-physician practice with an average patient load of 35 encounters per day, a registered family population of 1,600, with a growth rate of approximately 50 families per month. This model includes figures for a practice in close proximity to the computer center and also a practice using long distance leased lines. The second model is a two-physician practice seeing an average of 70 patients per day, with a registered family population of 2,800 and an average growth rate of 75 families per month. This, too, reflects both an intown and long distance relationship to the computer center. The assessment of staff time needed for registering new families and putting them into the data system, and making receipt and adjustment entries was calculated by observing staff at prac-

tices using the FMIS. The cost of staff time was calculated using average 1978 salaries.

Table 1 reflects comparative costs for an on-line 35-patient per day practice and a 70-patient per day practice, also on-line. The doubling of volume illustrates the economies of scale experienced by greater utilization of fixed cost categories such as: computer charge, terminal and printer rental, and the leased line charge. A 35-patient per day practice using batch processing on the FMIS would cost $692 per month, 90 cents per encounter per month, and 43 cents per registered family per month. The 70-patient per day practice would cost $1324.25 per month, 88 cents per patient encounter, and 47 cents per registered family per month.

At this time, the FMIS is competitive in cost with commercial systems in the region, while offering increments in: access to information on the part of the practice (23 hours per day); family orientation; flexibility in cross relating patients, services, providers, diseases, and costs; and ready comparisons across teaching, nonteaching, urban, and rural settings.

Comment

Kerr White[3] described a renaissance of clinical research in which research is "conducted with the cooperation of ambulatory patients in the doctor's office, the health center, the clinic, the outpatient department and in the home." As articles by Smith,[4] Braunstein,[5] and Rodnick[6] confirm, the FMIS is but one of several innovative systems assisting such investigation. However, the implementation of the FMIS into practices: (1) in diverse settings, (2) without disrupting the practice of family medicine, and (3) at affordable cost, may be particularly useful in the further development of family medicine. Already, physicians using the system express their pleasure at having an effective tool to review their own behavior. They also emphasize the importance of being part of a larger

Table 1. *Comparative Costs*

	35-Patients/Day*			70-Patients/Day*		
Staff Time						
New families	50/month × $1.00 =		50.00	75/month × $1.00 =		75.00
Encounters	770/month ×	.20 =	154.00	1,500/month ×	.20 =	300.00
Receipt and adjustments	350/month ×	.05 =	17.50	700/month ×	.05 =	35.00
Subtotal			$221.50			$410.00
Forms						
Encounter forms	770/month × $	.10 =	77.00	1,500/month × $	.10 =	150.00
FIS	50/month ×	.12 =	6.00	75/month ×	.12 =	90.00
Statements	800/month ×	.25 =	200.00	1,300/month ×	.25 =	325.00
Insurance	260/month ×	.10 =	26.00	500/month ×	.10 =	50.00
Aged accounts	1,600/month ×	.01 =	16.00	2,500/month ×	.01 =	28.00
Master patient list	1,600/month ×	.01 =	16.00	2,500/month ×	.01 =	28.00
Subtotal			$341.00			$671.00
Computer						
Computer charge	$350/month		350.00	$350/month		350.00
Terminal and printer	$105/month		105.00	$105/month		105.00
Leased line	$ 35/month		35.00	$ 35/month		35.00
Subtotal			$490.00			$490.00
Total (in-town site)			$1,052.50			$1,571.00
Registered family/month (in-town site)			$ .66			$ .56
Each encounter (in-town site)			1.36			1.05
Rural site additional leased line cost	$190/month		190.00	$190/month		190.00
Total (rural site)			$1,242.50			$1,761.00
Registered family/month (rural site)			$ .78			$ .63
Each encounter (rural site)			1.61			1.17

* Average.

system that helps them avoid a sense of professional isolation and encourages a sense of belonging to family medicine as an important, growing discipline.

Tables 2, 3, and 4 summarize the reports produced by the FMIS. Those marked with an asterisk are still developmental and are not yet functional. The listings imply where the system has been and where the system will go. Initially, the assurance of cash flow was paramount, but future developments will be toward: (1) additional practices using the FMIS, (2) more intelligent automated analysis (for example, Fubar's opinion), (3) applications directly into the physician/patient encounter, (4) the exercise of its research potential, and (5) learning to maintain the data bank.

Table 2. *Patient Accounts Module*

Patient/family statement
Insurance claims forms
  Blue Shield
  Medicare
  Medicaid
  AMA Universal
  Prepaid
  Commercial
  Workman's Compensation
Ledgers
Aged accounts receivable reports
  Complete
  Modified (patient's address and telephone number
    for delinquent accounts)
Monthly summary of accounts receivable
Daily charge and receipt list
Special reports

Table 3. *Practice Analysis Module*

Master patient list (monthly)
Family registration and activity report (quarterly)
Age/sex registry (quarterly)
Age/sex distribution of visiting patients quarterly)
Morbidity report (quarterly)
Service reports (quarterly)
  Practice service summary
  Provider service summary
  Provider service detail
Fubar's opinion
Special report

Authors' Update

This system continues to grow in size (it included over 50,000 different patients and processed almost $3.5 million in charges from July 1, 1979 through June 30, 1980). It also continues to evolve.

Current developments emphasize quality assurance efforts through "exception reports" and "tracking systems." Continuing efforts are being directed toward managing information in the office setting such that provider-patient encounters are enhanced.

Additional work is also underway to develop educational packages for patients and other educational packages for providers—as part of an office information system. The system at its current state of development is currently being tested on small computers suitable for operation within physicians' offices.

Table 4. *Patient Management Module*

Family profile
Patient profile
Problem surveillance and follow-up
Patient education assistance package
Special reports

REFERENCES

1. Geyman JP: On the need for critical inquiry in family medicine. J Fam Pract 4:195, 1977
2. Froom J, Culpepper L, Boisseau V, et al: An integrated medical record and data system for primary care: Parts 1-8. J Fam Pract 4:951, 1149; 5:113, 265, 427, 627, 845, 1007, 1977
3. White K: Primary care research and the new epidemiology. J Fam Pract 3:579, 1976
4. Smith HT, Schroer BJ, Bynum JD: Combining medical information with a business data system. J Fam Pract 2:365, 1975
5. Braunstein ML, Schuman SH, Curry HB: An online clinical information system in family practice. J Fam Pract 5:617, 1977
6. Rodnick JE: The use of automated ambulatory medical records. J Fam Pract 5:253, 1977

A Comparison of the Morbidity Recorded in Two Family Practice Surveys*

S.J. Kilpatrick, Jr., Maurice Wood

Crombie and his associates have recently summarized the results of their National Morbidity Survey in general practice in England.[1] The current paper presents a comparison of one year's data from Virginia with Crombie's study. The Virginia Family Practice Record System is modeled on the Second National Morbidity Survey with minor modifications. In order to use a problem-oriented medical record, our diagnostic coding utilizes a modified RCGP classification (RCGP [US]). There is no provision in our system for changing diagnosis as there is in the National Morbidity Survey.

Family practitioners in the Virginia study summarize each face-to-face contact by listing the problems presented on a worksheet. This procedure and the contents of these records have been described by Marsland et al.[2] Since problems are coded by the physician as new or old problems, we can count the number of episodes of disease brought by a given patient to his family practitioner in a given year. An episode is a period of disease during which there has been one or more visits to the family practitioner for that problem. For the most part this paper deals with episode rates per 100 patients per year, that is, the number of new problems brought to the family practitioner by 100 patients in a year. The episode rate per 100 patients is closer to the incidence of morbidity in the community. The physician can influence this rate by the number of new problems he codes during a visit. However, it is felt that the episode rate per 100 patients per year is less sensitive to physician influence than, say, total visits per 100 patients per year, a large component of which is repeat visits initiated by the physician rather than the patients.

Results

Table 1 summarizes the two studies. Note that we have further divided our data into the seven community and three teaching practices. In one year, we recorded about one third of the number of patients in the English study. Family practitioners in the community practices see about twice as many patients as do their peers in England.

Since age and sex affects the episode rate per 100 patients and since the composition of patient populations varies from practice to practice, we standardize episode rates per 100 patients by age and sex. In fact, the Virginia FY (Fiscal Year) 75 study had 8.5 percent more persons aged 15 to 44 years than did the English study (NMS 2).

Each of the seven community practices and three teaching practices in Virginia FY 75 and the 53 practices in NMS 2 can therefore be represented by a standardized episode rate per 100 patients. This information is summarized in Table 2, which shows the median adjusted rate for each group of practices together with the maximum and minimum around that value. There is a clear gradient from community practices to teaching practices to the English practices, which have the highest episode rates after standardization. There is very little overlap between the

* Reprinted by permission from *The Journal of Family Practice*, 4(5):972–973, 1977.

Table 1. *Comparison of English and Virginia Morbidity Surveys*

	Virginia FY 75 (July 1, 1974–June 30, 1975)			England and Wales NMS 2 (July 1, 1974–June 30, 1975)
	Community	*Teaching*	*Total*	
Number of practices	7	3	10	53
Number of patients*	37,240	28,123	65,363	196,292
Number of physicians (FTE)†	10.5	18	28.5	110+
Patients per physician (FTE)†	3,547	1,562	2,293	1,784−

* A patient is a person who has reported at least one episode of illness to the doctor in disease groups 1–18 of the RCGP (US) or RCGP classifications.
† Fulltime equivalent.

Virginia community practices and the English general practices, the maximum (227) of the community practices being higher than only four of the 53 English practices considered. Our teaching practices, on the other hand, are comparable to some of the English practices recording lower morbidity.

Since our teaching practices have rates falling between our community practices and English general practice, and since they are composed of family doctors at different stages in training, it was considered necessary to further subdivide according to the status of the recorders. Table 3 shows a clear gradient in the episode rates per patient from the least-experienced to the most-experienced physician. Faculty members would appear to record about 41 more episodes per 100 patients than do first-year residents. An attempt is also made in this table to show the workload of these different groups in terms of the number of patients per full-time equiva-

lent (FTE). Since there was no obvious association between workload and episode rate, we sought an explanation for this gradient in the characteristics of patients seen by different types of recorders.

This examination revealed that the faculty members tend to see older patients on average. Thus, Table 4 shows that the faculty saw patients 26 percent of whom were over 65, compared with seven percent for first-year residents. Accordingly, the episode rates per patient for each type of recorder has been adjusted for the age/sex of the patients seen. After standardization, there is little difference in the episode rates recorded by second and third-year residents and faculty. First-year residents still record a lower episode rate per patient, but this may have been caused by an inaccurate conversion of 37 first-year residents into three FTEs.

Discussion

Exact comparisons between Virginia and England are impossible due to differences in the health-care systems, to say nothing of the differences between the two recording systems. With that caveat, the English general practitioner has a greater workload from a smaller number of patients. Thus, he records 2.71 episodes presented by each of 1,800 patients on average com-

Table 2. *Episode Rates per 100 Patients per Practice (Adjusted for Age and Sex)*

	Virginia FY 75		England and Wales NMS 2
	Community	*Teaching*	
Median	158	248	271
Maximum	227	253	414
Minimum	151	248	205

Table 3. *Episode Rate and Workload by Status of Recorder in Three Virginia Teaching Practices*

Status of Recorder	Number of Recorders (FTEs)	Patients per FTE Recorder	Episode Rate per 100 Patients
First year	37 (3)	1028	233
Second year	26 (6)	2060	248
Third year	31 (5.5)	1705	257
Faculty	8 (3.5)	944	274

pared with 1.58 episodes for each of approximately 3,500 patients per family practitioner in our community practices. Each community physician in Virginia records 5,500 episodes per year compared with 4,900 episodes by his English counterpart but records fewer episodes per patient. This perhaps reflects the different health-care systems; the English GP is the only source of primary care and a visit to him involves no direct cost to the patient.

The finding that, in teaching practices, faculty members tend to see older patients is not unexpected. It is natural for incoming residents to be assigned new patients who will, in general, tend to be younger than the practice population. The need to use age and sex specific rates or rates standardized for age and sex differences is obvious. Such standardization has largely explained an apparent gradient in episode rates per patient which would otherwise have appeared to have been associated with experience.

Acknowledgments

The authors are indebted to their colleagues in the participating practices for this data and to Russell Boyle for his painstaking tabulations. This paper was supported by Grant Number 1 RO1 HS 01899-01 from the National Center for Health Services Research (HRA).

Authors' Update

A recent study of non-attenders in registered practices ("The Non-attending Patient in Denmark and England" by P. Krogh-Jensen and S.J. Kilpatrick: presented at W.O.N.C.A., October 1980 in New Orleans) demonstrated that rates per patients attending can give radically different comparative results than do rates per patients registered.

Since patient populations are unregistered in Virginia, we are forced here to use

Table 4. *Age and Sex Adjusted Episode Rates by Status of Recorder in Three Virginia Teaching Practices*

Status of Recorder	Average Age of Patients	Percentage of Patients over 65	Standard Episode Rate per 100 Patients
First year	25.3	7	240
Second year	29.8	8	250
Third year	31.1	9	254
Faculty	47.0	26	252

the number of attending patients as a denominator when comparing registered and unregistered practices. We cannot however, assume that the same relationships would hold if we were able to compare practices on the basis of the total practice population served.

Indeed, the finding that episode rates per 100 patients attending are lower in Virginia than in England and Wales may simply mean that patients in Virginia attend more than one doctor.

REFERENCES

1. Crombie DL, Pinsent RJFH, Lambert PM, et al: Comparison of the first and second National Morbidity Surveys. J R Coll Gen Pract 25:874–878, 1975
2. Marsland DW, Wood M, Mayo F: A data base for patient care, curriculum, and research in family practice. J Fam Pract 3:37–68, 1976

Reliability of Morbidity Data in Family Practice*

John E. Anderson

Because of its relative youth, family practice research has not yet developed a tradition of proven research techniques. New techniques, even those already proven effective in other disciplines, must be evaluated in the family practice setting if the results that they generate are to have any credibility. The collection of morbidity data has become a major activity in family practice research, but this has occurred without sufficient examination of its reliability. Several problems, both potential and real, exist requiring more detailed scrutiny, discussion, and possibly action. These problems of recording, diagnosis, coding, and population, and their ramifications, are explored with the aim of stimulating such action and encouraging a rigorous approach to the collection, publication, and interpretation of morbidity statistics.

Just as family medicine is a relatively new academic discipline, so is family practice research a relatively new activity. Both the discipline and its research arm have been the subject of discussions about the knowledge base that they should teach and study. Geyman has described the scope of potential research in and into family medicine.[1] Although this huge, exciting panorama creates considerable enthusiasm, it must be approached with caution.

As a new field, family practice research has not developed a stock of tried and proven methods. New tools are necessarily being developed while others are being adopted and/or adapted from other disciplines, notably epidemiology and the behavioral sciences. Caution is required to ensure that these new or borrowed methods function accurately in the family medicine setting and that they are applied appropriately. The reliability and precision of each method must be evaluated if the results of its employment are to be credible.

For example, difficulties with the denominator problem and with morbidity classification have been recognized already and are under review,[2-11] but another activity appears to have achieved major

prominence in family practice without sufficient consideration of its validity and reliability. This is the collection of diagnostic information for the compilation of morbidity statistics. Descriptive reports of disease distribution are seen as useful in examining differences in morbidity patterns between areas or jurisdictions, but their use—and the interpretations that flow from them—are based on the assumption that they are reliable. This assumption deserves critical attention because continuing unquestioned reliance on potentially faulty data can harm the whole of family practice research and not only the individual studies involved. Only when deficiencies have been sought, recognized, and assessed can the reliability of morbidity statistics be determined. This paper will review several real and/or possible deficiencies as an initial step in this process.

Mortality Statistics

Morbidity statistics are really an outgrowth of mortality statistics and, as such, they should be examined both for the known weaknesses of their progenitor and for any inherent flaws. There are certainly proven deficiencies in mortality data. There are problems in the registration process itself, in the application of rules for selecting the

* Reprinted by permission from *The Journal of Family Practice*, 10(4):677–683, 1980.

cause of death from a list of diagnoses, in diagnostic accuracy, and in coding.[12-16]

Mortality statistics are based on a well-circumscribed event, death, and on diseases that are usually definable and, thus, diagnosable with some accuracy. In contrast, morbidity statistics are based on what is usually a continuing event of variable length and with blurred onset and termination—the illness "episode." These latter events are more often poorly defined and less amenable to accurate diagnosis. Given that there is a certain level of imprecision in the more precise area of mortality, what is the level of the problem in the realm of morbidity?

Problem Areas in Morbidity Statistics

Any problems with morbidity statistics, whether real or potential, are significant only to the extent that they affect the purposes for which the data are to be used. Obviously, the collection of information for morbidity registers cannot be ignored, but the major emphasis in this discussion will be on publication of morbidity rates.

The major purpose of such publications is for comparison, for demonstrating similarities or differences between groups or areas. Such a comparison demands that the sources have a certain basic level of similarity. In a case control study, the controls must match the cases as closely as possible, except for the study variable. So too with comparisons of morbidity data. If there are too many confounding variables (differences between the data sources), then it is virtually impossible to determine the role of the study factor (eg, geographic location) in causing differences in rates.

Problems with morbidity statistics fall into four groups: problems of recording, diagnosis, coding, and population. Many of the problem areas are potential, rather than proven. Such is the current state of the art that the significance, indeed the reality, of some of these problems cannot be assessed.

Recording

1. The *purpose of the recording* may have some effect on the reliability of the results. For example, bias may be introduced if a prime purpose of a system is to facilitate billing procedures. Since the purpose of reporting is to justify payment of a fee, that justification will be paramount and accuracy may become a secondary consideration. Physicians may substitute more medically acceptable diagnoses for some social situations, such as housing problems, to justify payment from a "medical" insurance scheme. They may also make substitutions for other diagnoses, such as venereal diseases or therapeutic abortion, to keep such confidential information out of the hands of third parties. Obviously these substitutions lead to under-reporting of the problems in question and to over-reporting of the substituted labels. By the same token, physicians may record only one of multiple illnesses dealth with, since one diagnosis is sufficient for payment. These possible difficulties dictate special caution when examining data from the files of medical insurance plans.

2. The *frequency of recording* undoubtedly has an effect on the quality of the final data. Systems in which physicians report the same problem every time that they see it are more prone to inconsistent reporting and therefore to error. The likelihood of having the same illness reported under more than one diagnostic heading will result in an underemphasis of the correct diagnosis and an overemphasis on the others. The reporting of every encounter with patients having hypertension was one factor that led to an error of more than 50 percent in the apparent prevalence of hypertension in one data set.[11] On the other hand, physicians who only report an illness once during its course run the risk of forgetting to report some episodes.

3. The *recorders themselves* cannot help but have an effect on the resultant picture of illness distribution. Thus, one should not attempt to compare data from centers that include reports from nurses and social

workers with data from centers that specifically exclude such sources from their reporting. The data bases will obviously be different.

Differences between individual physicians can cause apparent incongruities in resultant morbidity distributions. The dedication of individual reporters to their task, and the volume of the rest of their workload can affect the accuracy and completeness of their reporting. In one family practice residency program, it has been demonstrated that residents actually reported, on average, one problem less than was actually dealt with.[17] Recording losses may well be higher in less motivated settings. Physicians having special clinical interests report higher frequencies of morbidity within those spheres of interest,[18] whether from the provision of consultative services, heightened sensitivity, or diagnostic prejudice.

4. The *geographic location* in which the physician practices has a bearing on reported morbidity distributions. Urban/rural differences are a case in point. Three Canadian studies have shown that urban physicians report higher rates of emotional illness than their rural colleagues.[18,19,20] Other differences were less consistent. This potential for regional variation was recognized in recruiting recorders for the National Morbidity Surveys in Great Britain.[21]

While this particular factor is often the study variable in comparing two sets of morbidity data, the two sets must come from similar sources to make the comparisons valid. For example, no conclusions on national differences in Canadian and British illness rates should be based on a comparison of data from inner London with data from rural and remote northern Ontario.

5. The *physical setting* from which the report is generated will alter the type of morbidity reported. Reports from groups that have a high work load in student health services, emergency departments, chronic institutions, and industry will be at variance with data coming from practices that do not have similar involvement. Because of the special nature of morbidity requiring service outside the office, eg, home visits, those systems that report only office encounters will be biasing their results toward the under-reporting of some diseases.

6. The *date of recording* is important. Diagnostic fashions change over time, whether because of new treatments, new information, or new emphasis. This temporal influence may have more effect on reported differences in rates than do actual changes in morbidity.

The two British national morbidity surveys contain examples of this phenomenon. Between surveys, the rate for hay fever doubled; that for the common cold increased by 25 percent; for acute sinusitis, the rate increased by 600 percent, and that for depressive neurosis by a startling factor of 22.[21] Objective analysis led to the conclusion that these changes were due to factors other than a real increase in the level of morbidity.[21]

7. The *number of diagnoses recorded* at an encounter will also have an effect on the final statistics. Those physicians that record only one diagnosis per encounter will show a lower total rate of morbidity in their practices. Since they usually record only the most important condition dealt with on any one encounter, this underreporting will be selectively biased towards the minor illnesses. Further, Bentsen found that experienced physicians disagreed on the major diagnosis in 15 percent of cases.[17] If only the major diagnosis is being recorded, this level of disagreement would result in important differences in ultimate data sets.

8. *Continuity of care* will encourage consistency of recording for the same problem in the same patient. Lack of such continuity was probably another factor that caused the problem with hypertension rates alluded to earlier.[11]

9. The *act of recording* may affect the accuracy of the report. Morrell has noted that "morbidity studies in some way constrain the doctor to make a diagnosis,"[22] ie,

to label a collection of symptoms with a definitive diagnostic tag of questionable veracity.

10. The accuracy of reports is inversely proportional to the *interval between service and recording*. It will, indeed, be the rare physician who does not remember leaving his patient records, insurance forms, or morbidity reports just a little too long to be totally positive about all of the details of a patient visit.

11. The *recording system* itself can have much to do with the accuracy and completeness of the reports. Systems that require little additional effort, that are seen as a part of a routine, and that have some perceived benefit to the recorders are likely to contain the more reliable data.

Diagnosis

1. *Diagnostic criteria* are poorly established for many of the more common problems encountered in family practice. The effect of this deficiency on morbidity statistics is clear. How can one really compare the incidence of an illness between two practices if one cannot be certain that the diagnostic label means the same thing in the two groups? This is a particular problem in the field of psychosocial illnesses. There is absolutely no guarantee that the diagnosis of anxiety neurosis means the same thing to different physicians, even if they practice in the same building.

During one 12-month period at this center, the prevalence rate of anxiety neurosis among females aged 15 to 64 years was 95.8/1,000 attending patients (of the same age and sex). The corresponding rate for men was 46.8. The female excess (by a ratio of 2.1:1) is quite in keeping with other studies,[18,23–27] but is the between-sex difference real?

How many of the recording physicians have definitive criteria for the diagnosis of anxiety neurosis? Probably very few, and even among those few, there is no assurance that the criteria are similar. Until such problems are dealt with, it will not be possible to look for the reasons behind the excess of reported psychiatric morbidity among women. Men may be presenting with similar problems, but being diagnosed as "chest wall pain" or "fatigue NYD" (not yet diagnosed).

To take another example, some physicians insist on obtaining a mid-stream urine culture with a colony count in excess of 10^5 before they will diagnose a urinary tract infection. Other physicians are content with a careful microscopic examination of the urine. Other again are less rigorous. What factors are really being compared when frequencies from these practices are studied? Differences in published incidence and prevalance rates may well be the result of physician factors and not of patient or population factors.

2. The *level of diagnosis* is a closely related problem. Where the difference has no real clinical significance, many physicians are satisfied to report manifestational diagnoses, eg, "tension headache" or "anxiety," as opposed to etiological diagnoses, eg, "sick child" or "marital problem." This aspect of clinical medicine is highly individualistic and there is no way of correcting the biases that it is bound to introduce once it becomes a part of a data reporting system. It can only be avoided by a prior agreement on the level of diagnoses to be reported, and an ongoing monitoring to be sure that the agreement is being lived up to—a cumbersome process. Perhaps pooling of results from several physicians will have some effect on smoothing out the differences, but the larger the number of recorders, the greater the difficulty in standardizing the data collected.[22]

3. The *importance of the diagnosis* may well affect the accuracy of the report. For many physicians, diagnostic accuracy is only important to the extent that it will assist them in helping the patient. Thus, for a self-limited illness of the respiratory tract, different physicians may label the same illness as "influenza," "bronchitis," "tracheitis," "pneumonia," or even "viral

illness NYD." Howie has shown the relatively greater significance of signs and symptoms, as compared to diagnosis, in the management of some respiratory illnesses.[28] If a physician can decide on the necessary treatment before gathering enough data to establish a firm diagnosis, diagnostic accuracy may suffer, although the patient will not.

4. Following this line of reasoning, *therapeutic decisions* may affect the diagnosis, rather than vice versa. Once again, reference to the British surveys will provide an example. A drop in the rates for menopausal symptoms paralleled the rise in neurotic depression, suggesting that the diagnosis of neurotic depression may have been used as an alternative diagnosis in the second survey.[21] This hypothesis was substantiated by the age and sex specific incidence rates for neurotic depression. If real, could this substitution have arisen because physicians perceived antidepressant therapy as more beneficial and/or safer than estrogen treatment?

Another possible example comes from data arising out of an unpublished study of the effect of patient gender on tranquilizer prescribing. Prescribing rates to men and women were reviewed for six psychiatric diagnoses and three psychosocial diagnoses. It was determined that there was a linear relationshp between the problem-specific prescribing rates and the prevalence rates of the psychiatric conditions. (The correlation coefficient was 0.98 for men and 0.95 for women.) The two diagnoses that appeared to have the greatest effect in causing this relationship (anxiety neurosis and unspecified anxiety) were the two with the least well-defined diagnostic criteria. Although this finding could well have been the result of chance or bias, other explanations are possible as well. One of the foremost of these must be that the physicians first determined the need for tranquilizer therapy and then assigned a diagnostic tag appropriate to the therapeutic decision. Howie has postulated the same phenomenon wherein the diagnosis

"will tend to be a justification for treatment, rather than the reason for it."[28]

5. The *definition of an episode* is confusing[29] but vital in the analysis of morbidity data. Should several related diagnoses be reported as a single illness, or should each be reported in its own right? A child presents with coryza, pharyngitis, and acute otitis media. Is this a single illness? If so, should it be reported with a single diagnosis? If yes, which one? Later the coryza and the pharyngitis resolve and the acute otitis subsides, but a serious otitis lingers. Is this a new illness or a new episode? Probably not, but how should it be reported?

There is also the elderly patient with hypertension. Are the hypertensive heart disease, the congestive heart failure, and the hypertensive retinopathy different problems or all a part of the same illness? Certainly they present quite different management problems to the physician. Therefore, they should probably be reported as separate diagnoses. Unfortunately, there is no convention for dealing with these problems. If all physicians were to report separate diagnoses, or all physicians report only the "root" diagnosis, it would at least be possible to know what is being dealt with and the data could be interpreted accordingly. Probably the current data contain a mixture of approaches, even from individual physicians.

Some agreement is required to be sure that everyone is reporting the same thing. Since family physicians deal with clinical problems, it would seem reasonable to make them the basis of reporting. For these purposes a clinical problem might be defined as any problem that requires individual investigation, therapy, or follow-up.

6. There is probably some confusion over *which diagnosis to report*. McWhinney has demonstrated the existence of a behavioral as well as a clinical diagnosis.[30] Within this model, patients may present identical symptoms for a variety of reasons; particularly significant here are the limits of tolerance and limits of anxiety.

If, for instance, a patient attends with chest pain, not because it is severe, but because he is worried about it, what is the diagnostic outcome? Some physicians will consider the anxiety as the major problem, concentrate their therapy on relieving the concern, and report the diagnosis as anxiety. Other physicians may recognize and deal with the anxiety, but really regard the "disease" as chest pain and report it as such. A third group of physicians may report both anxiety and chest pain, thus creating two illness episodes.

This difficulty arises because physicians do not differentiate between disease and response to disease (behavior). The result is that a certain number of behavioral diagnoses may be contaminating morbidity data. This may be a basic cause of the differences in psychiatric morbidity rates between practices, a difference that has caused some concern.[31] It may also account, in part, for the differences in reported psychiatric morbidity rates between men and women discussed earlier.

7. The *stage of diagnostic resolution* at which recording occurs is significant. The high presentation rate of undifferentiated problems is a hallmark of primary care. Frequently these problems remain nosologically unresolved at the end of the first visit and are recorded accordingly, eg, "cough NYD." If, as often happens, the problem resolves and there are no further visits, there is no difficulty. The diagnostic report of "cough NYD" is an accurate reflection of the illness episode. However, the process of health care frequently continues to a stage of higher resolution. The illness may persist and on a second visit there may be evidence to justify a diagnosis of "viral pneumonia." Not only are there now two diagnostic reports for the same episode, but one is highly inaccurate. While this problem can be overcome with close attention to detail in a manual recording system, its management is far more complex in a computerized system. Probably few, if any, computerized data systems have yet reached the level of sophistication required to overcome this difficulty.

Coding

1. A *standard system of classification* is essential for coding of information that is to be compared between centers. The advent of the ICHPPC has done much to alleviate this problem in family practice research. Unfortunately, even established systems of classification need to be revised periodically. These periodic revisions must be allowed for when comparing data sets collected and coded at different times.[21]

2. The *recombination of subdivision rubrics* can lead to inaccuracies. These are often developed to meet special local needs, then recombined for comparison of data with other centers. This process, however, requires considerable care. In one instance, faulty recombination of rubrics would have resulted in an 11 percent error in the reported prevalence rate of ischemic heart disease.[10]

3. The problem of *coding methods* has been discussed elsewhere.[11] Peripheral coding systems probably have a higher level of coding accuracy than central systems.[21]

4. *Inter-coder variability* may be a problem, despite the relatively concise nature of the ICHPPC. This factor has never been assessed in any detail. At this center, the coding accuracy varies from 92 to 97 percent among the eight members of the secretarial staff who are doing the coding. Unfortunately, very few reports of morbidity data actually mention any assessment of coding accuracy.

Population

"Rates are the hallmark of epidemiology, for they form the basis of comparisons. . . ."[32] To answer questions about causation, differences in disease frequencies, or success of intervention requires the "setting of two rates side by side and making some sense of comparison."[33] Thus far, this paper has discussed the effect that variability in the numerator can have on the feasibility of such a comparison. But rates, by definition, have a denominator as well, and it too can either help or hinder comparisons.

1. Patient *age and sex* are the strongest determinant of morbidity, yet how frequently does one find published descriptions of disease frequency with no mention of the age and sex distribution of the source population? These frequencies are, in fact, nothing more than crude rates and "crude rates must never be used to compare populations of different structure."[34]

This difficulty can be overcome by the relatively simple mathematical techniques of standardization.[15,16,34] This process could, however, be greatly facilitated if there were agreement about a uniform reference population for use with North American primary care data.

2. *Other population factors* are certainly important, but it would be too arduous to standardize for all of them, except in very special circumstances. As a basic rule, the population should be described. If certain variables, eg, race, education, social class, religion, are large enough (or atypical enough) to bias the results, this should be emphasized.

3. *Other denominators* may be more appropriate for some purpose, such as workload studies. They should receive the same rigorous attention as populations to ensure that the data will be comparable.

Discussion

The prime purpose of this paper is to stimulate concern about the reliability of morbidity statistics. It is hoped that this concern will precipitate dialogue and evaluation leading ultimately to resolution of some problems and proof that others are "non-problems." This list of potential weaknesses may not be complete and new ones may be found.

Some solutions are already being developed. The committee responsible for the ICHPPC is drafting a set of diagnostic criteria for each of the classification's rubrics.

The level of acceptance of these criteria remains to be seen. Automated coding of data should reduce inter-coder variation within any one center, but variation between centers will be dependent upon their use of the same program or on a rigid comparison and standardization of different methods. The publication of the "Glossary for Primary Care" has provided a provisional beginning to the standardization operational terms.[35]

Perhaps too, the same fortuitous circumstance will occur in morbidity statistics that has occurred in mortality statistics; that despite inaccuracies on the individual case level, the pooled data will have an acceptable level of reliability.[15]

When not controlled at the stage of data gathering, these problems introduce bias into the results, a bias that cannot always be corrected by post facto mathematical manipulation of the data. Even if the bias is controllable at the analytical stage, it must be recognized before action can be taken.

The possibility of so many sources of error, variability, and confusion in morbidity data should not be used as an argument to abandon their collection and use. Rather, it should be seen as stressing the need for disciplined activity and scientific interpretation. Descriptions of morbidity frequencies are useful for determining similarities and differences in rates. These, in turn, may be the signposts to areas for fruitful research. However, if the source data are not accurate and comparable, there is a major risk that the signposts will indicate only a maze going nowhere.

Finally, morbidity statistics from family practice should be seen for what they are, a reflection of the physicians' diagnostic opinions about the problems that patients bring to them. They are a picture of only a small portion of illness and disability in the community. Even the portion that they represent may be pictured in a biased fashion because of reliance on the process of diagnostic labeling—a highly individualized and often subjective process in primary care.

REFERENCES

1. Geyman JP: Research in the family practice residency program. J Fam Pract 5:245, 1977
2. Bass M: Approaches to the denominator problem in primary care research. J Fam Pract 3:193, 1976
3. Kilpatrick SJ: On the distribution of episodes of illness: A research tool in general practice. J R Coll Gen Pract 25:158, 686, 1975
4. Garson JZ: The problem of the population at risk in primary care. Can Fam Physician 22:871, 1976
5. Westbury RC, Tarrant M: Classification of disease in general practice: A comparative study. Can Med Assoc J 101:608, 1969
6. Bentsen BG: Classifying of health problems in primary medical care. J R Coll Gen Pract Occasional Paper 1:1–5, 1976
7. International classification of health problems in primary care. Report of the Classification Committee of the World Organization of National Colleges, Academies, and Academic Associations of General Practitioners/Family Physicians. Chicago, American Hospital Association, 1975
8. Froom J: International classification of health problems for primary care. Med Care 14:450, 1976
9. Working Party Report: International classification of health problems for primary care. J R Coll Gen Pract, Occasional Paper 1:6–10, 1976
10. Anderson JE, Lees REM: Optional hierarchy as a means of increasing the flexibility of a morbidity classification system. J Fam Pract 6:1271, 1978
11. Anderson JE: Centralized morbidity coding: International classification of health problems in primary care. Int J Epidemiol 8:257, 1979
12. The accuracy and comparability of death statistics. WHO Chron 21:11, 1967
13. McKenzie A: Diagnosis of cancer of lung and stomach. Br Med J 2:204, 1956
14. Alderson MR, Meade TW: Accuracy of diagnosis on death certification compared with that in hospital records. Br J Prev Soc Med 21:22, 1967
15. Barker DJP, Rose G: Epidemiology in Medical Practice. London, Churchill-Livingstone, 1976
16. MacMahon B, Pugh TF: Epidemiology: Principles and Methods. Boston, Little, Brown, 1970
17. Bensten BG: The accuracy of recording patient problems in family practice. J Med Care 51:311, 1976
18. Anderson JE, Lees REM: Patient morbidity and some patterns of family practice in southeastern Ontario. Can Med Assoc J 113:123, 1975
19. Greenhill S, Singh HJ: Comparison of the professional functions of rural and urban general practitioners. J Med Educ 40:856, 1965
20. Bartel GG, Waldie AC, Rix DB: Rural and urban family practice in British Columbia: A comparison. Can Fam Physician 16(6):121, 1970
21. Trends in national morbidity: A comparison of two successive national morbidity surveys. J R Coll Gen Pract Occasional Paper 3:1–43, 1976
22. Morrell DC: Now and then. J R Coll Gen Pract 29:457, 1979
23. Morbidity statistics from general practice: Second National Morbidity Survey 1970–1971. In Office of Population Censuses and Surveys: Studies on Medical and Population Subjects, No. 26. London, Her Majesty's Stationery Office, 1974
24. Marsland DW, Wood M, Mayo F: Content of family practice. Part 1: Rank order of diagnoses by frequency; Part 2: Diagnoses by disease category and age/sex distribution. J Fam Pract 3:37, 1976
25. Dixon AS: Survey of a rural practice: Rainy River, 1975. Can Fam Physician 22:693, 1976
26. National ambulatory medical care survey: 1973 summary: United States, May 1973–April 1974. In National Center for Health Statistics (Rockville, Md): Vital and Health Statistics, series 13, No. 21. DHEW publication No. (HRA) 76-1772. Government Printing Office, 1975
27. Rowe IL: Prescription of psychotropic drugs by general practitioners: Part 1: General. Med J Aust 1:589, 1973
28. Howie JGR: Diagnosis: The Achilles heel. J R Coll Gen Pract 22:310, 1972
29. Eimerl TS, Laidlaw AJ: A Handbook for Research in General Practice. London, E & S Livingstone, 1969
30. McWhinney IR: Beyond diagnosis: An approach to the integration of behavioral sciences and clinical medicine. N Engl J Med 287:383, 1972
31. Warrington AM, Ponesse DJ, Hunter ME, et al: What do family physicians see in practice? Can Med Assoc J 117:354, 1977
32. Rose G, Barker DJP: Epidemiology for the uninitiated: Rates. Br Med J 2:941, 1978
33. Rose G, Barker DJP: Epidemiology for the uninitiated: Comparing rates. Br Med J 2:1282, 1978
34. Hill AB: A Short Textbook of Medical Statistics. London, Hodder and Stoughton, 1977
35. Report of the North American Primary Care Research Group (NAPCRG) Committee on Standard Terminology: A glossary for primary care. J Fam Pract 5:633, 1977

Multipractice Studies: Significance of the Information Given to Participating Doctors*

Carl Erik Mabeck, René Vejlsgaard

A total of 1,176 general practitioners were asked to take part in a multipractice study. One group of 568 practitioners was given very detailed information about the study and 19.7 percent agreed to take part. The remaining 605 practitioners were given only a brief introduction to the study. Of this group 33.4 percent agreed to take part. Two thirds of the doctors participating in the trial were sent weekly reminders about the study while the remaining third were not. We found that the reminders did not affect the number of patients registered by the practitioners.

Introduction

Multipractice studies are commonly used in research in general practice. However, this method raises several theoretical and practical problems.

Aims

In this study we examined two problems in connection with the organization of multipractice studies. First, to what extent does the amount of information about the study influence a potential participant's decision about taking part; secondly, how far do regular reminders during the study influence the participating practitioners' activity in the study?

Method

A multipractice trial was designed to investigate the effect of sulphonamide and trimethoprim in the treatment of urinary tract infections in general practice.

All the general practitioners in six counties were invited to take part. The doctors in three counties (group A) received a detailed description of the project, including background, methodology, practical aspects, and formulas, in a 16-page booklet. The doctors in the other three counties (group B) were told about the study and invited to take part in a two-page letter. Furthermore, meetings about urinary tract infections in general practice were arranged in the three counties belonging to group A in order to stimulate interest in the trial. No meetings were arranged in the counties of group B.

The study was carried out between 15 October and 15 December 1977. All participating doctors were to fill in a form for any patient suspected of urinary tract infection during this period. In each case urine was cultured, using a dip-slide medium. The forms were sent to the organizing group as they were completed.

In order to encourage the participants, all doctors in group A and 96 doctors in one county in group B received information once a week about how many patients each participating doctor in the county had examined, and how many had been included in the trial. The doctors were listed anonymously, but each doctor could identify himself.

The remaining 106 doctors in group B did not receive any reminders during the trial period.

* Reprinted by permission from the *Journal of the Royal College of General Practitioners*, 30:283–284, May, 1980.

Table 1. *Number of General Practitioners Agreeing to Take Part in a Multipractice Study in Relation to the Extent of Information about the Project Given Before the Study (Percentages in Brackets)*

Group	Type of Information	Number of Doctors Contacted	Number of Doctors Agreeing to Take Part
A	Extensive	568	112 [*19.7*]
B	Brief	605	202 [*33.4*]

$P < 0.02$.

Results

A total of 568 general practitioners in group A received a detailed description of the study. Out of these 112 (19.7 percent) agreed to take part (Table 1).

In group B, 605 received a brief description of the project and an invitation to take part; 202 (33.4 percent) agreed to take part.

All 112 doctors in group A and 96 in group B were informed each week about the number of patients included in the study. Table 2 shows no difference between the number of patients examined by the doctors kept regularly informed and the doctors who were not sent reminders during the study. The number of patients included in the trial was a little higher in the first group.

Discussion

Very little is known about the factor's which motivate general practitioners to take part in multipractice studies.

For planners of multipractice studies it is of practical value to know about the effect of different ways of informing potential participants.

Cartwright (1978)[1] found that the response rate for questionnaires was affected by both the length of the questionnaire and the sponsoring organization. However, participation in surveys based upon questionnaires is different from participation in clinical trials.

In this study we found that a detailed description of the study before the trial reduced the number of general practitioners who agreed to take part. The reason is

Table 2. *Patients Examined and Included in the Trial in Relation to the Extent of Information Before the Study, and Reminders During the Study. The Figures Show the Number of Patients Examined and Included per 1000 Patients on Each Participating Doctor's List*

Group	County	Total Number of General Practitioners	Total Number of Participants	Regular Reminders	Patients Examined per 1000	Patients Included per 1000
A	Copenhagen city	342	41	yes	8.1	3.7
A	Roskilde	92	20	yes	7.6	3.6
A	West Sealand	134	51	yes	6.5	3.2
B	Copenhagen county	297	96	yes	7.7	3.6
B	Fr.-borg	161	48	no	7.6	2.4
B	South Sealand	147	58	no	7.0	2.7

probably very simple: a busy doctor has no time to read a full project protocol. Therefore he does not answer or accept.

Drop-out among doctors who initially agree to take part is a great problem in multipractice studies. Furthermore, many general practitioners have difficulty in changing their daily routine to suit the trial. The number of patients registered and included in the study are therefore generally a minimum.

It was our hypothesis that having received detailed information about the study, those who agreed to take part would be more likely to register all patients. Consequently, we had expected that such doctors would register a higher number of patients than the other group of doctors who agreed to take part after only a brief introduction to the study.

Sooner or later some doctors forget, probably because of the daily workload and lack of enthusiasm, that they are participants in a multipractice trial. In order to avoid this, two thirds of the participating general practitioners were reminded about the study every week.

It was therefore surprising that neither the extent of information given before the study, nor the current reminders, had any influence on the number of patients registered by each doctor.

REFERENCE

1. Cartwright, A: Professionals as responders: Variations in and effects of response rates to questionnaires 1961–1977. British Medical Journal, 2, 1419–1421, 1978

Multipractice Studies: How Representative Are the Participating Doctors?*

Carl Erik Mabeck, René Vejlsgaard

General practitioners participating in a multipractice study were compared with those who refused to participate. We found that younger doctors, doctors in partnerships, and doctors with many patients were represented more among participants. However, no correlation was found between the number of patients examined for urinary tract infection in connection with the study.

Introduction

Multipractice studies are necessary in order to compare and evaluate different aspects of general practice such as procedures and treatment. Results from hospital studies cannot always be applied to general practice, mainly because hospital patients differ from patients in general practice. They are specially selected for hospital treatment by general practitioners, because of the nature of their problems.

In general, a single practitioner is not able to collect enough patients with a defined disease or condition to conduct a controlled clinical trial within a reasonable period of time. Therefore clinical trials in general practice are usually planned and conducted as multipractice studies.

Among the problems involved is the question of how representative the participating practitioners are. They differ from their colleagues in one respect—they have a different attitude towards research in general practice. However, this does not necessarily mean that their patients, their treatment, and their results would differ from those of non-participating doctors.

Method

In this study the general practitioners who agreed to take part in a multipractice study

* Reprinted by permission from the *Journal of the Royal College of General Practitioners*, 30:285–287, May, 1980.

were compared with their colleagues who refused to participate. We also examined the correlation between the participating practitioners' activity within the study in relation to various sociological variables, such as graduation year, type of practice, numbers of patients registered in the practice, and membership of the Danish College of General Practitioners.

We asked 1,176 general practitioners to take part in a controlled clinical trial on the treatment of urinary tract infection in general practice. Of these, 314 agreed to take part.

Information about the 1,176 practitioners was obtained from the Danish Medical Association register. Participants were asked to state practice size and a statistical comparison of practice size by county was obtained from the Public Health Service.

Results

A strong correlation was found between the practitioners' seniority and their willingness to participate (Table 1). In the six counties, only 10 percent of the 153 practitioners who had graduated before 1940 agreed to participate, compared with 43 percent of the 201 practitioners who graduated after 1970.

In the six counties there were 353 members of the Danish College of General Practitioners. Among these, 38 percent agreed to take part, whereas only 23 percent of the 821 non-members agreed.

Table 1. *Participation in Relation to Graduation Year*

	Year of Graduation							
	Before 1940	*1940 to 1944*	*1945 to 1949*	*1950 to 1954*	*1955 to 1959*	*1960 to 1964*	*1965 to 1970*	*After 1970*
Total number of general practitioners*	153	125	109	120	130	151	185	201
Number of participants	15	17	21	31	29	46	68	87
Percentage	*10*	*14*	*19*	*26*	*22*	*30*	*37*	*45*

* Information was unavailable for two doctors.

Further analysis revealed that this difference was caused to some extent by the difference in seniority between members and non-members. In Figure 1 the participants are classified according to year of graduation and membership of the College. College members predominate in all age groups except for those graduating after 1970. Our data indicate that College members are more likely to participate in multipractice studies (Fischer's omnibus test: $p < 0.01$).

In Denmark 42 percent of practitioners work in single-handed practice, 12 percent in group practice, and 46 percent in partnerships. Only 20 percent of practitioners in single-handed practice or group practice took part in the study, compared with 46 percent of practitioners in partnerships.

Table 2 shows the number of patients examined for urinary tract infection during the study by practitioners working in the different types of practice. These figures are made comparable by correcting for practice size. There were no differences worth mentioning in activity between the different types of practice.

Table 3 shows the proportion of participants in relation to the number of patients registered per practitioner. Only patients aged 16 years or more are registered. It was found that only 15 percent of the practitioners with fewer than 1,000 patients on their list took part, compared with 39 percent of practitioners with more than 1,500 registered patients. However, the activity among the participants was nearly the same in all groups regardless of practice size (Table 2).

Discussion

The validity of conclusions drawn from results obtained from multipractice studies largely depends on how representative the participating doctors are.

Cartwright (1978)[1] reported that younger doctors are more likely to reply to questionnaires than older ones. In general practice single-handed doctors are less likely to take part than those working with others.

We confirmed that younger practitioners were much more likely to respond and take part. This study does not give any explanation for this phenomenon. In a fu-

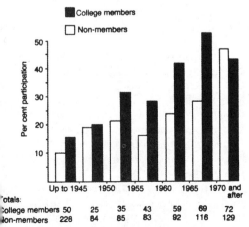

Fig. 1. Percentage participation of doctors by year of graduation.

Table 2. *Number of Patients Examined for Urinary Tract Infection in General Practice in Relation to the Seniority of the Doctor, Practice Type, and Practice Size*

	Number of Participants	Percentage of Participants			
		Number of Patients Examined per 1000 Patients Registered			
		(0)	*(1–3)*	*(4–12)*	*(>12)*
Graduation year					
Before 1945	32	*6*	*34*	*53*	*6*
1945–1954	52	*8*	*21*	*54*	*17*
1955–1964	75	*5*	*13*	*56*	*25*
After 1964	155	*7*	*26*	*45*	*22*
Practice type					
Single	128	*11*	*23*	*46*	*21*
Group	38	*11*	*21*	*47*	*21*
Partnership	148	*2*	*23*	*55*	*20*
Practice size*					
<1000 patients	35	*17*	*14*	*49*	*20*
1000–1250 patients	54	*4*	*13*	*50*	*33*
1251–1500 patients	82	*5*	*18*	*62*	*15*
>1500 patients	127	*2*	*28*	*48*	*21*

* Sixteen respondents did not report practice size.

ture study we plan to examine the attitudes towards research in different groups of general practitioners.

It has always been assumed that College members are more interested in research than non-members and our results support this assumption. A result of this assumption has been that in the past only College members have been asked to take part in many multipractice studies. However, the fact that only one third of practitioners are members of the College and that a relatively high proportion of non-

members took part leads to the conclusion that non-members as well as College members should be asked to take part in multipractice studies.

We found that practitioners in partnerships were over-represented. A possible explanation might be that if one doctor in a partnership suggests taking part, his partners are usually easily persuaded. It should also be mentioned that there is some overrepresentation of younger doctors in group practice and in partnerships.

It was surprising that practitioners with a large number of registered patients were overrepresented. It might be expected that the practitioners with the heaviest workload would have difficulty in finding extra time to take part in a multipractice study. However, it seems that those who have a great capacity within their daily work also have greater reserves and interests in other activities.

A total of 314 practitioners took part in a study of urinary tract infection in general practice. This group was not representative of general practitioners in relation t

Table 3. *Participation in a Multipractice Study in Relation to Practice Size*

Number of Patients Registered	Number of General Practitioners	Participants	
		N	*Percentage*
<1000	233	35	*15*
1000–1250	185	54	*29*
1251–1500	271	82	*30*
>1500	329	127	*39*
Not known	158	16	*10*

seniority, practice type or size. This does not necessarily mean, however, that their methods of diagnosing urinary tract infection would differ from nonparticipating practitioners.

This fundamental question can only be answered indirectly, because voluntary participation in multipractice studies precludes our learning what non-participants are doing—and what participants will do when the study is over. In this study we have investigated whether a specified activity, namely the number of urinary tract infections diagnosed during a two-month period, would vary with sociological variables such as seniority, practice type, and practice size. As no correlation was found between these variables and despite the unrepresentative sample of doctors, it seems justifiable in some cases to draw general conclusions from multipractice studies. The problem of whether a project will change the interest and daily routine of a practitioner during the study period is not considered in this context.

REFERENCE

1. Cartwright, A: Professionals as responders: Variations in and effects of response rates to questionnaires 1961–1977. British Medical Journal, 2, 1419–1421, 1978

A Comparison of Workload and Morbidity Recording by Partners in a Group Practice*

T. A. Carney

A survey was carried out of one year's workload and morbidity recording by three partners in a semi-rural teaching practice. Despite an equal workload of patient contacts, there were shown to be statistically significant differences between the partners in the number of return consultations, the sex and age of the patients seen, and in nine diagnostic groups. The statistically significant differences in the latter groups appear to have been caused by variations in policy for recalling patients and the different sex and age groups of the patients consulting the partners, not by diagnostic preferences. A lack of previous experience affected one group. The partners did not find the discussion of these differences to be threatening.

Introduction

The workload of individual general practitioners has been studied on many occasions. However, lack of comprehensive knowledge about it has been emphasized by the Seventh Report of the Review Body (1977), and the medico-political importance of the subject has been discussed fully by Ball (1978).

Fry (1972, 1975, 1978) and Marsh and Kaim-Caudle (1976) have shown falling workload and called for a radical review of medical manpower, although they acknowledge the great differences between countries, areas, and even practices in the same area.

Buchan and Richardson (1973) and Richardson and colleagues (1973) examined the consultation and the various factors that influence it, such as the patient's sex, the doctor's age, and the morbidity recorded. Buchan and Richardson found a degree of homogeneity within practice groups but did not explore the intrapractice characteristics.

The morbidity of general practice has been examined nationally (OPCS *et al*, 1974) and individually (Morrell, 1971),

and many of these papers also give information about workload.

The Second National Morbidity Survey (OPCS *et al.*, 1974) analysed the morbidity of self-selected practices and found differences in many factors between practices, such as home visiting, but did not look at the differences in individual recording, although this information was provided to the participating practices (Curtis Jenkins, 1977).

Morrell (1971), in a survey of his own three-man practice, found differences in the morbidity recorded in patient-initiated and doctor-initiated consultations, and described two contrasting groups of diseases presented to general practice:

1. Diseases for which a large number of consultations were initiated by a large number of patients demanding an episodic type of medical care with a high diagnostic content.
2. Diseases for which a relatively small number of patients consulted with a high frequency, many of these consultations being initiated by the doctor.

Valentine (1975) comments on the great variations within certain disease groups in many morbidity surveys. He found a variation in the respiratory group from 32.6

* Reprinted by permission from the *Journal of the Royal College of General Practitioners*, 30:271–277, May, 1980.

394

percent (Last and White, 1969) to 9.7 percent in his own.

It is clear that variations in workload and morbidity recording are influenced by many factors: list size (Bridgstock, 1976), patient's sex (Moorhead, 1975), doctor's age (Richardson et al., 1973; OPCS et al., 1974), country of practice (Berber, 1974; Valentine, 1975; Gibson, 1977; Colditz and Elliott, 1978), areas of the same country (OPCS et al., 1974; Fry, 1978), differing areas of the same practice (Hardman, 1965); but, what of partners in the same practice covering the same area?

Only Gibson (1977) seems even to have attempted to look at partner differences and Curtis Jenkins (1977) has called for more information on this topic because he feels that it is so threatening to the partners concerned. Only by open discussion of the differing workload with the factors that influence it can we learn to cope with this threat.

Aims

The aims of this study were to examine the workload and morbidity recording in our three-partner practice, to explore any differences between partners, and to see if they were correlated with the sex or age of the patient, a preferred diagnosis, or our previous clinical experience.

Method

The Practice

The practice, founded in 1869, is a three-man partnership in a market town in rural Northumberland. It has been associated with the Northumbria (Newcastle) Vocational Training Scheme since it began in 1969 and has taken trainees regularly since. The total list size at the mid-point of the study was 7,216 (males 46.6 percent and females 53.4 percent). It has an elderly population, 18.4 percent being over 65, and has an average social class distribution. Twenty percent of the patients live over three miles from the practice in a rural area covering 200 square miles.

The Partnership

The present partnership was formed in 1973. The senior partner (Dr A) holds a three-session appointment as Regional Adviser (Postgraduate Tutor) in General Practice at the University of Newcastle, and has a special interest in medical education. The middle partner (Dr B) has three clinical assistant sessions in geriatric medicine and a special interest in pediatrics. The junior partner (Dr C), formerly Dr A's trainee, is now an approved trainer with a special interest in family planning.

The three partners had a degree of experience before becoming principals which ranged from military service and formal assistantship to self-selected hospital posts and a formal three-year vocational training programme.

Practice Management

The practice employs a practice manager/secretary, two full-time and three part-time receptionists, and has an attached district sister, a nurse midwife and a health visitor.

A full appointment system operates for all surgeries, antenatal clinic, cervical smear clinic, well baby clinic and family planning clinic, the last two clinics being started by Drs B and C three months before the survey. Surgeries for all partners are booked at a rate of three patients per 20 minutes and last for one and a half hours. Dr A provides 10 hours' surgery time per week, Drs B and C $11\frac{1}{4}$ hours per week.

New home visits are selected by patient request. All follow-up visits are done by the doctor concerned unless the patient was seen as an emergency for another partner and, similarly, with all the chronic visiting.

Although the partners do not keep individual lists, it is practice policy that patients should always see one doctor, but that does not need to be the doctor with whom they are registered. They are encouraged to see the same doctor through any single episode of illness. They are further encouraged in a new illness, if their own doctor is not available, to see one of the other partners or the trainee in the practice.

The Survey

The survey was carried out during the year 1 March 1975 to 29 February 1976. The partners recorded every face-to-face patient contact (excluding telephone consultations and repeat prescriptions) by full name, date of birth, and diagnosis using the classification of morbidity recommended by the Second National Morbidity Survey (OPCS *et al.*, 1974). The partners discussed the use of this classification before the survey, after a pilot survey, and regularly from then on.

At each contact it was possible to record no diagnosis or multiple diagnoses.

An 'E' book provided by the Birmingham Research Unit of the Royal College of General Practitioners (Eimerl and Laidlaw, 1969) was used to record the diagnoses.

Each partner's workload figures were kept for new (patient-initiated) and return

(doctor-initiated) surgery and home contacts by the practice secretary.

The survey was undertaken in order to examine trainee/principal differences (Carney, 1979), to provide essential morbidity data for educational purposes, as an aid to practice management planning, and as a basis for future research. This paper is another outcome.

Results

The results were analysed using a two-by-three contingency table for each group. With 18 differing groups, it is possible that each of us would have one group with results significant at the $p < 0.05$ level, so only those categories which give $p < 0.01$ are considered.

Workload

The results for the practice as a whole show a nominal list size for each partner of 2,405. The total consultation rate was 3.8 patients per year: 2.7 at the surgery; 1.1 for domiciliary visits, including 0.45 for patient-initiated home visits.

The total workload figures for surgery and home consultations show the virtual equality of the partners' work (Table 1). However, these figures start to show differences when they are analysed.

Table 1. *Comparison of Consultations and Home Visits*

	Doctor	New	Return	New/Return Ratio	Total	Percentage
Consultations	A	3,415	1,464	1:0.4	4,879	31.1
	B	4,480	794	1:0.2*	5,274	33.5
	C	4,037	1,533	1:0.4	5.570	35.4
Total		11,932	3,791	1:0.3	15,723	100
Home visits	A	922	1,467	1:1.6	2,389	33.0
	B	902	1,534	1:1.7	2,436	33.5
	C	974	1,458	1:1.5	2,432	33.5
Total		2,798	4,459	1:1.6	7,257	100

* Significant difference $P < 0.001$.

Table 2. *Comparison of Total Consultations by Patient's Sex*

| Doctor | Male | Female | Total | Percentage | |
				Males	*Females*
A	2206	3659	5865	*38*	*62*
B	2723	3181	5904	*46**	*54*
C	2041	3685	5726	*36*	*64*

* Significant difference $P < 0.001$.

The new/return ratio of house calls for each partner is similar but the same ratio applied to the surgery consultations shows that one partner (Dr B) asks only half as many patients to return for review, and that he sees more new patients in total than either of his partners.

Sex of Patients

Dr B saw 46 percent males, Dr A 38 percent and Dr C 36 percent ($p < 0.001$) (Table 2).

If these are divided into diagnostic categories, Dr B sees fewer females in the endocrine, nervous system, and musculo-skeletal groups, and more males in the mental, circulatory, respiratory, digestive, skin, and accident groups.

Age of Patients

The results of a quarter sample of the survey for the age groups under 15 and over 65 are shown in Table 3. Dr A sees significantly fewer under 15s and Dr B significantly more in this age group. However,

Table 3. *Comparison of Total Consultations by Patient's Age*

Age	Dr A	Dr B	Dr C	Total
Under 15	198*	349*	230	777
Over 65	256	273	238	767

* Statistically significant $P < 0.001$.

both these figures are strongly influenced by the respiratory and accident groups.

There were no significant differences in the figures for the over 65s. However, Dr A saw fewer over 65s in the psychiatric category and Dr C saw more elderly in the musculo-skeletal group.

Morbidity

There are nine diagnostic groups in which a partner recorded a significantly different number of consultations (Tables 4 and 5). Dr A recorded less psychiatric illness and more diseases of the nervous system.

PSYCHIATRIC. He recorded fewer female patients and fewer return consultations. No differences were shown for psychotic illnesses either in the sex of the patients or by the three partners. However, Dr A recorded only half the number of consultations, new and return, of female patients in the diagnostic categories anxiety/neurosis and depressive neurosis than either of his partners.

NERVOUS SYSTEM. In contrast, Dr A recorded more female consultations, both new and return, than his partners in this disease group. It was not diseases of the cerebro-vascular system but diseases of eye (cataracts/glaucoma), ear (Menière's disease/deafness), and trigeminal neuralgia and brachial neuritis that showed marked differences between partners.

Dr B recorded less endocrine disease and more diseases of the respiratory system, digestive system, and accidents.

Table 4. *Comparison of Percentage Distribution of Consultations*

Classification of Morbidity	Dr A	Dr B	Dr C	Total Practice	Statistical Significance
1. Infective	4.0	3.7	4.8	4.1	NS*
2. Neoplasms	1.5	1.4	0.6†	1.0	$P < 0.001$
3. Endocrine	5.7	2.9†	5.3	4.1	$P < 0.001$
4. Blood	1.7	1.3	1.4	1.4	NS
5. Mental	11.0†	14.7†	15.3	12.9	$P < 0.001$
6. Nervous system	12.3†	9.3	9.1	10.7	$P < 0.001$
7. Circulatory	10.8	10.1	9.9	9.6	NS
8. Respiratory	13.1	16.8†	13.7	15.6	$P < 0.001$
9. Digestive	4.9	6.3†	4.8	5.5	$P < 0.001$
10. Genito-urinary	5.5	5.1	4.6	5.3	NS
11. Pregnancy	1.4	1.3	1.1	1.2	NS
12. Skin	6.4	7.3	4.8†	6.6	$P < 0.001$
13. Musculo-skeletal	10.8	8.4	13.5†	10.0	$P < 0.001$
14. Congenital	0.1	0.1	0.0	0.1	NS
15. Perinatal	0	0	0	0	NS
16. Ill defined	0.0	0	0.9	0.3	NS
17. Accident	4.9	6.3†	4.7	5.9	$P < 0.001$
18. Prophylactic	6.4	5.2	5.5	5.6	NS

* NS = Not significant.
† $P < 0.001$ for χ^2 is 13.8.

ENDOCRINE AND ALLERGIC. The hay fever, asthma, and allergy consultations were equal for all partners. However, only a small group of patients consulted Dr B for diabetes, thyroid disease, or gout, resulting in far fewer female and return consultations in this group for this partner.

RESPIRATORY SYSTEM. In this group Dr B recorded more patients, males and females equally, the increase being wholly attributable to upper respiratory tract infections. The under 15 age group significantly affects this group. He recorded less bronchitis and sinusitis.

DIGESTIVE SYSTEM. For Dr B the digestive group shows a strong predominance of males both with peptic ulceration and with acute diarrhoea and vomiting. The number of females is the same as his partners' but again acute diarrhoea and vomiting feature as a common diagnosis. This diagnosis caused a high number of single consultations.

ACCIDENTS. Similarly, Dr B recorded far more male consultations in this group and many single consultations, especially for sprains, strains and superficial injuries.

Dr C recorded less dermatological and neoplastic disease and more musculo-skeletal disease.

DERMATOLOGICAL DISEASES. In diseases of the skin Dr C recorded fewer consultations for male and female patients and made fewer diagnoses. He used the imprecisely diagnosed category twice as often as his partners and made fewer diagnoses in all the defined diagnostic labels in this group.

NEOPLASTIC DISEASE. Dr C recorded fewer episodes (13) compared with Dr A (43) and Dr B (28). Dr C had four terminally ill patients who died at home compared with eight recorded by both his partners.

MUSCULO-SKELETAL DISEASES. Dr C recorded far more arthritic diseases, especially osteoarthritis, but also cervical spon-

Table 5. *Factors Influencing the Diagnostic Groups*

Diagnostic Groups	Partner with Significantly Different Recording	All Consultations	Single Consultation Episodes	Return Consultations	Male Patients	Female Patients	Disease Categories
Mental	A	−	0	−	0	−	Psychotic equal < Neurotic diagnoses
Nervous system	A	+	0	+	0	+	
Endocrine/allergic	B	−	0	−	0	−	Allergic equal < Endocrine
Respiratory	B	+	+	0	+	+	>> Upper respiratory infection
Digestive	B	+	+	0	+	0	> Peptic ulcer > Diarrhoea and vomiting
Accidents	B	+	+	0	+	0	> Sprains and strains
Skin	C	−	0	0	−	−	>> Unspecified diagnoses < All specific diagnoses
Neoplasms	C	−	0	0	−	−	< Episodes < Terminal care
Musculo–skeletal	C	+	0	+	0	+	>> Osteo-arthrosis

dylosis and rheumatoid arthritis. He recorded far more female and return consultations.

The age and sex of the patient, single consultations, and return consultations are all identifiable factors which influence these morbidity differences.

Finally, Dr C recorded more contacts for oral contraception and Pap smears, and Dr B more routine developmental checks. This reflected their special clinics. The figures were not statistically different.

Discussion

The gross workload within the practice is distributed remarkably equally between the partners for both surgery and home consultations. Indeed the data have been available for the past nine years and have altered little despite outside commitments as regional adviser, clinical assistant, and trainer. Richardson and colleagues (1973) make the point that a harmonious partnership depends on an equitable sharing of work; they also found workload to be related to list size, high consulting rates, and a high proportion of return visits.

Our list size of 2,405 patients per partner is slightly larger than the 1976 national average of 2,351 (DHSS 1977).

The gross consultation rate of 3.8 per registered patient per year falls between the many reported figures: Morrell (1971) —4.7; Fry (1972)—2.1; Second Morbidity Survey (OPCS, 1974)—3.0 to 7.0; Marsh and Kaim-Caudle (1976)—2.3.

The return rate for all consultations was 36 percent compared with a mean of 56 percent quoted by Richardson and colleagues (1973) and 47 percent for Morrell (1971). Similarly, home visiting comprised 28 percent of our workload compared with Richardson's (1973) mean figure of 39 percent. Fry (1978) comments on the fact that Scottish practices and those in the North of England have higher home consultation rates.

Fry's (1972) home visiting rate of 0.1 per registered patient per year, which is the lowest that has been reported in England, and Marsh's (1976) of 0.3 per patient per year contrast with the figure for our practice which is 1.1 per year. However, the Second National Morbidity Survey (OPCS, 1974) showed a variation of between 0.1 and 1.5. Our higher rate is influenced by a high return visiting rate of 0.65 per patient per year which may be due to the semi-rural setting and the elderly population.

As Richardson and colleagues (1973) and Berber (1974) comment, first consultations are the product of a complex set of factors, but return consultations are controlled mainly by the doctor, who therefore determines his own workload. This is shown by Dr B, whose return rate is quite different from those of Drs A and C. This may reflect training differences. Dr B's much lower return consultation rate clearly causes less advance booking of surgery time and he is therefore more available for new acute patient-initiated consultations. The well baby clinic and the family planning clinic were both so new that the return rates they engendered were very small and not significant for either Drs B or C.

Morrell (1971) has shown that patient-initiated consultations are biased towards diagnostic categories of eye, ear, skin, digestive tract, and accidents and Dr B's figures show a higher rate for skin (not significantly), digestive tract, and accidents. The higher recorded level of respiratory illness is caused almost entirely by upper respiratory tract infection which is manifestly an acute presentation. Thus Dr B sees more of Morrell's first category and Drs A and C more of his second category.

It appears that males attend more often for patient-initiated consultations, as the groups of males seen more often by Dr B (mental, circulatory, respiratory, digestive tract, skin, and accidents) are similar to those of Morrell's patient-initiated group.

Each doctor influences his own workload and morbidity classification by the way in which he recalls female patients. Dr A had a very low rate in the neurosis group, Dr B a low level in the chronic illness group, (endocrine and arthritic conditions), and Dr C a very high rate in both neurosis and musculo-skeletal groups.

Many hypotheses can be put forward to account for these differences between the partners: perhaps Dr A is uninterested in emotional problems, or Dr B will not allow the development of dependency, or Dr C, because of his own anxiety, promotes dependency. However, none of these hypotheses are examined here. Further work is required in our own partnership and in others to allow partners to discuss such hypotheses between themselves without feeling threatened.

Buchan and Richardson (1973) and Westcott (1977) have both shown that length of consultation differs with morbidity classification but not with sex of the patient. Thus Dr B's different ratio of patients by sex should not affect the consulting time, while Dr C's large number of female chronic neurotic patients should lengthen his consulting time.

While the very different consultations in the under-15 age group may seem to reflect Dr B's previous experience in paediatrics, in fact the whole difference can be accounted for by the consultations for acute problems in the respiratory and accidents group and must again reflect his availability because of surgery booking rather than his special interest.

There is no obvious explanation why Dr A should diagnose more disease of the nervous system. If, as senior partner, he was consulted by the elderly then surely the cerebro-vascular element of this group would predominate, which it does not, and these differences would be shown in the over-65 age group, which they are not.

Dr C's low number of patients with neoplasms was influenced by his being a new partner; Drs A and B had a greater number both of episodes and terminally ill patients, which was related to their greater time in the practice.

It appears that the low level of skin diagnosis is caused by Dr C's lack of experience in this subject, with a much smaller number of definitive diagnoses, especially when it is contrasted with Dr B's higher total level and higher diagnostic level in this group. Dr B had a much lower level of imprecise diagnoses in this group than either Drs A or C and must reflect his previous experience in this subject.

Conclusions

The morbidity differences are caused not by partners' disease or diagnosis preferences but by a differing policy of recalling patients. The latter also results in significant differences in the age and sex distribution of the patients seen.

One partner, who had no postgraduate experience of dermatology and only two years as a principal at the time of the survey, showed a low level of diagnosis in the dermatological group of diseases.

The partners have not found discussion of these differences to be threatening. They think that they are healthy and complementary and do not detract from a shared philosophy of general practice.

Acknowledgments

My most sincere thanks are due to my partners Dr M. McKendrick and Dr P. Willis without whose sustained co-operation and encouragement this study could not have been undertaken; Mrs D. Fullard for typing the manuscript; Birmingham Research Unit of the Royal College of General Practitioners and Mr A. Metcalfe of the Medical Care Research Unit, Newcastle, for their help with the analysis of the results; and Mr R. Jacklin for his advice.

REFERENCES

1. Ball JG: Workload in general practice. Br Med J 1:868–870, 1978
2. Berber M: A survey of clinical activity in a Dublin general practice. J Irish Med A 67:169–172, 1974
3. Bridgstock M: General practitioners' organisation and estimates of their workload. J R Coll Gen Pract 26, Suppl. 1:16–24, 1976
4. Buchan IC, Richardson IM: Time Study of Consultations in General Practice. Scottish Health Services Studies 27. Edinburgh: Scottish Home and Health Department, 1973
5. Carney TA: Clinical experience of a trainee in general practice. J R Coll Gen Pract 29:40–44, 1979
6. Colditz GA, Elliott CJP: Workload in rural practice. Aust Fam Physician 7:571–575, 1978
7. Department of Health and Social Security: Health and Personal Social Services Statistics for England. London. HMSO, 1977
8. Eimerl TS, Laidlaw AJ (eds.): A Handbook for Research in General Practice. 2nd edn. Edinburgh & London: E & S Livingstone, 1969
9. Fry J: Twenty-one years of general practice— changing patterns. J R Coll Gen Pract 22: 521–528, 1972
10. Fry J: Work trends in general practice now and in the future. Update 11:13–16, 1975
11. Fry J: Home visiting—how much is necessary? Update 16:1119–1120, 1978
12. Gibson JF: A study of general practitioner consultations and work-load in a trainee practice in South-West Ireland. Irish Med J 70:174–180, 1977
13. Hardman RA: (1965). A comparison of morbidity in two areas. J R Coll Gen Pract 9:226–240, 1965
14. Jenkins G Curtis: How many patients? J R Coll Gen Pract 27:627–630, 1977
15. Last JM, White KL: The content of medical care in primary practice. Med Care 7:41–48, 1969
16. Marsh G, Kaim-Caudle P: Team Care in General Practice. London: Croom Helm, 1976
17. Morrhead R: A general practitioner's study of his own workload and patient morbidity. Med J Aust 2:140–145, 1975
18. Morrell DC: Expressions of morbidity in general practice. Brit Med J 2:454–458, 1971
19. Office of Population Censuses and Surveys, Royal College of General Practitioners, and Department of Health and Social Security: Morbidity Statistics from General Practice. Second National Study 1970–1971. London: HMSO, 1974
20. Review Body on Doctors' and Dentists' Remuneration: Seventh Report. Cmnd. 6800. London: HMSO, 1977
21. Richardson IM, Howie JGR, Durno D, Gill G, Dingwall-Fordyce I: A study of general practitioner consultations in North East Scotland. J R Coll Gen Pract 23:132–142, 1973
22. Valentine AS: What is family practice? Maybe the 'E' book can tell you. Can Fam Physician 21: 29–35, 1975
23. Westcott RH: The length of consultations in general practice. J R Coll Gen Pract 27:552–555, 1977

ABSTRACTS

McWhinney IR: The naturalist tradition in general practice. J Fam Pract 5(3):375–378, 1977

Medicine, like other branches of biology, is predominantly an observational science. The observations are made by clinicians, who are the field workers of medical science, just as the field naturalist and field anthropologist are the field workers of biology and anthropology. To say this is not to deny the importance of experiment in biology or medicine. In these sciences, however, an experiment usually follows and derives from a long period of observation. The distinction between observation and experiment is in any case artificial. The laboratory scientist and the naturalist both use experiments: One creates his own experimental conditions; the other uses the slow and massive experiments of nature.

The general practitioner has advantages as an observer which are shared by few other physicians. The general practitioner can follow illnesses from their beginning to their termination, even if the course is of many years duration; all variants of illness, from the mildest to the most severe, can be observed; and the physician can, if he/she chooses, observe patients in their own natural habitat.

This paper illustrates this theme by describing the work of three general practitioners—Edward Jenner, James MacKenzie, and William Pickles, who made their observations while practicing for most of their lives in one community.

These three examples represent a tradition which runs from the eighteenth century to our own times. Does the tradition continue? Assuredly it does. In men like Fry in Britain, Bentsen in Norway, Braun in Austria, and Hames in the United States, we see the same principles exemplified: long-term observations carried out by individual physicians who share the same habitat as their patients. And for each one who can be named, there must be many we will never know, whose observations enrich their own lives, but never come to publication. In recent years, also, the work of these individuals has been supplemented by collaborative studies in which many physicians pool their observations.

The beauty of studying natural history is that it needs so few instruments: the ordinary tools of our profession plus a notebook, a pen, and an indexing system for organizing our collection. We need no laboratory, for the practice and the community are our laboratory.

Gordon M: Research traditions available to family medicine. J Fam Pract 7(1):59–68, 1978

Family medicine has declared its territory to include the *psychological* and *physical* health of the *patient* in the context of his or her family and *community*. The underlined words suggest that the disciplines basic to family medicine must range far beyond the biological sciences usually taught in the medical schools. These disciplines certainly include psychology, sociology, anthropology, and epidemiology in addition to the biological sciences. Arguments can also be made to include economics, organizational development, education, and other disciplines.

The purpose of this paper is to present in broad strokes some of the major differences in orientation and methods of research which exist among family medicine's basic disciplines. That paper concludes with some suggestions for family medicine researchers who intend to work closely with researchers from these disciplines.

The biological sciences share enough in orientation and method to be considered as belonging to a single research tradition. There is no question that the practice of family medicine has been profoundly influenced by developments within anatomy, biochemistry, physiology, and other biological sciences, and will continue to be profoundly influenced by them in the future. A second tradition of research likely to influence family medicine is the agricultural tradition. Experimental methods and statistical analysis techniques developed for the scientific study of agriculture have permeated psychology, sociology, economics, and many areas of public health and clinical medicine. A third major tradition,

the epidemiologic tradition, is expected to play a major role in many concerns of vital interest to the family physician including prevention and control of chronic illness, community medicine, and development of a rational system of health care delivery. Finally, the ethnographic tradition, most closely associated with community sociologists and anthropologists, offers concepts and methods for the study of dynamic human relationships in communities, families, and other groups. This paper summarizes the aims, interests, methods, and assumptions of each of these four traditions.

Most research in family medicine will be applied rather than basic, with an emphasis on improving practical decisions of patient care and health care delivery. Such a real-world orientation can profit greatly from eclectic borrowing of well-established concepts and methods of related disciplines. Coherence of ideas and methods cannot be mandated. Every academic discipline and medical specialty has evolved and continues to evolve through both external influence and the accomplishments of its members. Family medicine will also evolve as its individual practitioners and scholars define their concerns and reach out to resolve them.

Geyman JP: Climate for research in family practice. J Fam Pract 7(1):69–74, 1978

The word "climate" has been defined by the *Random House Dictionary* in nonmeteorological terms as a particular set of "prevailing attitudes, standards, or environmental conditions of a group, period, or place." It is the premise of this paper that the climate within family practice in terms of attitudes, standards, and environmental conditions has an important bearing on the direction and success of its future development as an academic

discipline and specialized pattern of practice. It is the further premise of this paper that the climate within its field of birth, general practice, was generally unsupportive of the kind of vigorous intellectual and investigative efforts required to establish any specialty discipline, and that this deficiency must be corrected if family practice is to prosper and survive as a specialty in its own right.

The purpose of this paper is threefold:

(1) to outline the climate which prevailed within general practice in the past, (2) to suggest the elements of a new climate in family practice which can nurture its continued development and maturation as a specialty, and (3) to discuss the implications of this new climate in terms of patient care, practice satisfaction, and related factors.

Eight attitudes are proposed as important ingredients of this new "mind set" for the family physician, including (1) curiosity, (2) skepticism, (3) honesty, (4) awareness of limited knowledge, (5) interest in learning something from every patient, (6) appreciation of the role of the family physician in research, (7) valuing of own observations over time, and (8) acceptance of responsibility for advancing the field.

Since research in the other clinical specialties has been focused mainly on secondary and tertiary care settings, it is likely that more relevant standards to the primary care setting can be developed through family practice research. As this takes place, opportunities will increase for family practice to take greater responsibility for establishing standards of acceptable practice within the field based on supporting evidence. Such standards should relate to cost, morbidity, and patient care outcomes from diagnostic and therapeutic interventions. In the hospital, clinical (not administrative) departments of family practice can play a vital role in applying reasonable standards of care in collaboration with other clinical departments. In office practice, family physicians in partnership and group practice can establish similar standards acceptable to their colleagues and subject to periodic audit.

Six kinds of environmental conditions are necessary to facilitate research in family practice, including (1) the practice itself, (2) research tools, (3) stimulation by colleagues, (4) consultation and collaboration, (5) access to library services, and (6) a forum for communication.

While the numbers of family physicians willing to develop the clinician research style of practice may remain relatively small, many family physicians can make some kind of contribution to the field, and all can develop a more scholarly approach to their practices. The payoffs of such an approach are considerable—expansion of the body of knowledge which family physicians teach, an ongoing form of continuing medical education, increased practice satisfaction, and most importantly, improved quality of care for patients and their families.

Wood M, Stewart W, Brown C: Research in family medicine. J Fam Pract 5(1):62–88, 1977

In an attempt to assess some current activities in research in family medicine, this report reviews the research efforts of the following three university programs of family medicine: (1) the Family Medicine Program of the University of Rochester, New York, (2) the Department of Family and Community Medicine of the University of Utah at Salt Lake City, Utah, and (3) the Department of Family Medicine, University of Western Ontario, London, Ontario.

Research efforts have been divided into five areas. The first three are patient oriented. The last two areas are organizationally oriented.

1. *Patient care research.* Included here is work concerned with diagnosis, disease management, therapeutics, and the interface with other specialties and subspecialties. Also, work is included which deals with the natural presentation of disease in the office and in the community as well as work which deals with the whole area of patient education.

2. *Epidemiological and environmental research.* This includes work concerned with

health and disease in cohorts of patients and cohorts of families defined by demography, morbidity, geography, and environment. Also, work is included which is concerned with the incidence and prevalence of health and disease in communities and populations, including the patient populations served at primary care practice sites.

3. *Behavioral and social research.* Here are included those papers concerned with behavioral and social manifestations of disease in individual patient groups of all types; the problems of communication between patients and health care providers and among providers themselves; the behavioral and social patterns of providers of health care and among these providers at the individual and group (team) levels; and the patterns of relationships among providers of various types and backgrounds, both with each other and with patients at various patient care sites.

4. *Operational and managerial research.* This area consists of papers concerned with providers of all types in office and hospital practice, the rates of hospital admission and referral, and the evaluation of health care delivery systems of various types. Papers on the development, use, and evaluation of recording and retrieval methodologies in the primary care practice environment are also included.

5. *Educational research.* Here are included papers which are concerned with the measurement and evaluation of training programs for all types of providers of primary care: physicians at both undergraduate and graduate levels in addition to mid-level providers of care (e.g., nurses, nurse practitioners, physicians' assistants, Medex, etc.). Also, those papers are included which present and evaluate methods of auditing the process of training these providers of care, the appropriateness of their educational environment, and the evaluation of the records used in that process.

Table 1 shows a measure of the research effort of each of the three programs in terms of the number of published papers in five content areas.

The difficulties and time-consuming demands of behavioral and social research are epitomized by the comparative paucity of work in this area. This may be a reflection of the lack of precision of the taxonomy and classification systems in these areas and the general fuzziness of the concepts being evaluated.

The three programs vary in numbers of faculty and residents. The Family Medi-

Table 1. *Types of Research by Program*

		Patient Care Research	Epidemiological/ Environmental Research	Behavioral/ Social Research	Operational/ Managerial Research	Educational Research
Rochester	In family practice	3	5	1	17	5
	In other areas	0	0	0	2	0
University of Utah	In family practice	0	4	2	3	2
	In other areas	32	28	14	9	15
Western Ontario	In family practice	11	4	4	15	7
	In other areas	1	2	0	3	0

Reprinted by permission from Wood et al: J Fam Pract, 5(1):62, 1977.

cine Program at the University of Rochester employs the smallest number of faculty and residents and has only one Family Practice Teaching Center. The Department of Family Medicine at the University of Western Ontario is next in size and has three Family Practice Teaching Centers available to it. The largest of the three, the Department of Family and Community Medicine of the University of Utah, has three Family Practice Teaching Centers available and two Research Centers in the community. In the two smaller departments, it is obvious that most of their work in all areas has been carried out in the Family Practice Teaching Center or in community practices with which they have a formal association. Their research effort was concentrated largely in the area of practice organization and management, and scrutiny of the papers produced shows that the work is concerned with the creation of instruments and methodologies to define and describe the demand in the family practice environment. The research efforts of the Department of Family and Community Medicine of the University of Utah was spread over the whole of community medicine, with particular focus on community practice situations in Vernal, Ogden, Salt Lake City, and the offices of resident graduates of the department.

This investigation into three leading programs leads one to believe that at this still very early stage of development, only seven years after reaching specialty status, family medicine is still in its late childhood. However, the early influences were good, excellent habits were established, and the discipline is now about to embark on a journey through a highly active adolescence.

Hesbacher P, Rickels K, Zamostien B, Perloff M, Jenkins B: A collaborative research model in family practice. J Fam Pract 4(5):923–927, 1977

Clinical settings in family practice represent an important area for much needed research in various aspects of primary care which to date have been largely neglected. Such settings provide the research setting of choice for studies involving pharmacotherapy of the psychoneuroses. Neither the individual researcher in an academic center nor the busy practicing family physician can alone undertake meaningful research efforts of this kind.

A collaborative research organization has been developed at the University of Pennsylvania which involves resources of the university medical center as well as practicing family physicians and psychiatrists in the area. Through the Private Practice Research Group, the clinical skills of family physicians are combined with the technical competence of professional researchers. The collaboration of physicians in family and psychiatric practice (currently about 40) and a central research unit, with personnel trained to design clinical trials and to collate, process, and analyze the trial data, has been shown to yield findings that will ultimately be of use to other clinicians, researchers, and the public at large.

Drug studies are initiated by the research unit. The principal concern is to obtain clinical data of good quality relating to the efficacy and safety of a particular medication. Other studies are initiated because clinicians and researchers have spotted a gap in our knowledge of available treatments.

While the collection of trial data occurs solely within the physician's office, it is the central research unit which trains him/her in clinical research procedures and which receives and processes the data collected in

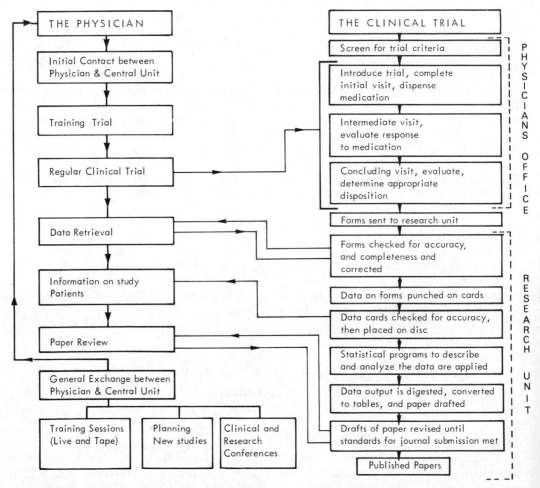

Fig. 1. Private practice research group operation. (Reprinted by permission from Hesbacher, Rickels, Zamostien et al: J Fam Pract, 4(5):923, 1977.)

his/her practice. The physician's role within the total research operation is shown in greater detail in Figure 1. This diagram follows the physician's various contact points with the research unit and traces all the steps involved in the conduct of a clinical trial as it progresses from the physician's office to the research unit.

The ultimate improvement in medical care, specifically regarding the selection of appropriate agents for the treatment of the symptoms of emotional illness, is un-doubtedly the most important objective being met through clinical drug trials. For the family physician, however, participation in a program of clinical research like the one we have described offers additional benefits as well. Involvement in a university-affiliated research effort is certainly an educational experience of the first order, and the instruction received at research meetings and conferences may be used to acquire postgraduate education credits.

Report of the North American Primary Care Research Group (NAPCRG) Committee on Standard Terminology: A glossary for primary care. J Fam Pract 5(4):633–638, 1977

The recent upsurge of interest in primary health care within the academic medical community and government agencies has underscored the need for accurate ambulatory health care data. Essential to collection of such data are precise definitions of terms describing the process of primary care. Whenever possible, uniform, unambiguous definitions are required by research workers as well as by agencies concerned with reimbursement and health care planning.

In response to these needs in North America, an ad hoc committee of the North American Primary Care Research Group (NAPCRG) was formed in 1976. The product of the collaborative efforts of this committee, with suggestions from the general NAPCRG membership, is presented in this paper in the form of a glossary of terms defining the process of primary health care delivery.

The definitions are intended as guidelines rather than absolute dicta for primary care providers and researchers who desire comparability. New knowledge, drifts in use of language with time, and new processes will inevitably require revision of definitions and the addition of new terms. Countries other than the United States and Canada may wish to make use of the glossary with certain modifications, or they may feel that differences in definition of included terms are sufficient to preclude its use. A comprehensive dictionary is, however, beyond the scope of this work. Included are terms most commonly used in the United States and Canada.

Martini CJM, Clayden AD, Turner ID: A comparison of three systems of classifying presenting problems in general practice. J R Coll Gen Pract 27:236–240, 1977

There is increasing interest in the study of the presenting symptoms, signs, and complaints that motivate demand in primary medical care. This paper compares the results of using three different systems of classifying presenting problems in primary medical care.

Three internationally recognized systems have been devised for classifying presenting problems in general practice. They are the Royal College of General Practitioners' (RCGP, 1963) classification, the U.S. Ambulatory Medical Care Classification of Symptoms (NAMCS), and the World Organization of Colleges and Academies of General Practice/Family Medicine

(WONCA, 1976) classification which is known as An International Classification of Health Problems of Primary Care (ICHPPC). These three systems were compared in over 8000 consultations conducted by 81 randomly selected British general practitioners in Nottinghamshire.

Each presenting problem (if there was more than one, only the first was considered for this exercise) was classified as either "specific," "general specific," "general," or "other" using the following definitions:

1. *Specific.* If there was a proper label in the classifications for the statement

Table 1. *Classification of Presenting Problems of New and Old Patient/Doctor Contacts (all ages)*

Classification Criteria	NAMCS		RCGP		ICHPPC	
	Number	*Percent*	*Number*	*Percent*	*Number*	*Percent*
Specific	7847	98.1	4865	60.8	6958	87.0
General specific	106	1.3	2393	29.9	989	12.4
General	3	0.04	674	8.4	—	—
Other	46	0.6	70	0.9	55	0.7
Total	8002	100.0	8002	100.0	8002	100.0

Reprinted by permission from Martini et al: J R Coll Gen Pract, 27:236, 1977.

written by the doctor in the encounter forms (for example, vomiting: 303 in the RCGP classification, 184 in the ICHPPC, and 572 in the NAMCS).

2. *General specific.* If the presenting problem could be classified within a group of conditions but among the remainders only, for example, as part of the group including diseases of the circulatory system but only as "other symptoms, signs, or incompletely diagnosed disease in this group." Two hundred and thirty-seven were recorded in the RCGP (Group 7), either 429 or 459 in the ICHPPC (Group 7), and 216 or 220 in the NAMCS (Group 4).

3. *General.* Presenting problems that could not be located within a group of conditions, but could be classified as "other signs, complaints, or symptoms" in general (999 in the ICHPPC, 464 in the RCGP, and 990 in the NAMCS).

4. *Other.* For all statements not considered within the classification systems. None of the three classifications had more than 70 statements of a possible 8,002 (0.9 percent) attributed to this group.

The results of classifying all "new" and "old" patient/doctor contacts together are given in Table 1, but only the first problem recorded which was the most significant from the doctor's point of view has been taken into account. It can be seen that NAMCS has a greater proportion of problems classified as specific (98.1 percent) compared with 87 percent in the ICHPPC and 60.8 percent in the RCGP, the least specific classification. This last system also had a much greater proportion of problems classified as general (8.4 percent), while in the other two classifications there was practically no need to use this label.

No judgment is made, needless to say, about the value of the RCGP and the ICHPPC in coding medical diagnosis, nor of the many other and different advantages both systems have. If, however, it is felt that the classification of presenting problems is an important issue, the RCGP system is clearly less than satisfactory and the ICHPPC would benefit from further development.

Schneeweiss R, Stuart HW, Froom J, Wood M, Tindall HL, Williamson JD: A conversion code from the RCGP to the ICHPPC classification system. J Fam Pract 5(3):415–424, 1977

The Royal College of General Practitioners Classification of Diseases was first established in the 1950s and its modification for use with problem-oriented medical records (RCGP) was introduced into the United States in 1970 (RCGP-US). It was used to classify morbidity in numerous ambulatory care settings including practices associated with family medicine training programs. The most extensive report using morbidity data generated by the RCGP classification was that emanating from the Medical College of Virginia. Although there was no frank discontent with the RCGP-US classification during the 1970s, there later developed a growing feeling that a simpler, international classification specifically designed for use within the primary care setting would be desirable. Thus, the International Classification of Health Problems in Primary Care (ICHPPC) was developed by the World Organization of National Colleges and Academies of General Practice/Family Medicine (WONCA).*

RCGP contains 22 categories with 628 diagnostic titles compared with the ICHPPC's 18 categories and 371 diagnostic titles.

Faculty members of four family medicine training programs were chosen to in-

dependently produce a diagnostic title conversion from the RCGP to the ICHPPC. When the four preliminary translations were considered together there was concern over the subtleties of conversion of several diagnostic titles. By discussion and reference to the International Classification of Diseases—Eighth Revision (ICD-8 and ICDA-8) mutually agreeable titles were established.†

At the level of specific diagnostic titles there are some differences which warrant description. As shown in Table 1, several diagnostic titles from RCGP are combined into a single title in ICHPPC. Conversely, in other instances (see Table 2), a single rubric from RCGP has been expanded to several rubrics in ICHPPC. In most of the latter instances the "Other Diseases" rubric was used.

The importance of ICHPPC as a new international classification for primary care physicians cannot be underestimated. It has been produced under the auspices of the World Organization of National Colleges and Academies of General Practice/Family Medicine (WONCA) and is endorsed by the North American Primary

† A detailed translation with the appropriate ICHPPC equivalent for each RCGP diagnostic title and code number is available on request from Dr. Ronald Schneeweiss, Department of Family Medicine RF-30, School of Medicine, University of Washington, Seattle, Washington 98195.

* ICHPPC is published by the American Hospital Association, 840 North Lake Shore Drive, Chicago, Illinois 60611.

Table 1. *Examples of Several RCGP Titles Converted to One ICHPPC Title*

RCGP		ICHPPC	
Code	*Title*	*Code*	*Title*
240	Coryza (common cold)	460	Upper respiratory tract infection, acute
241	Pyrexial cold		
242	Acute pharyngitis		

Table 2. *Examples of One RCGP Title Expanded to Several ICHPPC Titles**

RCGP		ICHPPC	
Code	Title	Code	Title
112	Other specific anemias	281	Macrocytic anemias
		282	Sickle cell anemia, sickle cell trait, thalassemia, other hereditary hemolytic anemias
		*285	Other anemias
335	Vulvitis, vaginitis, non-venereal with or without discharge	1121	Urogenital moniliasis, proven
		131	Urogenital trichomoniasis, proven
		*6221	Vaginitis NOS

Reprinted by permission from Schneeweiss, Stuart, Froom et al: J Fam Pract, 5(3):415, 1977.
* The "other diseases" title was preferred in the conversion. A detailed listing of these titles is available from Winston Stuart, MS, Department of Family Practice, Medical College of Virginia, Richmond, VA 23298.

Care Research Group (NAPCRG) and by the Central Office of the International Classification of Diseases—Adapted (ICDA). The classification will receive widespread use in numerous and diverse ambulatory care settings. Although problems are inevitable with conversion from one classification to another, the authors strongly recommend this change and are, therefore, presenting this detailed rubric-by-rubric conversion table to facilitate the change from RCGP to ICHPPC.

Cole WM, Baker RM, Twersky RK: Classification and coding of psychosocial problems in family medicine. J Fam Pract 4(1):85–89, 1977

Disease and problem classification systems for primary care have recognized that psychosocial problems are integrally related to more traditional medical problems which patients present to physicians. These classification systems remain inadequate for the description of primary care problems, especially as several disciplines interrelate in primary care, such as medicine, nursing, and social work.

This paper presents a classification and coding system of psychosocial problems gleaned from a number of existing coding systems.* The application of this coding system in family practice is discussed.

The psychosocial classification and code has been used in the Family Medical Center to report monthly the problems seen by our social workers. From an educational standpoint, the reports indicate why physicians refer patients to the social worker. These monthly reports serve as a teaching tool to residents, faculty, and nurses, illustrating the kinds of problems in which the social worker can be involved as a member of the health care team and what agencies in the community can be called upon to help provide comprehensive patient care. In addition, the social worker has begun to charge for services rendered and the coding system is being used to identify problems handled for billing purposes. In the realm of patient care, process and outcome audits of psychosocial problems in the office and evaluations of the performance of health professionals are facilitated. Finally, the expanding coding system will pave the way for research on psychosocial problems.

* Available on request from Reva K Twersky, MSW, Department of Family Medicine RF-30, School of Medicine, University of Washington, Seattle, Washington 98195.

Hodgkin K: Diagnostic vocabulary for primary care.
J Fam Pract 8(1):129–144, 1979

The concept of a diagnostic vocabulary helps both to understand and to teach primary care. Most practicing clinicians, when presented with any patient's complaint, automatically recall from their diagnostic vocabulary about two to four (rarely more) diagnostic possibilities, which they rank in order of probability. This list then guides their further questions and other actions which are aimed at refuting or confirming their initial ranking. As the clinician collects further information the rank order may be changed, or some items on the list replaced. In the primary care setting, few physicians appear to manipulate more than four diagnostic hypotheses at any one moment, but during a long clinical history they may have considered a much greater number of diagnostic possibilities.

The diagnostic vocabulary used in this way by most clinicians appears to have the following significant characteristics:

1. It forms the basis of the physician's clinical actions.
2. The effective recall and manipulation of this vocabulary is the basis of the physician's skill and is the essential element that must be taught to students.
3. The range of each clinician's working vocabulary is a measure of previous clinical experience.
4. The character of the diagnostic vocabulary used by primary care physicians is similar to primary care morbidity surveys.
5. The individual items of each experienced physician's vocabulary and the frequency of their usage are specific for the discipline practiced by the physician.
6. "Disuse atrophy" of a physician's range of vocabulary appears to follow: (a) diminished clinical experience, (b) lack of adequate continuing medical education, or (c) aging of the physician.

In this study, 11 general practitioners at the end of every consultation reviewed their actions and recorded every diagnosis (suspected or firm) which had formed the basis for any action taken after the consultation. Thus, if the physician had prescribed a tranquilizer and ordered a chest x-ray for an anxious middle-aged female smoker, the physician might record the following: Anxiety and smoker's cough/?? Ca lung.

The 11 physicians were distributed as follows: two urban practices—7 physicians; one rural practice—2 physicians; and one dormitory/resort town—2 physicians.

The study covered four years, 1969–1973, and the population cared for varied between 22,000 and 25,000 National Health Service patients in the Northeast area of Britain between the rivers Tees and Tyne.

For every 1000 patients cared for, each physician made, on average, 2691 diagnoses every year, representing a diagnostic vocabulary of 475 different clinical entities. This paper presents an analysis of this vocabulary according to frequency of usage and clinical decision making. The clinical, teaching, and administrative implications of this analysis are discussed.

Freer CB: Description of illness: Limitations and approaches. J Fam Pract 10(5):867–870, 1980

The collection of health information by diaries has raised questions about the limitations of existing diagnostic terms and taxonomies in describing ill health in a holistic fashion. Despite the advantage of the problem oriented medical record system in recognizing the social and psychological dimensions of illness, problem lists do not communicate the unique mix of problems for any individual.

This paper uses health information from a recent community based study to illustrate the shortcomings of the conventional diagnostic approach to clinical data and suggests areas which require more attention and experimentation. An argument is made for more anecdotal description of illness in medical records and more research to develop a systems approach to describe ill health.

An example of the problem of incomplete description of illness is illustrated by a patient noted to have "headache" and "menstrual cramps." Of course, many physicians make such notes in their records. What is being suggested, however, is that a summary statement should be structured into our record keeping, particularly for those patients with multiple and/or psychosocial problems. The entry could be underlined or highlighted by colored pen and provide an instant and up-to-date reminder at the next visit. This would not replace but supplement the problem list. The use of anecdotal diagnostic summaries would free us from the pressure and the temptation to force available clinical information into a firm problem label while providing the opportunity to include the whole-person dimensions of the problem in a more realistic way.

Systems theory recognizes the existence of an organized whole with overlapping, interacting systems. Unfortunately, to date its applications to the diagnostic method have been purely theoretical and the continuing inability to describe and measure these interactions necessitates the analytic and organic description of illness. Nevertheless, it is in this area that more intensive thought and work are required.

Froom J: An integrated medical record and data system for primary care, Part 1: The age-sex register: Definition of the patient population. J Fam Pract 4(5):951–953, 1977

An age-sex register is an essential part of a practice data system. The manual register used by the Family Medicine Program at the University of Rochester consists of a file of 3 × 5-inch cards. The cards are color coded (blue for male, pink for female) and contain the following information: patient's name, date of birth, sex, marital status, race, address, census tract, date of entry into the practice, date and cause of removal from the practice, the physician's code number, and a specific identification number (Figure 1).

To permit family linkage each family is assigned a five-digit number and individuals within the family a two-digit modifier which describes his/her position within the family. The following modifiers are used:

01   Head of household (HOH)
02   Spouse

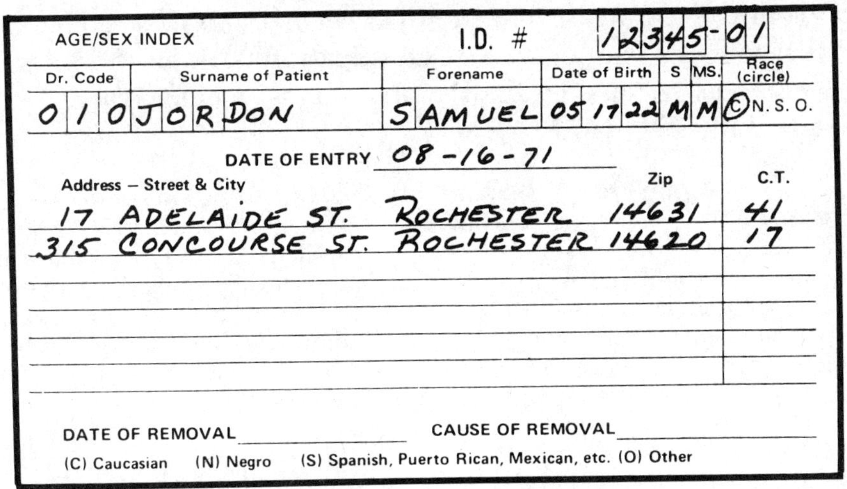
AGE/SEX INDEX   I.D. # 12345-01

Dr. Code	Surname of Patient	Forename	Date of Birth	S	MS.	Race (circle)
010	JORDON	SAMUEL	05 17 22	M	M	Ⓒ N. S. O.

DATE OF ENTRY 08-16-71

Address – Street & City	Zip	C.T.
17 ADELAIDE ST. ROCHESTER	14631	41
315 CONCOURSE ST. ROCHESTER	14620	17

DATE OF REMOVAL ______ CAUSE OF REMOVAL ______

(C) Caucasian (N) Negro (S) Spanish, Puerto Rican, Mexican, etc. (O) Other

Fig. 1. Sample age-sex index card. (Reprinted by permission from Froom J: J Fam Pract 4(5):951, 1977.)

03–30 Children numbered consecutively with "03" as oldest
31 Father of head of household
32 Mother of head of household
33 Father of spouse
34 Mother of spouse
35–40 Unrelated persons living with family
41–50 Other relatives living with family
61–63 Reassigned HOH
64–66 Reassigned spouse
99 One-time only patient coming in with family patient

Age-sex cards are filed by year of birth; males are grouped separately from females; and cards are arranged alphabetically within each section. Cards are maintained for active patients only.

Age-sex data may also be maintained by computer storage on magnetic tape or disc. Monthly reports may then be easily generated which analyze the practice by age, sex, race, and socioeconomic status.

Some of the uses of the register which have been found practical in this program include the following: (1) Analysis of data from the register to permit rational planning for additional personnel. (2) Use of the age-sex register to identify patients within specific age groups with special health needs. Appropriate patients were invited to partake of influenza immunization (age over 65) and blood level screening (ages one to six). (3) Use of the register to identify charts of males aged 40 to 60 in order to audit the assessment of risk factors for ischemic heart disease. Children's charts have been audited for completeness of immunization and those of 30-year-old women for performance of cervical cytology. (4) Research involving morbidity data requires accurate information about the population from which those data were derived. An age-sex register provides this important denominator information.

Froom J: An integrated medical record and data system for primary care, Part 2: Classifications of health problems for use by family physicians. J Fam Pract 4(6):149–151, 1977

Health problems encountered in the ambulatory setting differ from those of hospitalized individuals. For that reason disease classifications of morbidity devised for inpatient categorization are not totally applicable in the ambulatory setting. Numerous classification systems have been devised to overcome this discrepancy and have enjoyed varying levels of success.

At the 1972 meeting of the World Organization of National Colleges and Academies of General Practice/Family Medicine (WONCA), a working party with international representation was established. This international group was charged with establishment of a field-tested international classification to be presented at the next international meeting of WONCA in 1974. By 1973 the WONCA Committee on Classification had developed a list of 407 diagnostic titles suitable for testing. This trial version was tested in nine countries by over 300 physicians in varying types of ambulatory care settings. Analysis of data derived from the more than 100,000 doctor-patient contacts as well as comments from involved physicians led to production of the final version of the International Classification of Health Problems in Primary Care (ICHPPC).*

ICHPPC is an accurate reflection of the unique health problems frequently encountered by the primary care provider. It is not intended as an abbreviation of ICD but has of necessity incorporated appropriate modifications to accommodate different patient problems. Some of the advantages of ICHPPC may be briefly summarized:

* Published by the American Hospital Association (AHA) and available from their Chicago Headquarters, 840 North Lake Shore Drive, Chicago, Illinois 60611.

1. ICHPPC has, by comparison to other ambulatory classification systems, more closely adhered to the widely used hospital classifications, ICD and ICDA. By this means comparison of hospital and ambulatory morbidity is facilitated.
2. Extensive field testing in numerous countries and varied health-care delivery situations has provided a relatively universal choice of diagnostic titles.
3. Its 371 diagnostic titles allow it to be more wieldy for the busy practitioner while maintaining specificity of health problem classification.
4. Residual titles account for less than five percent of recorded health problems as determined statistically by the extensive field trials mentioned above and corroborated by subsequent review.

The 371 diagnostic titles contained in the final version of ICHPPC are divided into 18 sections. These sections are compatible with those of ICD, ICDA, and the H-ICDA classifications. The number of diagnostic titles within each section varies from one (1) in Section 15 to 35 in Section 16.

There exist a myriad of classification systems for the physician, each with its specific advantages and orientation. The type of practice, administrative and health-care delivery needs of the individual provider, and the population served will be important considerations in his or her choice of classification method. The ICHPPC classification combined with a procedure classification seem, at this time, to most appropriately meet the needs of the family physician. Although a reason-for-visit classification appears to be an interesting innovation, its practical value in the primary care setting has yet to be demonstrated.

Froom J, Culpepper L, Kirkwood CR, Boisseau V, Mangone D: An integrated medical record and data system for primary care, Part 4: Family information. J Fam Pract 5(2):265–270, 1977

The gathering of family information has numerous advantages in a family practice setting. This paper describes methods which not only allow description of family structure but also permit identification of each individual family member and his/her relationship to the family as a unit. The value of filing individual medical records in family folders is detailed.

The University of Rochester Family Medicine Program uses a family information sheet (FIS) to collect family information (Figure 1). This is a three-part NCR (no carbon required) form, one part of which is filed with the family folder. The other parts produce alphabetic and numeric files. The FIS is completed at the time of initial visit from the first member of a family to register with the practice. At that time, information is collected on all household members whether or not they intend to receive care at the Health Center. If they do intend to receive care there it is further determined whether they will receive total care or prefer to receive some of their care elsewhere. Thus, an active patient need not receive every portion of his/her medical care within this family practice. At the time of interview a unique five-digit family number is assigned and each household member is identified with an additional two-digit modifier which describes his/her position in the family. Data from the FIS are entered and stored in the

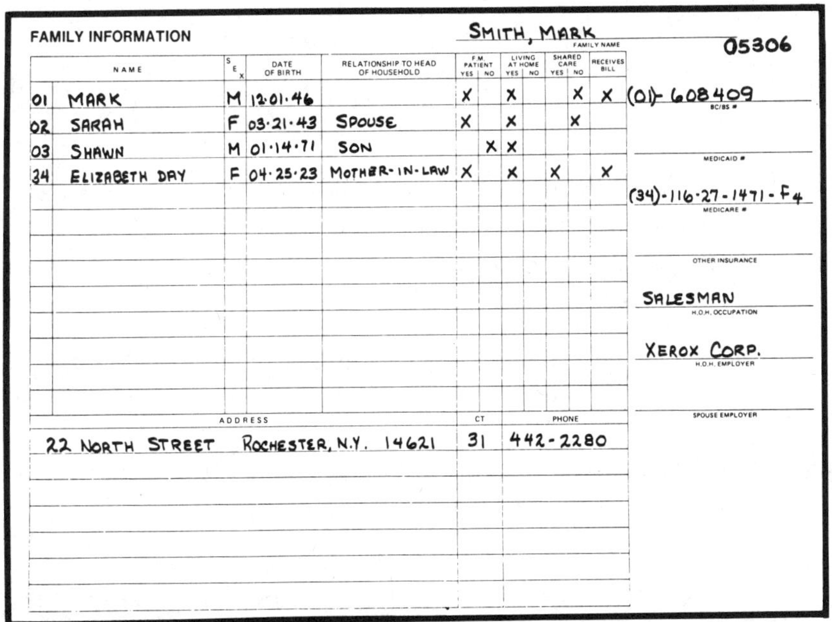
FAMILY INFORMATION

SMITH, MARK
FAMILY NAME

05306

	NAME	SEX	DATE OF BIRTH	RELATIONSHIP TO HEAD OF HOUSEHOLD	F.M. PATIENT YES	F.M. PATIENT NO	LIVING AT HOME YES	LIVING AT HOME NO	SHARED CARE YES	SHARED CARE NO	RECEIVES BILL
01	MARK	M	12·01·46		X		X			X	X
02	SARAH	F	03·21·43	SPOUSE	X		X			X	
03	SHAWN	M	01·14·71	SON		X	X				
34	ELIZABETH DAY	F	04·25·23	MOTHER-IN-LAW	X		X		X		X

(01)-608409
BC/BS #

MEDICAID #

(34)-116-27-1471-F4
MEDICARE #

OTHER INSURANCE

SALESMAN
H.O.H. OCCUPATION

XEROX CORP.
H.O.H. EMPLOYER

SPOUSE EMPLOYER

ADDRESS	CT	PHONE
22 NORTH STREET ROCHESTER, N.Y. 14621	31	442-2280

Fig. 1. Sample family information sheet. The family identification number appears in the upper right-hand corner. In the left-hand column appear the individual identifying numbers. In the address row, CT refers to census tract. (Reprinted by permission from Froom, Culpepper, Kirkwood et al: J Fam Pract, 5(2):265, 1977.)

computer. A single family folder is set up. This becomes the repository for all records on each family member.

Folders containing charts of all members of a family permit and implement a coordinated and comprehensive approach to the management of health problems within the family. The folders are convenient and time-saving for the physician. At the time of a patient visit, questions concerning diagnosis and therapy of other family members frequently arise. Additional time spent retrieving and replacing charts is saved by reference to the family folder. The patient at hand can often contribute additional information on other family members and frequently such information can contribute also to the analysis of the problems of the patient presenting at that visit. Although the family folder has more bulk and is somewhat more difficult to handle than the individual chart, the disadvantage can be minimized to some extent by careful pruning of reports and the use of flow sheets to record laboratory data.

Examples of some aspects of family data compilation and evaluation are drawn from the University of Rochester-Highland Hospital Family Medicine Center (FMC). As of January 1977 the FMC had 11,748 active patients. There are a total of 5,897 families in the practice register. Complete-care families are considered to be those families of which every member is a registered patient within the FMC. There are 3,440 of such complete-care families, or, complete care at the FMC is received by 58.3 percent of all registered families. There are two spouses in 46.3 percent of the families, and grandparents live in the households of 1.9 percent of the families.

Important studies to be performed by full utilization of these data systems include the relationship of morbidity in the individual to family structure and its reverse, the effect of family structure and family dynamics upon individual morbidity; patterns of morbidity within families; the effect of morbidity and utilization of health services by other family members; and many others.

Farley ES, Boisseau V, Froom J: An integrated medical record and data system for primary care, Part 5: Implications of filing family folders by area of residence. J Fam Pract 5(3):427–432, 1977

Simple alphabetic or numeric filing systems allow rapid chart retrieval but give no indication of the geographic location of the family in question. These filing systems give no information about local community resources, neighborhood problems, or socioeconomic status (SES) of the family. For purposes of outreach into the community to screen children for lead levels, for example, it is necessary to know where the family resides as an indicator of the age of the dwelling with the probability of the presence of lead-based paint. Outbreaks of communicable diseases may be more easily identified and controlled if the area of residence is known. Also, specific medical problems have been shown to correlate in incidence with SES and demographic characteristics, as have levels of prophylactic immunization.

This paper describes some advantages of filing patients' charts by area of residence. Experience indicates that the measurement of several factors can give insights into the health-care behavior of the practice population. Some of these are (1) geographic boundaries, (2) neighborhood and ethnic factors (particularly in urban areas), (3) distance from practice site, (4) accessibility of other health-care facilities, and (5) socioeconomic factors.

There are numerous ways to file charts by area of residence. In an urban area, census tracts offer feasible boundaries. However, although census tracts describe the neighborhoods, geographic barriers may limit the predictability of estimations of health service utilization based upon distance from practice. In more rural areas other geographic boundary descriptors may be more useful. In a small town, railroad tracks may be an important determinant of neighborhood boundaries. In some areas, "on the hill," "the other side of the hill," "across the creek," and sometimes school districts may be useful in studying the epidemiology of common diseases. Although census tract boundaries are generally good geographic demarcations, some practices should establish unique systems to describe the geographic boundaries of the practice setting.

Although it is possible to establish socioeconomic status (SES) of each family in a practice by any of several methods, it is more efficient to define clusters of SES groups by location of patients' residence. No census tract is completely homogenous in economic, ethnic, and social composition but similar families tend to live in close proximity.

Once a means for definition of area of residence has been established and an index of SES incorporated into the information base, maintenance of a family chart filing system by area of residence and SES is not difficult. The Family Medicine Center uses a three-digit code to identify census tract, and the family folder itself is identified by the name of the head of household and census tract of residence. For further identification and to minimize misfiling, a ten-color digit code is used to describe census tract number. The folder itself is colored to represent the end digit of the census tract. On the upper right of the outside of the folder two color-coded tabs are affixed; the upper tab identifies the first and the lower tab the second census tract digit. Family folders are then filed alphabetically by HOH name within individual census tract sections in open-shelf file units. Total Practice File Cards are also maintained for all patients and are filed alphabetically. Included on these cards are: name, census tract, address, telephone number, name of HOH, and names of all family members if the patient is the HOH.

Filing patients' charts by area of residence has several advantages for family physicians. These include assessment of socioeconomic status and a visual picture of the practice population. Capacity for health service research and planning for developments such as satellite offices and outreach are enhanced.

Newell JP, Bass MJ, Dickie GL: An information system for family practice. J Fam Pract 3(5):517–520, 1976

In a series of four papers, an information system is described which has been developed for the Department of Family Medicine at the University of Western Ontario. This paper describes the background for the system and the methods used for gathering demographic data on the patient populations of the academic teaching practices.

On the first convenient occasion in which a responsible adult member of the household appears in the teaching center for a visit, the staff person responsible for registration completes a Household Data Sheet (Figure 1). No registration of any household takes place until either of the following conditions is satisfied: (1) at least one member of the household has been

INFORMATION ON MEMBERS OF YOUR HOUSEHOLD
(Include anyone who lives and eats with you for more than six months of the year)

Family No.
(OFFICE USE ONLY)
PLEASE PRINT EVERYTHING

Your surname

Your address

Phone No.

Date of First Contact with Family Medical Centre: _____

Date Questionnaire Completed or Updated: _____

	HEAD OF HOUSEHOLD 01	02	03	04	05	06	07
FIRST NAMES — Print							
DATE OF BIRTH — In this order Day 8 Month 12 Year 70							
SEX — M - Male F - Female							
SURNAME — give only if different from yourself.							
RELATIONSHIP TO YOURSELF — e.g., wife, father, boarder							
MARITAL STATUS — S - Single, M - Married, C - Common law, W - Widowed D - Divorced, Sep - Separated							
COUNTRY OF BIRTH. If Canada or USA print Province or State.							
EDUCATION — give highest grade completed.							
FURTHER QUALIFICATION, e.g. R.N., Grade A Mechanic, B.A.							
OCCUPATION — If student put S. If retired give last occupation, and put R beside it. If unemployed give usual occupation and put U beside it.							
PLACE OF WORK							
RELIGION							
Put a "Y" for "Yes" if person's regular doctor is at Family Medical Centre — "N" for "No".							
SOCIAL INSURANCE NUMBER (if any)							

OHIP NO.   Subscriber's Initials

Fill this square in only if another listed family member has own OHIP No.

Subscriber's Initials

☐ This No. covers ALL FAMILY MEMBERS listed above.

OR

☐ I do not have OHIP coverage at present.

☐ This No. only covers — _____

This OHIP No. covers — _____

NEXT OF KIN

NAME: _____

ADDRESS: _____

PHONE NO: _____

Fig. 1. Sample Household Data Sheet. (Reprinted by permission from Newell, Bass, Dickie: J Fam Pract 3(5):517, 1976.)

seen by a health-care professional at the center on at least two occasions, or (2) the household indicates its firm intention to make use of the facilities.

A vital part of the initial registration process is the assignment of unique identifying numbers to both the household and each individual within it. The household number is four digits in length, and the individual number is a two-digit suffix. Once assigned, neither of these can be altered or reassigned. Generally the head of the household gets the 01 suffix, but this is not a necessary convention. These numbers link together data in the Household Data System, the Encounter System, and the clinical record; the household number is used for filing clinical records, which are grouped into households.

Because the development of an appropriate age-sex baseline requires regular, accurate updating, provision has been made to ensure that this occurs annually for each household. A responsible adult is asked if changes have occurred on the Data Sheet since the last completion.

The newly completed or updated Household Data Sheet is separated, the top copy is affixed to the chart, and the duplicate copy goes to a coding clerk who ensures the completion of this sheet and then codes the information onto 80 column coding sheets. From these sheets, punched cards are created, and the cards are batch processed and update the Household Data File.

The Household Data System functions effectively and provides significant baseline information concerning the patient populations of the teaching centers. Its advantages are many, and relate to clinical, educational, research, and administrative activities in the Department. Its disadvantages stem from the time and personnel required to create and maintain an accurate and up-to-date file. A reduction in the amount of information gathered and some simplification of procedures for data acquisition would be necessary before such a system could be extended readily to a community practice.

Bass MJ, Newell JP, Dickie GL: An information system for family practice, Part 2: The value of defining a practice population. J Fam Pract 3(5):525–528, 1976

The gathering of information on the practice population is essential for practice monitoring, preventive medicine, and research.

Because illnesses and problems often tend to occur in geographic patterns, it was felt important to develop a denominator that could relate patients to their area of residence in the city. This geographic denominator would allow the determination of workload by area of the city, and would assist in answering questions relating to utilization, specific illness patterns, new patients' residences, and the feasibility of new programs for the patient population. When patients are registered, their home

addresses are recorded. This address is coded into one of the 51 census tracts of London.

The minimum necessary information is the age and sex of individuals cared for in the practice. This allows the expression of age-sex specific morbidity rates for the at-risk population. The age-sex register has been a useful aid in executing preventive programs. Each year an age-sex register is produced that groups all patients by year of birth, sex, and the practice that they attend. The physicians have used this listing to identify at-risk groups. In several practices, all those over 65 were invited to attend for influenza vaccine. In other prac-

Table 1. *1973 Midyear Registered Population by Age and Sex*

Age Groups	Victoria Centre	St. Joseph's Centre
Males		
0–4	205	331
5–14	451	766
15–24	424	678
25–34	312	708
35–44	231	401
45–54	211	307
55–64	148	139
65+	144	143
Unknown	5	27
Total	2131	3500
Females		
0–4	154	276
5–14	455	698
15–24	568	1088
25–34	368	831
35–44	255	430
45–54	253	351
55–64	191	191
65+	250	213
Unknown	11	28
Total	2505	4106
Overall totals (male and female)	4636	7606

Reprinted by permission from Bass, Newell, Dickie: J Fam Pract, 3(5):525, 1976.

tices, the computer listing of all those under five years was used as the starting point for a check of charts for immunization status. A similar approach has been used to determine the Pap smear status of all adult women in the practice.

To have a denominator that would allow the expression of rates for disease and symptoms was one of our major reasons for determining the practice population. The values in Table 1 are used as denominators for the calculation of incidence and prevalence rates for events occurring within the teaching centers.

Newell JP , Dickie GL, Bass MJ: An information system for family practice, Part 3: Gathering encounter data. J Fam Pract 3(6):633–636, 1976

It is important to realize that encounter information can be much broader in scope than morbidity information alone. A number of methods for gathering encounter data exist each with limitations. The E-book, for example, is a commonly used manual method and, though it lends itself to ready retrieval of limited amounts of information, extensive cross-analyses are not possible unless the data can be entered into a computer.

There is much more than morbidity information to be obtained from the encoun-

ter between the patient and the health-care professional. Certain aspects of problem solving, beyond diagnosis itself, may not only be more interesting, but may serve a wide range of purposes.

The initial version of the data-gathering form (Visit Data Sheet) was developed, and a pilot study implemented, in early 1972. On the basis of that experience, Version 1 of the Visit Data Sheet was implemented in all of the teaching practices in June 1972. Version 2 of the Visit Data Sheet (Figure 1) was implemented in April

---

TO BE COMPLETED BY RECEPTIONIST

SURNAME: _____

Date of Service: | 1 | 2 | 3 | 4 | 5 | 6 |

Day   Month   Year

Patient Number: 7 8 9 10 11 12

Sex: Male 13 □1
      Female □2

Date of Birth: 14 15 16 17 18 19

Day   Month   Year

Health-Care Professional Number: 20 21 22

F.M.C.: 23
SJH □1
VH □2
SWMHC □3

Firm: 24
A □1
B □2
C □3
D □4
E □5

Place of Service: 25
Office .... □1
Hospital....... □2
Emergency...... □3
Home .... □4

- -

TO BE COMPLETED BY HEALTH CARE PROFESSIONAL

PROBLEMS

| | N | C | R | | CODE |
| | 1 | 2 | 3 | | 26 27 28 29 |

1. _____

| | 1 | 2 | 3 | | 30 31 32 33 |

2. _____

| | 1 | 2 | 3 | | 34 35 36 37 |

3. _____

| | 1 | 2 | 3 | | 38 39 40 41 |

4. _____

| | 1 | 2 | 3 | | 42 43 44 45 |

5. _____

(a) List in order of importance.
(b.) Do not use the term "No Problem."
(c) Only Problem 1 may be referred to in Follow-Up or Referral/Consultation.
(d) Remember to check one of N, C, or R.

ORIGIN OF CONTACT (Only one box)
46
Health-Care Professional... □1
Patient...................... □2
Parent...................... □3
Other...................... □4
Specify _____

(a) H.C.P. —you asked the patient to return now.
(b) Patient—the patient came on his own.
(c) Parent —the patient was brought by a family member
(d) Other —the patient was advised to come in by another H.C.P., agency, etc.

INITIAL REASON FOR CONTACT
47
Consultation for Complaint(s) □1
Well Baby/Child............. □2
Prenatal................... □3
Well Female................ □4
Well Male.................. □5
Required Physical.......... □6
Allergy Shots............. □7
Other..................... □8
Specify _____

Most applicable reason, as you see it, prior to contact.

Only one box.

FOLLOW-UP
48
None............... □1
Deferred........... □2
≤1 week........... □3
>1 week - ≤1 month. □4
>1 month - ≤3 months □5
>3 months - ≤1 year □6
>1 year........... □7
As required........ □8

Based on what you told the patient.
"Deferred"—for special situations.
Only one box. Link to Problem 1.

REFERRAL/CONSULTATION
49
None........... □1
F.M.C. Physician □2
Consultant...... □3
Admit to Hospital □4
P.H.N........... □5
M.S.W. .... □6
Dietician....... □7
Physiotherapist. □8
Other........... □9
Specify_____

Only one box. Link to Problem 1.

Column 80:   Code 2

Fig. 1. Version 2 of the Visit Data Sheet. (Reprinted by permission from Newell, Dickie, Bass: J Fam Pract, 3(6):633, 1976.)

1973, and it added to Version 1 a mechanism for distinguishing the first visit in any episode from subsequent visits for the same episode. This is a most important requirement for the accurate calculation of incidence and prevalence rates.

The Visit Data Sheet is completed for every encounter between a patient and a health-care professional in the teaching practices, with the single exception of in-hospital visits. Figure 1 demonstrates the presence of the minimum data set. Surname is used for administrative purposes only. The Patient Number is a unique six-digit number (four-digit suffix identifying the individual within that family), and it permits linkage between the Household Data File and the clinical record for that patient. The Health Care Professional Number is assigned to that particular provider so long as he/she is responsible for the care of patients in one of the Departmental teaching practices. Below the dotted line, the Visit Data Sheet allows for the listing of more than one problem; up to five are permitted, though it is uncommon for this number to be reached. The form permits each problem to be further specified as to:

N—new: the first time this problem has been identified by any health care professional during the current episode.

C—continuing: the patient has been seen previously in this episode by this or by another health-care professional.

R—recurrent: the first time the patient has been seen for this episode of a problem which tends to recur (e.g., peptic ulcer). In practice, this category has proven difficult to capture accurately and will be dropped in future revisions of the form. N and R are generally added in order to arrive at incidence rates for any problem.

The person responsible for coding the Visit Data Sheet checks to make sure the Visit Data Sheet is complete, returning incomplete forms. Each problem is given a three-digit code; N, C, and R receive a one-digit code; the rest of the form is self-coding. Once coding is complete (every effort is made to keep it up on a daily basis), the Visit Data Sheets are handsorted in patient number order and are merged with sheets previously collected. At the end of a period of time, usually two weeks, the sheets are used to create punched cards, which are batch processed to update the Encounter Data File.

Dickie GL, Newell JP, Bass MJ: An information system for family practice, Part 4: Encounter data and their uses. J Fam Pract 3(6):639–644, 1976

This paper describes the ways in which encounter data from the family practice teaching units of the Department of Family Medicine, University of Western Ontario, have been used for teaching, service, and research.

On a day-to-day basis, the single most useful product of the information system is the "Disease Index." This is a computer printout which lists, under each diagnostic heading, the chart number, age, sex, and number of visits for each patient who has had that problem dealt with during the year. Visits are categorized as initial or subsequent visits for an episode. The Disease

Index permits the rapid identification of patients with specific conditions, and allows an age-sex analysis to be made. It has been used in patient recall—for example, juvenile asthmatics for a newly introduced exercise program. It is useful in teaching, since a group of patients' charts can be quickly accessed for the preparation of relevant material on specific diseases. It provides a starting point for descriptive research into the natural history of disease, and has been used extensively over the past two years by residents in family practice.

The information system allows examination of the morbidity patterns of registered teaching practices, which are generally representative of the city of London. Flexibility in the system permits the presentation of data in a variety of formats for service, educational, and research uses. The data have been used for internal comparison of the practice patterns of physicians at staff and resident levels. The data are useful as a resource in the preparation of teaching materials, both undergraduate and postgraduate. The possibilities for intercenter comparisons are now being explored. Patients with high-risk conditions can be identified. Future developments in computing techniques may allow direct recall of patients at predetermined intervals.

The availability of a registered patient population, from which control groups can be prepared without difficulty, makes the information system an ideal base for clinical, operational, and educational research. Perhaps one of the most significant aspects of the system is that it involves all residents and medical students who pass through the teaching practices. They can see at first hand the benefits of information which can be obtained by simple techniques of recording. It is hoped that they will be encouraged to institute similar inquiry in their own practices.

Boyle RM: Adding information and intelligence to a family practice data system. J Fam Pract 10(1):141–143, 1979

A recent and quite conspicuous trend in family medicine is the establishment of data systems, ranging in comprehensiveness from manual instruments in a solo office setting to a proposed regional primary care registry. In this communication a "data system" is an organized collection of a minimum set of data on family practice patients, using automated resources for storage and production of reports.

This paper describes approaches to add both information and intelligence to such systems: these are structured within the familiar patient care, research, and education triad. Methods outlined are presently being applied at the Medical College of Virginia (MCV) with the Virginia Family Practice Data System, a state-wide, continuous morbidity recording network.

A hierarchy of users can be identified, listed in order of understanding and actual application of data systems:

1. Faculty/researchers at health sciences institutions
2. Faculty and residents at teaching practices
3. Community family physicians

Reasons for these differences are intrinsic problems of most systems. For instance, the four essential tasks of administration—planning, facilitating, organizing, and controlling—break down at various points in the network. Failure to communicate among all levels is an equally substantial issue. Finally, the main problem may be inability to recognize that the most important element of any data system is the *people* involved.

Frequency and format of routine reports should be instructive, responsive to user needs, and should concisely cover the family practice experience. Pertinent reports should stimulate interest in both individual performance and comparisons with peers. A critical test of any data system is its relevance: more simply, reports must present what users want. That is, residents and physicians are interested in workload rates, such as visits/patient, and a delineation of diagnoses by frequency. Applications of these reports are organizational, comparative, and educational.

Anderson JE, Lees REM: Optional hierarchy as a means of increasing the flexibility of a morbidity classification system. J Fam Pract 6(6):1271–1275, 1978

The need for a suitable system of problem classification was quickly recognized when national primary-care (general practice or family medicine) institutions were established in many countries during the 1950s and 1960s. An evolution occurred from multiple regional and national systems, through recognition of the need for an international standard, to the testing and publication of the International Classification of Health Problems in Primary Care (ICHPPC). This evolution came about only after the establishment of the World Organization of National Colleges, Academies, and Academic Associations of General Practitioners/Family Physicians (WONCA) in which the interests of the several national bodies of primary care were represented.

The principal intent of ICHPPC was to provide a vehicle for the international comparison of morbidity data. Another major objective was that the system should be flexible enough to permit local adjustment to accommodate problems which were of local but not international importance. To meet with this objective, the principle of optional hierarchy was established, whereby a local rubric or subdivision code can be assigned to allow greater specificity of classification provided provision is made for its replacement in the parent ICHPPC, thus allowing comparison of data for other purposes.

Optional hierarchy is a mechanism that may be employed to achieve the desired specificity for local use while permitting recombination into parent rubrics for external comparisons. Optional hierarchy may be employed to develop subdivision rubrics when justified by the high incidence of specific problems, whether due to geographic or social circumstances or because of the special nature of individual practice(s). It may also be used to meet the sometimes esoteric needs of the researcher, the unique needs of the teacher, or the preferential needs of other individual recorders.

One example of the use of optional hierarchy is as follows: For academic reasons it was desirable to separate diagnostic data for postmenopausal bleeding and intermenstrual bleeding within the department. These are both included in rubric 6269 along with "other disorders of menstruation." Thus, three new rubrics were developed (Table 1), all identifiably related to the original. Identification and retrieval of the relevant patient records was facili-

Table 1. *Number of Patients Encountered, Number of Problem Contacts, and Prevalence Rate, Using Subdivisions of ICHPPC Rubric 6269**

	Patients	Problem Contacts	Prevalence (per 1000)†
Intermenstrual bleeding	56	65	1.9
Postmenstrual bleeding	10	14	0.3
Other menstrual disorders	4	4	0.1
Parent ICHPPC (#6269)	70	83	2.4

Reprinted by permission from Anderson, Lees: J Fam Pract, 6(6):1271, 1978.
* Table illustrates the usual simplicity of recombination to parent rubric.
† In attending population.

tated by the use of the more specific rubrics. For general ICHPPC reporting or comparisons of problems with other centers, however, simple addition of each sub-rubric provides the data covered by the original rubric, 6269.

Optional hierarchy is a logical, pragmatic system of increasing the flexibility and the practical value of morbidity or problem classifications. The use of optional hierarchy is simple, but its accuracy can be destroyed by failure to anticipate the pitfalls which can arise when parent rubrics are split and the subdivisions are subsequently combined to assign a value to the parent.

Culpepper L, Holler JW: Guidelines for the revision of practice data sets. J Fam Pract 11(3):437–442, 1980

In recent years, a constant debate has followed attempts to define the appropriate data base for ambulatory care. Such discussions have centered primarily on defining the *minimum* data appropriate for the informational needs of governmental agencies and reimbursement systems. Family medicine teaching programs and practices have information needs beyond these. As residencies and practices mature, a frequent undertaking is the revision of initial data sets and information systems. To facilitate this process, this paper presents an expanded data set and guidelines for the selection and implementation of a data set.

Patient related information consists of both registration and encounter information. Registration information is less likely to change once collected. It frequently is used at each encounter, and it should be checked periodically for updating purposes. Encounter data is new information which is likely to be different at each visit. Its collection is facilitated by use of the encounter form.

Within family medicine environments, information needs frequently include demographic, practice management, financial, educational, and research data. Suggestions are made in each area for specific items to consider in expanding a practice data set.

The careful selection of items for inclusion within a data set is essential for the proper performance of an information system. The following guidelines are suggested for avoiding problems which are often encountered:

1. Identify the uses for each data item.
2. Define items in writing.
3. Review the complexity of items.
4. Consider whether it is realistic to collect and update registration information.
5. Consider future information needs.
6. Consider whether the complete set of information desired is realistic.

The implementation of a revised data system requires careful planning and frequent involvement of staff to insure accurate collection of information and to assure proper management of workload. The implementation phase should not be considered complete until an ongoing system for reviewing and maintaining data is established.

Baker C, Schilder M: The "E-Box": An inexpensive modification of diagnostic indexing. J Fam Pract 3(2):189–191, 1976

The diagnostic indexing system developed by Eimerl in England several years ago has attracted wide interest among primary care physicians in a number of countries. The E-book is an elegantly complete, multiple-ring binder provided with indexing for each of the rubrics of the RCGP code. One limitation to its more extensive use in training programs has been the cost of the E-book itself. This paper describes an inexpensive modification of the E-book system involving the "E-box."

This modification consists of an "E-box," containing index guides which are numbered at intervals of 25, from zero through 950. These guides may be inexpensively prepared by photo-offset printing of the numerals on "Press-A-Ply" labels; the labels are cut apart and applied to blank index guides. There are loose data sheets on which patient information is recorded. Each sheet has space for the code number of that problem, and the sheets are filed numerically in the box. Also needed is a standardized ICHPPC code book, a convenience list of most frequently used index numbers, and a list of the "50 Most Common" problems encountered in ambulatory practice.

The data sheets are initially used to record the name of each patient, his or her social security number and year of birth, the condition for which the patient is seen, and any other information in which one is interested. It is not necessary to use data sheets for this purpose, but it is convenient to do so. At the end of the day, or at weekly intervals, this information is transcribed onto separate data sheets which are coded with the number of the appropriate problem. New data sheets are made out for each new problem not previously encountered, or the patient's name is added to a data sheet previously indexed. The front of the data sheets are printed in black and are used for recording male patients; the backs are printed in red and are used for recording female patients. This system makes it easier to tabulate results later.

A wide space at the right of the data sheet is provided for whatever information one wishes to record, such as hospital chart number or the place where the patient was seen. When index numbers refer to a rubric beginning "Other diseases of . . . " the specific diagnosis should be recorded here.

This method is a valuable learning tool and provides a simple system for monitoring the clinical experience of students and residents in family practice.

Westbury RC: The analysis of family practice workloads by seriousness. J Fam Pract 4(1):125–129, 1977

Any effort to understand the mechanics of family medicine must focus on the doctor-patient contact. It was logical that attempts to quantify the workload of family physicians should begin by counting these encounters. However, it soon became apparent that not all encounters were equal; in order to quantify practice workloads and be able to compare one practice to another, it was necessary to subdivide doctor-patient contacts according to various criteria.

For example, doctor-problem contacts differ in terms of the amount of time they take, and in the amount of stress and worry they bring to the patient and his

Table 1. *Relation of Age and Sex to Seriousness**

Age-Sex Group		Serious		Nonserious		Index of Seriousness
		Number	*Percent*	*Number*	*Percent*	
<1	Male	9	1.3	162	23.2	(.055)
	Female	8	1.4	105	18.2	(.076)
	Total	17	1.3	267	20.9	(.064)
1–11	Male	149	2.1	1590	22.3	.094
	Female	96	1.6	1540	25.8	.062
	Total	245	1.9	3130	23.9	.078
12–20	Male	195	3.9	929	18.7	.210
	Female	176	3.3	1081	20.5	.163
	Total	371	3.6	2010	19.6	.184
21–64	Male	643	6.4	1406	14.0	.457
	Female	1243	7.4	1963	11.6	.633
	Total	1886	7.0	3369	12.5	.560
65+	Male	278	24.2	74	6.4	3.757
	Female	368	23.6	69	4.4	5.333
	Total	646	23.9	143	5.3	4.517
Total	Male	1274	5.3	4161	17.3	.306
	Female	1891	6.2	4758	15.7	.397
	Total	3165	5.8	8919	16.4	.355

Reprinted by permission from Westbury: J Fam Pract, 4(1):125, 1977.
* The seriousness of doctor-patient contacts by age and sex, showing (for each age and sex group) (1) the number of "serious" contacts, (2) this figure expressed as a percentage of all doctor-patient contacts in that group, (3) the number of "nonserious" contacts, (4) this figure expressed as a percentage of all doctor-patient contacts in that group, (5) the Index of Seriousness. The figures are for all doctor-patient contacts made by Drs. T. & W. over a five-year period.

family physician. It is to the latter consideration that this paper is directed; physicians think of some problems as being more serious and some as being less serious. The more serious ones require more diligence and more effort from the physician.

Thirty-five family physicians were invited to participate in the study. All had an interest in teaching and/or research. They were presented with 274 rubrics of the 389 rubrics in the "Canuck Book." This was an interim classification, created for use in Canadian general practice until an internationally acceptable classification could be agreed upon. From 1971 to 1975, it was found to be acceptable and was widely used by GP recorders in Canada. It shows a high level of concordance with the International Classification of Health Problems in Primary Care (ICHPPC).

The physicians were asked to go through the list and classify each rubric as to seriousness on the following scale: 0— usually not serious, 2—usually serious, 1—somewhere in between.

There was sufficient agreement on 96 rubrics for them to be used as indicators of the seriousness of workloads in general. It was found useful to have a "shorthand" summary of the seriousness of workloads; for this purpose, an "index of seriousness" can be calculated by dividing the number of "serious" contacts by the number of "nonserious" contacts. Table 1 demonstrates clearly the differences in seriousness of doctor-patient contacts grouped by the age and sex of the patient. The increasing seriousness of morbidity with increasing age is intuitively appreciated by all family physicians and, indeed, is tangibly recognized by the age-weighting of the capitation fees paid to British family physicians. The tendency for adult females to present with more serious problems than adult males is not so well known.

While the technique described has proved to be useful for various analyses within our practice, its potential for interpractice comparisons has not been achieved because it relates to an obsolete classification. It would be most useful if a similar weighting for seriousness were to be developed for ICHPPC, a classification which is likely to be used very widely.

Keller K, Podell RN: The survey in family practice research. J Fam Pract 2(6):449–453, 1975

The survey is a method that can be employed in family practice research. It is an adaptable tool that can be used with good results by those not sophisticated in research.

General guidelines for survey research are discussed in this article, including the following steps: (1) formulating the problem, (2) selecting a sample, (3) choosing the instrument, (4) constructing the questionnaire, (5) dealing with nonresponse; (6) processing the data, and (7) analysis and uses of results.

The question of sample size is one which often plagues beginning researchers. The investigator should be able to answer three questions:

1. What is your estimate of the actual variability of the target population?
2. How close must the results from the survey sample be to the frequencies which actually occur in the target population?

3. How confident must you be in the answer to Question 2? (Usually being right 95 times in 100 is quite acceptable.)

The researcher must decide which survey instrument will best serve the study's objective—the self-administered questionnaire or the interview. The advantages and disadvantages of each are discussed.

The organization of the questionnaire is important. It must be organized so that it can easily be handled by the respondent, the interviewer, and the investigators. From the respondent's point of view, the sequence of questions should be logical and nonthreatening. From the interviewer's point of view, the questionnaire should be designed for maximum ease of administration. It should be easy to read the questions and record answers. From the researcher's point of view, the questionnaire should be designed to facilitate editing, coding, and identification of the questionnaire.

Freer CB: Health diaries: A method of collecting health information. J R Coll Gen Pract 30:279–282, 1980

This paper reviews the use of health diaries, gives some examples of the type of information that can be collected by them, and discusses their potential in general practice research.

Table 1 illustrates the kinds of information which may be recorded in a health diary.

Health diaries provide the opportunity for a patient-centered approach to research. Since they are completed by the patients themselves and, although structured, permit freedom of expression, their content is less likely to be restricted to purely medical problems and provides more of the social aspects of a person's

Table 1. *Summary Extract of Recorded Information on Perceived Health Problems and Responses to Them on Four Consecutive Days from One of the Health Diaries*

	Continuing Problems	New Problems	Self-Care Response
Monday	Nervous and depressed	Argument with husband—gets mad when I go to bed before him Son mad with me	Valium Had a drink with neighbor Worked in garden
Tuesday	Depressed	Low backache—period due Headache Argument with husband	Coffee Wore more make-up
Wednesday	Depressed Headache Still having differences with husband	Period cramps	Had a few drinks with neighbor
Thursday	Depressed	Husband told me that house was a pig-sty Husband drank all night	Valium Drank too much myself

Reprinted by permission from Freer: J R Coll Gen Pract, 30:279, 1980.

day-to-day health, which is important for a holistic appreciation of health. A further advantage of health diaries is that they provide a time frame for the various components of the process of an illness. The sequence of events and responses, especially for common and ill-defined problems, is unlikely to be recalled with any degree of accuracy by the more traditional research methods. The diary method minimizes the problem of factual recall and it has been shown to provide more accurate information than the retrospective studies. As a prospective method, diaries reproduce health problems and related events as they happen and can be used to study such processes as patient decision making.

While no single research method can produce all the answers, health diaries seem to have particular advantages for the study of the distinctive clinical content of general practice. In addition, their clinical and educational potential may warrant further exploration and experiment.

Stamps PL: Toward the evaluation of family practice: Development of a family utilization index. J Fam Pract 7(4):767–779, 1978

There is no lack of description of the model of family practice. However, most of this has concentrated on definitional and philosophical issues. Few studies have empirically assessed how patient care is delivered within that model and how patients react to the care. As in the case of many theoretical models, there are numerous problems with implementation and evaluation of results.

This paper describes a project that establishes criteria for utilization patterns of a family practice that could be used to develop evaluation techniques for family practice as a method of delivering primary medical care. The criteria are summarized in a Family Utilization Index, which measures the utilization patterns of a family unit.

The Family Utilization Index provides a means of summarizing patterns of utilization. Since the Index is weighted, it also provides a means of comparison of actual patterns to expected or ideal patterns. The Index contains four components:

1. The number of persons in the family with medical records at the Family Medicine Clinic compared to the total number of persons in that family.
2. A description of the persons within the family unit who are active patients.
3. The length of time the family has used the clinic.
4. Total number of visits made by the family.

To create one summary figure for the Family Utilization Index, each component was granted a total number of points and the points were added together for one score.

The Family Utilization Index is an attempt to document the relationship of behavior (i.e., utilization) and attitudes toward family practice as a model and one specific family practice as a provider site. In this study, it has been treated as an independent variable. Realistically, of course, the relationship between utilization and attitudes is much more complex and multidimensional.

The Family Utilization Index itself is not suggested as the only or as a final evaluation technique. It should be validated as a measurement instrument in other family practice settings, with special attention paid to the weighting of the components and to the computation of the Index. It should then be used in a prospective study so we can determine the causal effect of a family practice site on a patient's utilization. It should also be used to compare utilization patterns in other sites of primary care. By developing comparative evaluations, it will be possible to more accurately assess the impact of the model of family practice on the health care delivery system.

Stein REK, Reissman CK: The development of an impact-on-family scale: Preliminary findings. Med Care 18(4):465–472, 1980

To date, no comprehensive measure exists which can quantify the impact of childhood illness on a family and which delineates the many facets of this complex domain. None of the measures meet rigorous scientific criteria, e.g., demonstrable reliability and validity.

The purposes of this report are (1) to describe the development of a new measure of impact of chronic illness in childhood on the family, (2) to discuss the methods used in its development, and (3) to suggest some of the uses for this new measure.

Four dimensions emerged as central to the domain and therefore needing systematic measurement: (1) *economic burden*, or the extent to which the illness changes the economic status of the family, drawing resources away from other areas; (2) *social impact*, or the quality and quantity of interaction with those outside the immediate household; (3) *familial impact*, or interaction within the family unit including parental and sibling relationships; and (4) *subjective distress*, or the strain experienced by the primary caretaker that is directly related to the demands of the illness. The four-factor derived scales are not completely independent. This is understandable, since a family experiencing impact in one area will be more likely to experience impact in other areas as well. Therefore, the decision was made to employ a total score as a general measure of impact, as well as four component scores.

As it now stands, the instrument should prove useful in describing the impact on a family of an ill child along four dimensions of response. The total score yields a general measure of this impact. The scale and subscales elicit sufficient variability in response to different subjects. As the instrument has sufficient reliability to detect change, the measure may be used to assess family response at the onset of an illness and over its course. The differential impact of illnesses which vary in the kind of demands they make of families also could be addressed. Finally, the measure may prove useful in evaluation research designed to test the relative efficacy of psychosocial intervention programs in reducing the impact of chronic illness on family life.

Bruhn JG, Trevino FM: A method for determining patients' perceptions of their health needs. J Fam Pract 8(4):809–818, 1979

Success or failure in establishing a meaningful relationship between physician and patient depends to a large extent on how fully the patient communicates, and the physician understands, his/her health needs. Return visits, compliance with the physician's prescribed regimen, and the effectiveness of the treatment and rehabilitation are also closely related to the disclosure and assessment of the patient's health needs.

No simple method has been devised to determine how patients see their health needs other than through a dialogue between patient and physician. During this exchange, patients may omit information that the physician might consider important, or the physician may not be aware of the significance of some information in the life of a particular patient. This encounter between physician and patient can be marred by a mismatch between conceptions of what constitutes important information and behavior. Full disclosure in a frank, open manner may be hampered by the restricted time that the physician has to give to each patient and the patient's sensitivity to this.

The authors believe that with enough time and with some avenue available, patients can provide much information about their health needs at the time of the initial meeting with a physician, and that the physician can use this information to make a sensitive and comprehensive assessment of why the patient came and what he expects. The authors recognize that determining health needs is not a simple matter. Indeed, health needs change and must be reassessed periodically. Nonetheless, the authors feel that a practical method can be developed to assist physicians in determining the health needs of their prospective patients. The purpose of this paper is to propose such a method for use, testing, and refinement. This method, or a variation of it, could enhance patient-physician communication and interaction.

The behavioral options that are in effect when a person considers a health problem and the outcome of following each path have been designed into a flow chart (Figure 1). Based on this model, a method is described that can be used by physicians to obtain a better grasp of patients' needs at the first encounter. The method is based on written information provided by the patient. The prospective patient is asked to answer 30 questions relating to health needs while waiting to see the physician. This information is then given to the physician to use as a part of the history taking process; the patient's responses to the questions serve as cues for physician

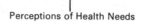

Some Factors Influencing Perception of Health Needs

Age	Knowledge of health care system	Economic situation
Education	Previous experience with illness	Access to health care
Religious beliefs	Rank of health in personal value system	Attitudes of family and friends
Knowledge of illnesses	Cultural values	Present life situation
Fear	Availability of health care and kind available	Degree of hopefulness

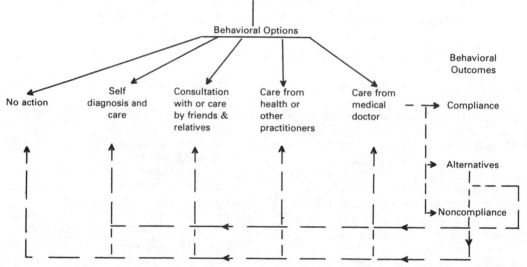

Perceptions of Health Needs

Identification and Verification: "I need to know whether I'm sick or not"
Knowledge: "I need to know what I can do to get well, and the implications of my illness"
Treatment: "Can my illness be treated"
Support: "I need to talk to someone who understands"

Fig. 1. Flow chart of behavioral options and outcomes based on patients' perceptions of health needs. (Reprinted by permission from Bruhn, Trevino: J Fam Pract, 8(4):809, 1979.)

discussion in the initial interview. The Health Needs Assessment Questionnaire was modeled somewhat after the Cornell Medical Index, which is a self-administered review of personality characteristics and physical symptoms.

Dickinson JC, Gehlbach SH: Process and outcome: Lack of correlation in a primary care model. J Fam Pract 7(3):557–562, 1978

The assumption underlying "process" audits of health care is that physicians who demonstrate high adherence to established criteria, e.g., performing fundoscopic examinations, obtaining urine cultures, ordering antibiotics, are providing good care. However, there is a growing concern that adherence to process criteria may not be the best measure of quality of care. All that physicians do to and for patients does not necessarily improve the patients' well-being. Favorable patient outcome is probably a more important index of successful medical care, and the question remains: Does correct process necessarily result in good patient outcome?

To explore the validity of the process audit a chart review was conducted of 87 hypertensive patients in a family practice. The study population was the registered patient population of the Duke-Watts Family Medicine Residency Program. This group practice serves a population of approximately 8000.

Although a significant reduction in mean diastolic blood pressures was found at two follow-up intervals, physician performance scores showed no significant correlation with this outcome. Nor could an association between medical process and outcome be demonstrated when control of blood pressure to less than 95 mmHg was used as an outcome measure. The reliability between two chart auditors was poor, with complete agreement being achieved in only 29 percent of cases.

Despite the overall improvement in blood pressures, physician adherence scores were not particularly high. On the average, only 59 percent of criteria were fulfilled overall and only 43 percent of history items. Furthermore, the authors were unable to demonstrate that successful blood pressure reduction was related to the degree of adherence to the protocol. No correlation could be found even for the cohort of patients who were diagnosed for the first time at the index visit and should have shown most improvement.

The absence of association between recorded process and adequate outcome raises serious questions about the validity of the standardized process audit as a predictor of patient improvement. The problem may lie in the discrepancy between recorded and actual process. Physicians may comply with criteria but fail to record their adherence in the chart. Accurate quality assessment will require more practical methods of review which relate directly to patient outcomes.

Gehlbach SH: Comparing methods of data collection in an academic ambulatory practice. J Med Educ 54:730–732, 1979

Collecting patient morbidity information in academic ambulatory practice is useful for research, practice management, and evaluation and planning of educational programs. Diagnostic data commonly are collected from log books or encounter sheets and then encoded a batch-entered into computer storage for later processing and retrieval. Unfortunately, errors in this process can reduce the accuracy of the data. Providers underrecord the patient problems that are encountered, problems are incorrectly coded, and transcribing errors occur.

In the Duke-Watts Family Medicine Program, medical services are offered to 11,000 patients by 47 providers. Informa-tion on demographic characteristics and diagnoses of patients is collected and stored by computer. Since 1977 three alternate methods of data collection evolved in an attempt to improve the accuracy of the system. In this study three methods of morbidity data collection were compared to determine which was most accurate: (1) Write-in encounter form, (2) Checklist encounter form, and (3) Direct entry from the medical record.

Coding errors occurred in 5.5 percent of the 216 entries on the written encounter forms. The number of these mistakes was reduced by the checklist method as only 61 (28 percent) of the problems had to be coded. However, two new errors occurred.

With the checklist format providers could accidently check the wrong box or could inappropriately force diagnostic impressions into precoded categories. For example, a patient with gastritis (which was not precoded) could be incorrectly labeled as having peptic ulcer disease (which was on the list). These additional mistakes nullified the gains of reduced coding and left an error rate identical to that of the write-in form (5.5 percent).

As might be expected, encounter forms were more likely to reflect the medical record when fewer problems were recorded in the progress notes. When single problems were noted in the chart, concordance with the encounter form was found over 90 percent of the time. When there were three or more problems, agreement between the medical record and encounter form dropped to 10 percent. With the direct coding method more than 70 percent agreement was maintained even when there were multiple problems.

The high rate of errors that occurs when data, especially multiple problems, are collected by encounter forms suggests that caution must be exercised in interpreting information gathered in this fashion. Given the greatly improved accuracy of direct medical record entry, it is the preferred method of morbidity data collection in academic ambulatory practices.

Wiegert HT, Wiegert O: The impact of disease prevalence on the predictive value of laboratory tests in primary care. J Fam Pract 8(6):1199–1203, 1979

The physician's interest in the usefulness of a diagnostic test depends upon how accurately the test predicts the presence or absence of disease. That is, if given a normal result, what are the chances that the patient is free of the disease, and if given an abnormal result, what are the chances that disease is actually present? An additional consideration is whether the cost of doing a test yields an equivalent value in knowledge on which to base the management of the condition under consideration. If several tests can be accomplished to increase the probability of correctly determining the existence of a disease state, the physician must determine if the marginal increase in predictive value gained from doing each additional test is likely to result in a change in the management of the disease. The cost of doing the test must accrue equivalent expected benefit to the patient or society.

Probability calculations permit physicians to make better decisions about the efficacy of a laboratory test in confirming or excluding a diagnosis, and provide a predictive value of a positive or negative test result. The predictive value of test results is important to determine the probability of the presence or absence of the disease and to assess the extent of possible benefit, psychological trauma, or economic burden that could ensue from embarking on a particular mode of management.

The predictive value of any diagnostic process is related to the sensitivity and specificity of the test and the prevalence of the underlying pathology for which the diagnostic testing is accomplished. Prevalence is the most important, but least understood, factor affecting the usefulness of a test result.

This paper illustrates the effect of prevalence, sensitivity, and specificity on the predictive value of a positive test result by considering two commonly used tests in the family physician's office: the Monospot test and the throat culture.

If physicians will estimate accurate probabilities of positive results before ordering diagnostic tests, the quality of medical care will improve and the cost of medical care incurred as a result of laboratory testing will decrease.

Index

Page numbers in *italics* indicate illustrations.
Page numbers followed by *t* indicate tables.